Immunological and Clinical Aspects of Multiple Sclerosis

Published in cooperation with
ARS MEDICI
International Journal for Practical Therapy

Medical Media International
Avenue A. van Beceleare 28B
1070 Brussels
Belgium

Editor-in-chief **J. de Castro** MD

Immunological and Clinical Aspects of Multiple Sclerosis

The Proceedings of the XXV Anniversary Symposium of the Belgian Research Group for Multiple Sclerosis

Edited by
R. E. Gonsette and
P. Delmotte

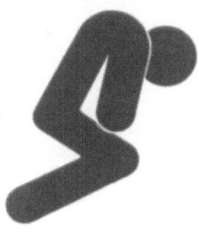

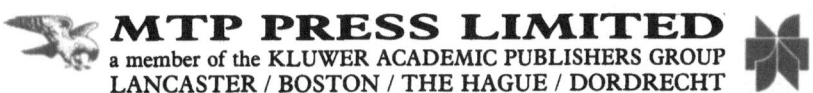

MTP PRESS LIMITED
a member of the KLUWER ACADEMIC PUBLISHERS GROUP
LANCASTER / BOSTON / THE HAGUE / DORDRECHT

Published in the UK and Europe by
MTP Press Limited
Falcon House
Lancaster, England

British Library Cataloguing in Publication Data

Immunological and clinical aspects of multiple sclerosis.
   1. Multiple sclerosis
   I.Delmotte, P.   II. Gonsette, R.E.
   III. Belgian Research Group for Multiple Sclerosis
   616.8′34   RC377

   ISBN-13: 978-94-011-6354-5   e-ISBN-13: 978-94-011-6352-1
   DOI: 10.1007/978-94-011-6352-1

Published in the USA by
MTP Press
A division of Kluwer Boston Inc
190 Old Derby Street
Hingham, MA 02043, USA

Typeset by Georgia Origination, Liverpool
Printed by McCorquodale (Scotland) Ltd.

Contents

CONTENTS

CONTENTS

Section II Treatment of the Disease

CONTENTS

CONTENTS

CONTENTS

Section VI Free Communications

CONTENTS

Section VII   Posters

CONTENTS

CONTENTS

List of Participants

G. ALEMA
Ospedale San Camillo
Circonvallazione Gianicolense 73
I–00153 Rome
Italy

R. ALLAN
Pharmaceutical Division
Clinical Research
Sandoz Basle
CH–4002 Basle
Switzerland

E. ALVORD
University of Washington
Hospital Mail Stop RJ 05
Seattle WA 98195
USA

L. AMADUCCI
Clinica Malattie Nervose e Mentale
Università di Firenze
Firenze
Italy

O. ANDERSEN
University of Gothenburg
Department of Neurology
Sahlgrenska Hospital
S–413 45 Gotenburg
Sweden

C. ARFAIOLI
Università di Firenze
Firenze
Italy

G. AVANZI
Centro Transfusione Sague e
Immuno-Ematologia
U.S.L. 10 D
Ospedale de Careggi
Firenze
Italy

A. BARCLAY
4me Avenue
Parc Du Centenaire 22
B–1320 Brussels
Belgium

D. BATES
The Royal Victoria Infirmary
Queen Victoria Road
Newcastle upon Tyne
NE1 4LP
Great Britain

R. BENECKE
Department of Clinical Neurophysiology
University of Göttingen
Robert Koch St 40
D–39 Göttingen
West Germany

C. BENETON
Centre Medical Germaine Revel
Saint Maurice sur Dargoire
F–69440 Mornant
France

S. BERVOETS
Avenue P. Bols, 114
B-1020 Brussels
Belgium

F. BOLLENGIER
Labo. voor Fysiopathologie
van het Zenuwstelsel V.U.B.
Fak. Geneesk. en Farmacie
Gebouw D/R1
Laarbeeklaan 103
B-1090 Brussels
Belgium

S. BORENSTEIN
Hôpital Erasme
Service de Neurologie
Route de Lennick 808
B-1070 Brussels
Belgium

B. BORNSTEIN
Department of Neurology
Albert Einstein College of Medicine
1300 Morris Park Avenue
Bronx, New York 10461
USA

TH. BOUZIN
Trumelet Faber Straat 9
BP 8
Oost-Duinkerke
Belgium

C. J. J. BRINKMAN
Radboud University Hospital
Department of Neurology
Reinier Postlaan, 4
NL-6525 GC Nijmegen
The Netherlands

J. M. BRUCHER
Laboratoire de Neuropathologie
Cliniques Universitaires St Luc
Av. E. Mounier 52
B-1200 Brussels
Belgium

H. BRYON
KU. Leuven
Dienst Neurologie
St. Rafaël Kliniek
B-3000 Leuven
Belgium

F. CAMBI
Eunice Kennedy Shriver Center
for Mental Retardation, Inc.
200 Trapelo Road
Waltham, Mass. 02254
USA

A. CAPON
Hôpital Brugmann
Revalidation Neurologique
4 Place van Gehuchten
B-1020 Brussels
Belgium

R. CAPPARELLI
Clinica Malattie Nervose e
Mentali
Università di Firenze
Firenze
Italy

D. CAPUTO
Centro Studi Sclerosi Multipla
Ospedale Civile
Via Pastori 4
I-21013 Gallarate
Italy

G. CARELS
Laboratory of Neurophysiology
Department of Molecular Biology
University of Brussels
B-1640 Rhode-Saint-Genèse
Belgium

D. C. CARROLL
University of Alberta Hospital
112th Street & 84 Avenue
Edmonton, Alberta T6G 2B7
Canada

H. CARTON
Nat. Centrum M.S.,
Vanheylenstraat 16
B-1910 Melsbroek
Belgium

I. CATZ
Department of Medicine
W.W. Cross Cancer Institute
Edmonton, Alberta
Canada

C. L. CAZZULLO
Piazza Duse 1
Milan
Italy

W. S. CENDROWSKI
Institut Psychoneurolocany
U. Partysantow nr. 63 Pruszkov k
Warsaw
Poland

J. A. CERF
Laboratory of Neurophysiology
Department of Molecular Biology
University of Brussels
B-1640 Rhode-Saint-Genese
Belgium

F. CLAESSEN
Kul Leuven
Dept. Neurologie
St Rafael Kliniek
B-3000 Leuven
Belgium

M. CLANET
Centre Hospitalier Regional de Toulouse
Place du Dr. Baylac
11059 Toulouse Cedex
France

J. CLAUSEN
Neurochemical Institute
58 Rudmansgade
DK-2200 Copenhagen N
Denmark

G. CLINET
Institut Pasteur de Brabant
B-1040 Bussels
Belgium

B. CONRAD
Dept. Clinical Neurophysiology
University of Göttingen
Robert Koch St 40
D-3400 Göttingen
West Germany

R. CROLS
Laboratory of Neurochemistry
Born-Bunge Foundation U.I.A.
Universiteitsplein 1
B-2610 Antwerp
Belgium

A. CZLONKOWSKA
Psychoneurological Institute
Sobieskiego 1/9
02957 Warsaw
Poland

P. DAEMS
Koningsstraat 37
B-8400 Ostende
Belgium

M. K. DASGUPTA
University of Alberta
Department of Medicine
Edmonton, Alberta T66 2E2
Canada

H. DASSEL
Poorthofsweg, 14
NL-9751 CE Haren
The Netherlands

R. DECLERCQ
Rerum Novarumlaan 35
B-2110 Wijnegem
Belgium

T. DECOSTER
Hôpital St Luc
Service Neurologie
Woluwe
Belgium

W. DE COSTER
Dienst Neurologie
Akademisch Ziekenhuis
De Pintelaan 185
B-9000 Gent
Belgium

P. DELMOTTE
Nat. Centrum MS
Vanheylenstraat 16
B-1910 Melsbroek
Belgium

P. DELTENRE
Kleine Wouwerlaan 52/4
B-1860 Meise
Belgium

P. J. DELWAIDE
Departement de Neurologie
Hôpital de Baviere
Boulevard de la Constitution, 66
B-4020 Liege
Belgium

L. DEMONTY
Nat. Centrum M.S.
Vanheylenstraat 16
B-1910 Melsbroek
Belgium

LIST OF PARTICIPANTS

J. DE REUCK
Dienst Neurologie
Academisch Ziekenhuis
De Pintelaan 185
B–9000 Gent
Belgium

J. de SAEDELEER
K.U. Leuven
St. Rafael Kliniek
Neuropathology Unit
Kapucijnenvoer 33
B–3000 Leuven
Belgium

H. de SAXCE
Clinique de Neurologie et de
    Neuropsychologie
Hôpital de la Salpétrière
47 boulevard de l'Hôpital
75651 Paris Cedex 13
France

E. de SCHUTTER
Neurochemistry
Born-Bunge Foundation U.I.A.
Universiteitsplein 1
B–2610 Antwerp
Belgium

J. E. DESMEDT
Avenue Boetendael 69
B–1180 Bruxelles
Belgium

Y. DE SMET
Nat. Centrum M.S.
Vanheylenstraat 16
B–1910 Melsbroek
Belgium

D. DOMMASCH
Max Planck Institut
Klin. Forschungsgruppe MS
Wurzburg
West Germany

J. B. DOSSETOR
Department of Medicine
University of Alberta
Edmonton, Alberta
Canada T6G 2E2

M. DUPUIS
Clin St Pierre
Neurologie
B–1340 Ottighies
Belgium

P. EIBEN
Neurol. Univ. Klinik
Robert Koch strasse 40
D–3400 Göttingen
Germany

J. M. ESPADALER
Medina
Hospital de la Cruz Roja
Barcelona
Spain

K. FELGENHAUER
Neurologische Klinik der Universität
Robert Koch strasse 40
D–3400 Göttingen
Germany

E. J. FIELD
Crossley House
Neurological Research Centre
17 Brighton Grove
Newcastle upon Tyne NE4 5NS
England

W. FIRNHABER
Neurol. Klinik der Städt. Kliniken
    Darmstadt
Heidelberger Landstrasse 379
D–6100 Darmstadt Eberstadt
West Germany

M. FRANCESCHINI
Via Coste S. Paolo
Trevi Perugia
Italy

C. FRANCO
Centro Transfusione Sangue
e Immuno-Ematologia
U.S.L. 10 D
Ospedale de Careggi
Firenze
Italy

H. FRIEDRICH
Dept. Medical Sociology
University of Göttingen
Humboldtalle 1 d
D–3400 Göttingen
Germany

N. GENETET
Centre Regional de Transfusion Sanguine
Rue Pierre Jean Gineste
F–35000 Rennes
France

J. GEUTJENS
MS en Revalidatiecentrum
Boemerangstraat 2
B-3583 Overpelt
Belgium

J. GHEUENS
Laboratory of Neurochemistry
Born-Bunge Foundation – U.I.A.
Universiteirtsplein 1
B-2610 Wilrijk
Belgium

C. GILLAIN
Clinique St Pierre
B-1340 Ottighies
Belgium

R. GONSETTE
Nat. Centrum M.S.
Vanheylenstraat 16
B-1910 Melsbroek
Belgium

B. M. GUARNIERI
Clinica Malatti Nervose e
Mentali
Università di Firenze
Firenze
Italy

W. GUENTHER
Neurological Clinic
Klinikum Grosshadern
Marchioninistr 15
D-8000 Munich 70
Germany

L. GUILLAUMAT
Centre National d'Ophthalmologie des
   Quinze Vingts
22 Place des Vosges
F-75004 Paris
France

A. GUSEO
Central Hospital of Cty Fejér
Skekesfehervar
Seregélyesi u. 3
Hungary 8001

J. GYBELS
A.Z. St Rafael
Kliniek voor Neurologie en Neurochirurgie
Kapucijnenvoer 33
B-3000 Leuven
Belgium

J. F. HALLPIKE
Royal Adelaide Hospital
North Terrace, Adelaide, SA 5000
Australia

J. J. HAUW
Hopitâl de la Salpetrière
47 Boulevard de l'Hopitâl
F-75654 Paris Cedex 13
France

S. HAWKINS
Institute of Neurological Sciences
Department of Neurology
Ward 21, Royal Victoria Hospital
Grosvenor Road
Belfast BT12 6BA
Ireland

A. HELTBERG
Kommunehospitalet
Neuromedicinsk Afdeling
DK-1399 Copenhagen K
Denmark

A. HERODE
Hopital Erasme
Service d'Ophthalmologie
Route de Lennick 808
B-1070 Brussels
Belgium

M. HEULLE
Clin. Univ. St. Luc
Service de Neurologie
Av. Hippocrate 10
B-1200 Brussels
Belgium

H. HEYLIGEN
Dr. L. Willems Instituut
Universitaire Campus
B-3610 Diepenbeek
Belgium

L. A. H. HOGENHUIS
Department of Neurology
Hospital 'De Goddelijke Voorzienigheid'
Walramstraat 23
NL-6131 BK Sittard
The Netherlands

O. R. HOMMES
Sint Radboudziekenhuis
Institute of Neurology
Catholic University
Reinier Postlaan, 4
Nijmegen
The Netherlands

R. HOOGHE
S.C.K.–C.E.N.
Steenweg op Retie
B–2440 Geel
Belgium

E. HOOGHE–PETERS
Metabolism & Endocrinology
Medical School VUB
B–1090 Brussels
Belgium

M. HUTCHINSON
St Vincent's Hospital
Elm Park
Dublin 4
Ireland

P. INDEKEU
Rue de la Tannerie 4
B–7000 Mons
Belgium

D. KARCHER
Lab. of Neurochemistry
Born-Bunge Foundation U.I.A.
Universiteitsplein 1
B–2610 Antwerp
Belgium

R. E. KELLY
Head, Dept. of Neurology
St Thomas' Hospital
Lambeth Palace Road
London SE1 7EH
Great Britain

B. KENNES
C.G.T.R. 'Le Rayon de Soleil'
706 Route de Gozée
B-6110 Montigny-le-Tille
Belgium

P. KETELAER
Nat. Centrum M.S.
Vanheylenstraat 16
B–1910 Melsbroek
Belgium

N. KOENIG
Neurological University clinic
Klinikum Grosshadern
D–8000 Munich
West Germany

J. C. KOETSIER
Valerius Kliniek
Free University
Amsterdam
The Netherlands

E. KRATZENBERG
Blvd. Joseph II
1840 Luxembourg

K. J. B. LAMERS
Radboud University Hospital
Department of Neurology
Reinier Postlaan, 4
6525 GC Nijmegen
The Netherlands

X. LATASTE
Sandoz Medical Research Dept
Sandoz Ltd
CH–4002 Basle
Switzerland

E. C. LATERRE
Service de Neurologie
Cliniques Universitaires St Luc
Avenue Hippocrate, 10
B–1200 Brussels
Belgium

K. LAUER
Klinik für Neurologie
Heidelberger Landstrasse, 379
D–61 Darmstadt
Germany

H. LISKA
Immunolog. Institut
der Universität Wien
Borschkegasse 8
A–1090 Vienna
Austria

F. LISSOIR
Nat. Centrum M.S.
Vanheylenstraat 16
B–1910 Melsbroek
Belgium

LIST OF PARTICIPANTS

A. LOWENTHAL
Dienst Neurologie
U.I.A.
Universiteitsplein, 1
B–2610 Wilrijk
Belgium

O. LYON-CAEN
Hôpital de la Salpétrière
47 Boulevard de lHôpital
F–75651 Paris Cedex 13
France

L. NOEMI
Inst. neurol. Psychiat.
O.P. 61, CP. 6180, R–75622
Bucharest
Romania

Ch. MAERE
Schinkelkade 17
NL–1075 VG Amsterdam
The Netherlands

ANTONIO MAGALHAES
Centro de Estudos Egas Monis
Hospital de Santa Maria
Lisbon
Portugal

A. MAHLER
LABO voor Fysiopathologie van het
Zenuwstelsel V.U.B.
fak. Geneesk. en Farmacie
Gebour D/R1
Laarbeeklaan 103
B–1090 Brussels
Belgium

A. M. MALFROID
Laboratory of Neurophysiology
Department of Molecular Biology
University of Brussels
B–1640 Rhode-Saint-Genese
Belgium

R. MARTEAU
Clinique de Neurologie et de
  Neuropsychologie
Hôpital de la Salpétrière
47 Boulevard de l'Hôpital
F–75651 Paris Cedex 13
France

T. A. McPHERSON
Department of Medicine
WW Cross Cancer Institute
Edmonton, Alberta
Canada T6G 1Z2

R. MEDAER
Boemerangstraat 2
B–3583 Overpelt
Belgium

J. MERTIN
University Dept. of Clinical
Neurology
The National Hospital
Queen Square,
London WC1
Great Britain

M. F. MILLET
'Les Amis de Chanta-Corio'
Centre Germaine Revel
69440 Saint Maurice Sur Dargoire
France

J. M. MINDERHOUD
Department of Neurology
State University Groningen
Groningen
The Netherlands

G. MONSEU
Zevengatenlaan 24
Alsemberg
Belgium

R. MONTANINI
Neurological Department
Ospedale Civile
I–21013 Gallarate
Italy

J. M. MUSSINI
Service de Clinique Neurologique
C.H.R.
44000 Nantes
France

I. NEU
Neurologische Klinik
Klinikum Grosshadern
Ludwig-Maximilians Universität
D–8000 Munich 70
West Germany

D. NIJST
Dr. L. Willems Instituut
Universitaire Campus
B-3610 Diepenbeek
Belgium

M. NOPPE
Laboratory of Neurochemistry
Born-Bunge Foundation U.I.A.
Universiteitsplein 1
B-2610 Antwerp
Belgium

H. OFFNER
Institute of Neuropathology
University of Copenhagen
Frederik V's Vej 11
DK-2100 Copenhagen Ø
Denmark

E. PEDERSEN
Head of Department of Neurology and MS
  Hospital
Kommunehospitalet
DK-8000 Aarhus C
Denmark

I. R. PEDERSEN
Institute of Medical Microbiology
University of Copenhagen
Juliane Mariestej 22
DK-2100 Copenhagen
Denmark

R. PIPERNO
Via Montebello 6
Trevi Perugia
Italy

CHARLES M. POSER
Dept of Neurology
Boston Univ. School of Medicine
80 East Concord St
Boston, Mass 02118
USA

S. POSER
Department of Neurology
Univ. of Göttingen
Robert Koch Strasse 40
D-3400 Göttingen
Germany

J. PRANGE
Dept. Neurology
State University Groningen
Groningen
The Netherlands

M. PROSTEGEL
Max Planck Institute for Psychiatry
Department of Neurology
Kraepelinstrasse 10
Munich
West Germany

A. RASCOL
C.H.U. de Toulouse
Purpan
31000 Toulouse
France

J. P. H. REULEN
Institute of Medical Physics
Vrije Universiteit
Vander Boechorststraat 7
NL-1081 BT Amsterdam
The Netherlands

I. RISTIC
Proleterkih Brigada 47
4000 Belgrade
Yugoslavia

E. ROULLET
Clinique de Neurologie et de
  Neuropsychologie
Hôpital de la Salpétrière
F-75651 Paris Cedex 13
France

P. RUDGE
National Hospitals for Nervous Diseases
Maida Vale Hospital
London W9 1TL
Great Britain

Z. RZEPECKI
22 Lipca 24/2
65510 Konin
Poland

O. SABOURAUD
Hopital de Pontchaillou
Service de Neurologie
Rue Henri le Guillou
35033 Rennes Cedex
France

M. SAMPSON
Dept of Medical Sociology
University of Göttingen
Humboldtallee 1 d
D-3400 Göttingen
West Germany

E. A. C. M. SANDERS
Academic Hospital
University of Leyden
Department of Neurology
Rijnsburgerweg 10
NL–2333 AA Leiden
The Netherlands

Ch. Y. Th. SANDERS-BOZON
Department of Neurology
Academic Hospital
University of Leiden
Rijnsburgerweg 10
NL–2333 AA Leiden
The Netherlands

F. SCHELLING
Strahlehmedizinisches Institut
Arlbergstr. 3
A–6850 Dornbirn
Austria

H. I. SCHIPPER
Neurologische Universitäts-Klinik
Robert Koch Strasse 40
D–3400 Göttingen
West Germany

R. SCHIPPER
Multiple Sklerose Informations u.
  Beratungsstelle
Zentrum f. Neurol. Medizin
Gosslerstrasse 10 E
D–3400 Göttingen
West Germany

P. SEELDRAYERS
Department of Neurology
Hopital Erasme
808 Route de Lennick
B–1070 Brussels
Belgium

I. L. SIMONE
Department of Neurology
University Piazza G. Cesare
Policlinico
I–70124 Bari
Italy

C. J. M. SINDIC
Laboratoire de Neurochimie
Avenue Mounier, 53
B–1200 Brussels
Belgium

E. SLUGA
Neurologisches Institut Der Stadt Wien
University of Vienna
Schwarzspanierstrasse 17
A–1000 Vienna
Austria

M. SOEUR
c/o Dr R Soeur
Rue Marie Thérèse 102
B–1040 Brussels
Belgium

W. SOUKOP
Neurologisches Krankenhaus
Rosenhügel
1 Neurolog. Abteilung
Riedelgasse 5
A–1130 Wien
Austria

E. E. STADLAN
Neurological Disorders Program
NINCDS–NIH
7550 Wisconsin Avenue
Bethesda
Maryland 20205
USA

S. STECCHI
Ospedale M. Malpighi
Divisione Recupero e Rieducazione
  Funzionale
Via Albertoni 15
Bologna
Italy

B. TAVOLATO
Ospedale Civile de Padova
Clinica delle Malattie Nervose e Mentali
Via Giustiniani
I–33107 Padova
Italy

E. TOKARZ
Department of Neurology
School of Medecine
Poznan
Poland

R. TOLA
Neurological Clinic of the University of
  Ferrara
Corso della Giovecca, 203
I–44100 Ferrara
Italy

LIST OF PARTICIPANTS

W. W. TOURTELLOTTE
Department of Neurology
V. A. Wadsworth Medical Center
Los Angeles
CA 90073
USA

H. TSCHABITSCHER
Neurologisches Krankenhaus
Rosenhügel
*.Neurolog. Abteilung
A–1130 Vienna
Austria

A. A. VANDENBARK
Dr. L. Willems Instituut
Universitaire Campus
B–3610 Diepenbeek
Belgium

R. VAN DEN BERGH
Heidebergstraat 248A
B–3200 Leuven
Belgium

V. VAN DEN BERGH
K.U. Leuven
Dienst Neurologie
St. Rafael Kliniek
B–3000 Leuven
Belgium

H. vander EECKEN
Dienst Neurologie
Akademisch Ziekenhuis
De Pintelaan, 185
B–9000 Ghent
Belgium

J. H. van der HOEVEN
Department for Neurology
State University
NL – Groningen
Nederland

L. VANDERHOVEN
A.Z. St. Rafael
Kliniek voor Neurologie en Neurochirurgie
Kapucijnenvoer 33
B–3000 Leuven
Belgium

H. Van HAVER
A.Z. St Rafael
Kliniek voor Neurologie en Neurochirurgie
Kapucijnenvoer 33
B–3000 Leuven
Belgium

M. van ORSHOVEN
Mechelsestraat 20/3
B–3000 Leuven
Belgium

H. van POPPEL
Nat. Centrum MS
16 Van Heylenstraat
B–1910 Melsbroek
Belgium

F. VAN ROMPAEY
Dr. L. Willems Instituut
Universitaire Campus
B–3610 Diepenbeek
Belgium

D. van ROOST
A.Z. St. Rafael
Kliniek voor Neurologie en Neurochirurgie
Kapucijnenvoer 33
B–3000 Leuven
Belgium

P. van SANDEN
MS en Revalidatiecentrum
Boemerangstraat 2
B–3583 Overpelt
Belgium

M. van USSEL
Kloosterstraat 42
B–2750 Beveren
Belgium

H. K. van WALBEEK
Alexander v.d. Leeuw Kliniek
Overtoom 363–365
1054 JN Amsterdam
The Netherlands

E. VERJANS
A.Z. St. Rafael
Kliniek voor Neurologie en Neurochirurgie
Kapucijnenvoer 33
B–3000 Leuven
Belgium

R. VERMOTE
A.Z. St. Rafael
Kliniek voor Neurologie en Neurochirurgie
Kapucijnenvoer 33
B–3000 Leuven
Belgium

LIST OF PARTICIPANTS

D. VERVERKEN
Dienst Neurologie
St Joseph Kliniek
Roeselaarsestr. 47
B-8700 Isegem
Belgium

G. VERVLIET
University of Leuven
Campus Gathuisberg
Laboratory of Neurochemistry
B-3000 Leuven
Belgium

A. WAJGT
Department of Neurology, Medical School
Przybyszewskiego 49 Str
60-355 Poznan
Poland

K. G. WARREN
Clinical Sciences Building
University of Alberta
83 Rd Ave at 112 Street
Edmonton, Alberta T66 2G3
Canada

M. WEGGE
Nat. Centrum MS
Vanheylenstraat 16
B-1910 Melsbroek
Belgium

H. WEKERLE
Max Planck Institute
Klin. Forschungsgruppe MS
Wurzburg
West Germany

M. WENDER
Klinika Neurologiczna
Akademii Medycznej w Poznaniu
Prybyszewskiego 49
Poznan
Poland

K. WESTELINCK
Sandoz N.V.
Haachtse Steenweg 226
B-1030 Brussels
Belgium

U. WURSTER
Labor der Neurologischen Klinik
Medizinische Hochschule Hannover
Postfach 610180
D-3000 Hannover 61
West Germany

B. YORDANOV
Medical Academy
Clinic of Neurology
1 G. Sofinski str
1431 Sofia
Bulgaria

A. ZANEN
Hôpital Erasme
Service d'Ophthalmologie
Route de Lennick 808
B-1070 Brussels
Belgium

I. E. ZEEBERG
Department of Neurology (N2081)
Rigshopitalet
9 Blegdamsvej
DK-2100 Copenhagen
Denmark

D. ZEGERS DE BEUL
Beiaardlei 22
B-1850 Grimbergen
Belgium

Foreword

Looking back is a luxury for which scientists normally have little time. This XXV Anniversary Symposium, however, gives the opportunity of reminding us that in Belgium, where the risk of developing multiple sclerosis is among the highest in the world, a great man to whom we all pay tribute, I mean Dr Ludo van Bogaert, in 1957, took the initiative in founding the Belgian Research Group for Multiple Sclerosis.

It may sound immodest but since that time members of the Belgian Research Group happen to have an honourable record of important contributions to MS research, quite out of proportion to the financial support they received for it. Indeed, when compared to the situation in English speaking countries, funding of MS research has always been neglected in our country in spite of the fact that in 1958, acting on the advice of the Belgian Research Group, the Belgian National MS Society was founded with the specific object of collecting money for research as well as for social care.

At that time, the difficulty in raising funds for research was partly due to the fact that solving the problem of MS appeared almost impossible. Scientists could apparently only too slowly improve their ability to prevent and cure the disease. Media were indifferent to MS which was considered to have no news value, and the public remained uninformed.

Over the last few years, however, there have been new and exciting findings in MS. Perhaps the most important progress is our realisation that MS research is research pure and simple, and that everything is interrelated. We must thus be able to look for and exploit all new leads coming from other medical fields.

The tremendous development of immunological studies in MS is a good example. Basic immunological research in the field of tissue transplantations as well as treatment of autoimmune diseases with immunosuppressors have doubtless accelerated the pace of advance in MS.

Nearly two-thirds of this symposium is confined to immunology, probably the field in which there is the greater chance of finding a way of changing the course of the disease. Recent clinical studies, conducted in different countries, seem to indicate that 'immunomodulation' in a broad sense could influence the evolution of MS and provide grounds for supporting more extensive trials.

Recent progress in MS research and a better understanding of some of the biological mechanisms associated with the disease have attracted scientists who were not previously familiar with the problem. Multidisciplinary meetings like this congress enable the biomedical community to enlarge its areas of interest, and also highlight the international nature of the battle against MS.

We were therefore particularly delighted to welcome speakers coming from more than 20 different countries, and they must know that their important scientific contribution to this congress has been deeply appreciated.

The editing performed to a strict timetable has been possible through the outstanding cooperation of all the participants and the unstinting helpfulness of P. Delmotte, PhD, Secretary of the Belgian Research Group for Multiple Sclerosis.

R. E. Gonsette MD
Chairman of the
Belgian Research Group
for Multiple Sclerosis

Section I
Immunological Aspects
of Multiple Sclerosis:
Basic Observations

1
Auto-immunity

E. HOOGHE-PETERS and R. J. HOOGHE

'The similarity of some lesions in multiple sclerosis (MS) to those of experimental allergic encephalomyelitis suggests an auto-immune origin of MS, attacking first myelin-forming cells and following presumably a viral infection contracted early in life'. This statement, adapted from R. Adams in Harrisson's *Textbook of Internal Medicine* clearly summarizes the current interest of neurologists for immunology.

In this introductory chapter, we will briefly review some basic concepts in immunology and theories about auto-immunity.

IMMUNE REACTIONS

An immune reaction usually requires

(1) an antigen,
(2) antigen-processing cells, accessory cells such as macrophages,
(3) antigen-reactive cells, the lymphocytes.

There are several lymphocyte subpopulations which are not easily recognized at first sight. They include effector lymphocytes (B and T effectors) and regulatory T lymphocytes (T helper and T suppressor).

B effector lymphocytes will secrete antibodies (immunoglobulins) upon stimulation and differentiation into plasma cells (humoral immunity). T effector lymphocytes are involved in the cutaneous reaction of delayed hypersensitivity, for instance, in cytotoxic reactions (including graft rejection, tumour rejection, destruction of virus-infected cells,...) and in cellular reactions against pathogens such as *Listeria monocytogenes* (cellular immunity). Regulatory T lymphocytes modulate the activity of effector lymphocytes (both B and T effectors), through the production of helper or suppressor factors.

Efficient immune reactions occur only after contact with a suitable antigen (i.e. an antigen in a suitable form administered in an adequate amount, by a favourable route). A foreign protein, injected intramuscularly, several times,

3

might be a good vaccine. Porcine insulin is too small a molecule and too related (not different enough) to human insulin to regularly induce the formation of good antibodies even after 10000 injections. For reasons that are poorly understood, some antigens such as mycobacteria stimulate cellular immunity, while others, such as tetanus toxin, easily induce the production of humoral antibodies.

AUTO-IMMUNITY

Whether humoral or cellular, immune reactions should not be directed against auto-antigens: 'horror auto-toxicus', said Ehrlich. Yet, antibodies as well as cellular responses can be generated against auto-antigens upon appropriate stimulation. For instance, during a normal humoral immune response, in addition to antibodies reacting with the antigen, other antibodies reacting with these antigen-specific antibodies are also generated (anti-idiotypic antibodies). Self-recognition (of histocompatibility antigens) is also required when virus-infected cells are lysed by cytotoxic T lymphocytes. Macrophages, helper, suppressor and effector cells must also share antigens of the major histocompatibility complex as a prerequisite for their collaboration: thus recognition of auto-antigens is not forbidden but mandatory for normal immune responses.

Simple experiments can account for the failure to observe reactions to auto-antigens in several situations. It is now possible to fractionate subpopulations of lymphocytes. If pure B cells are cultivated in the presence of auto-antigens, it is easier to demonstrate the production of auto-antibody than when mixtures of B and T lymphocytes (as found in normal lymphoid tissues such as spleen and lymph nodes) are cultivated with the auto-antigen. It could be demonstrated that in many cases the absence of detectable immune reactions was due to regulatory T suppressor lymphocytes, rather than to an inability of effector lymphocytes to generate auto-immune reactions.

The three partners of normal immune reactions have to be discussed here, since they have all been implicated in auto-immune reactions.

Antigen

The pathogenic role of antigen has received much attention in the past. It was assumed that the immune system was unable to react against unmodified auto-antigens. However, auto-immune disease might result from the immune response against modified auto-antigens. For instance, patients taking α-methyl-dopa for hypertension may acquire auto-immune haemolytic anaemia, because the drug coats autologous (the patient's own) erythrocytes and stimulates the formation of antibodies against erythrocytes which are no longer 'seen' as auto-antigens.

Another way foreign antigens induce the formation of auto-antibodies is through cross-reaction with auto-antigens. A well-known example is the *Streptococcus*, which mimics a normal brain antigen. Therefore, after streptococcal tonsillitis, patients may have anti-brain antibodies. The latter are

4

responsible for auto-immune Sydenham's chorea.

A third way antigen may induce auto-immune disease is by polyclonal stimulation. Some antigens stimulate immune responses against themselves but also against a large variety of unrelated antigens, including auto-antigens. Among known polyclonal activators are Epstein-Barr virus (EBV) and measles virus.

Macrophages

Only recently have macrophages been implicated in the onset of auto-immune disease. They are responsible for the clearance of antigens including auto-antigens, and might contribute to auto-immunization if auto-antigens are presented to lymphocytes in adequate concentrations or in immunogenic (stimulatory) forms, for instance as large catabolic fragments.

Lymphocytes

The delicate balance between T helper and T suppressor lymphocytes may be disrupted. Whenever effector lymphocytes reactive against auto-antigen receive more help or less suppression than in the normal situation, auto-immune reactions may be generated. This model has received experimental confirmation in cases of humoral and cellular auto-immunity. Auto-immune allergic encephalomyelitis can be induced by immunization protocols that result in the stimulation of T helper cells collaborating with T effector cells that will destroy myelin-forming cells. Different immunization protocols favour the emergence of T suppressor cells. These cells can be separated, and upon transfer they will prevent the induction of auto-immune allergic encephalomyelitis. Thus, purified immune T suppressor cells protect against certain auto-immune diseases.

Neoplastic transformation is an extreme case of escape from regulatory influences. When plasma cells undergo neoplastic transformation, large amounts of antibodies are produced in an uncontrolled manner, in the absence of antigenic stimulation or help from regulatory T cells. We have observed the occurrence of paraproteins (myeloma proteins) reacting with neurons and probably responsible for the neuropathy complicating myeloma in these patients. In other patients, the neuropathy has been ascribed to the reaction of the paraprotein with myelin-forming cells.

THERAPEUTIC APPROACH

Classical treatments include the control of metabolic defects caused by the auto-immune disease: thyroid hormone in Graves' disease, insulin in juvenile diabetes, anticholinesterase in myasthenia, vitamin B12 in pernicious anaemia, ...

Anti-inflammatory drugs such as corticosteroids, indomethacin, ibuprofen have been largely used. Antimalarial drugs, penicillamine and gold salts may well belong to this group, although their mode of action is not clearly understood. Cytostatic drugs and irradiation are immunosuppressive and thus reduce inappropriate immune responses.

Plasmapheresis and lymphoplasmapheresis have been tried too, but usually with limited success. Treatment was often followed by a quick rebound of auto-immune responses. Feasible new approaches include:

(1) Manipulation of the stem cell compartment, by thymus or bone-marrow graft or with thymic extracts.

(2) Manipulation of the lymphocyte populations, by T-cell suppressor factors, with idiotypic or anti-idiotypic antibodies, with anti T-cell, or blast specific antibodies, possibly monoclonal, possibly tagged with a bacterial toxin or a radioactive isotope that would destroy effector cells responsible for the disease.

(3) Alternatively, antigen could also be injected after coupling to a tolero-genic carrier or to a bacterial toxin or a highly radioactive isotope so that the clones of antigen reactive cells would be selectively hit and depleted.

CONCLUSION

Antigen, macrophages and lymphocytes are the main factors involved in normal and pathological immune responses.

In many cases, auto-immune disease probably results from an imbalance between help and suppression. Therefore, current interest is largely focused on regulatory (helper and suppressor) T lymphocytes.

References

1. Bona, C. Hooghe, R., Cazenave, P.A. and Leguern, C. and Paul, W.E. (1979). *J.Exp.Med.*, **149**, 815
2. Hooghe-Peters, E., Fowlkes, B.J. and Hooghe, R. (1979). *Nature*, **281**, 376
3. Hooghe-Peters, E., Rentier, B. and Dubois-Dalcq, M. (1979). *J. Virol.*, **29**, 666
4. Steck, A.J., Murray, N., Meier, C., Page, N. and Perruisseau, G. (1983). *Neurology*, **33**, 19
5. Theofilopoulos, A.N. and Dixon, F.J. (1982). *Am. J. Pathol.*, **108**, 319

2
Occurrence of an internal image of measles haemagglutinin in an anti-idiotype immune response

J. GHEUENS and A. LOWENTHAL

The increased antibody titres to measles virus in multiple sclerosis (MS) patients were first described in 1962 by Adams and Imagawa.[1] Initially, this was believed to indicate an aetiological role for measles virus in MS, but it is safe to say that the evidence that measles virus causes MS has grown weaker and weaker over the years. The increased antibody titres to measles and to other viruses in MS are now thought by many to reflect a disturbed immunoregulation in this disease.

It is now well recognized that idiotype–anti-idiotype interactions in the form of immune networks are the basis of antigen specific immunoregulation[2-4]. Therefore, we are interested in the role of idiotypes in MS, and in anti-viral immune responses, and we have chosen measles virus as a model to study.

An assembled measles virion is a complex particle. There are six major structural polypeptides in the virus[5,6]. Each of these polypeptides can be immunogenic, and the immune response against measles virus will therefore be complex and heterogeneous. In order to study the immune response against measles virus we have, therefore, initially focused on the viral haemagglutinin. This is a glycoprotein, with a molecular weight of 76 000, which is expressed on the surface of the virion and of acutely and persistently infected cells[7,8]. The haemagglutinin is known to be a major target for the immune response against the virus[8]. In order to further simplify the situation, we have begun by studying the idiotypes of different monoclonal antibodies to the viral haemagglutinin[9]. This provided simple systems of one antibody, directed against one epitope, or antigenic determinant on a surface antigen of the virus. In these systems several aspects and implications of a network idiotypic regulation of an anti-viral immune response could be examined. For instance, because BALB/c mouse immunoglobulins were studied, experiments could be done in syngeneic conditions, in BALB/c mice. It is a precondition of any form of idiotypic network regulation that idiotypes are recognized by the immune system in which they are expressed. Syngeneic anti-idiotype, and anti–anti-idiotype to the anti-haemagglutinin antibodies have been produced. This demonstrated that a limited network of specific and anti-idiotypic antibodies could be induced originating from a single epitope on the surface of a pathogen, such as measles virus. Results were obtained with this system that suggested a possible direct role of anti-idiotype in the pathogenesis of viral infections[9].

In this communication, we present new results that further illustrate the implications of a network regulation of the immune response against viruses. In his original formulation of the network theory, Jerne[10] proposed that the antibodies that were directed to the antigen, would also recognize the idiotype of a set of antibodies, that were therefore said to present an 'internal image' of the antigen. We now have experimental results that support the existence of such internal images of measles haemagglutinin in the anti-idiotypic immune response to anti-haemagglutinin antibodies. Vero-cells were incubated first with different dilutions of normal BALB/c or anti-idiotypic sera, and then with 100 plaque forming units of the Edmonston strain of measles virus. A standard plaque assay was then performed. It was found that, in two out of the three systems tested, anti-idiotypic sera were capable of inhibiting the infection with measles virus. Normal serum did not affect the infection. This phenomenon was specific for measles virus. The infection with Vesicular Stomatitis Virus was not inhibited by those same antisera. It was shown that the effect was not due to measles neutralization by the anti-idiotype. These results suggested that an internal image of measles haemagglutinin existed in anti-idiotypic sera, and that this internal image inhibited infection through competition with the virus for binding to the viral cell receptor.

It was then examined if human sera, containing anti-measles antibodies, would bind to these anti-idiotypes, that presumably expressed an image of measles virus. This was assessed by a radioimmunoassay, in which human sera were reacted with solid-phase affinity-purified anti-idiotypic antibodies. The sera from three normal adults, four MS and eight subacute sclerosing panencephalitis (SSPE) patients were tested. Significant binding, which was at least twice the binding to other BALB/c immunoglobulins, was found to one anti-idiotype in almost all of the human sera, and to another anti-idiotype in some of the sera. No human serum reacted with the third anti-idiotype. The two anti-idiotypes that reacted with the human serum were also the ones that inhibited the infection. It was shown that this binding was not due to a cross-reacting idiotype in human sera with the idiotypes against which these anti-idiotypes were raised. The results, therefore, support the idea of an internal image of an epitope of measles virus in those anti-idiotypic sera. This internal image would then be mistaken for the virus by the human anti-measles antibodies.

These results point out the possible implications of an idiotype specific regulation of an anti-viral immune response. Auto-anti-idiotype that occurs during an immune response to a pathogenic virus may interfere directly with the viral infection, apart from having an immunoregulatory role. We are currently pursuing this work, and are trying to extend this fully to humans. Insight in immune networks involved in regulation of anti-viral immune responses will surely contribute to our understanding of the immune disturbances in multiple sclerosis.

ACKNOWLEDGEMENTS

This work was supported by grants from the National Fund for Scientific Research (Belgium), and the WOMS. J. Gheuens is Senior Research Assistant with the National Fund for Scientific Research (Belgium).

References

1. Adams, J.M. and Imagawa, D.T. (1962). Measles antibody in multiple sclerosis. *Proc. Soc. Exp. Biol. Med.*, **111**, 562
2. Golub, E.S. (1980). Idiotypes and the network hypothesis. *Cell*, **22**, 641
3. Bona, C. (1981). Regulation of clonal expression through immune network (limited network model). *Compendium in Immunology*, **2**, 223
4. Urbain, J., Wuilmart, C. and Cazenave, P.A. (1981). In Inman, F.P. and Mandy, W.J. (eds). Idiotypic regulation in immune networks. *Contemporary topics in molecular immunology*, **8**, pp. 113–148
5. Mountcastle, W.E. and Choppin, P.W. (1977). A comparison of the polypeptides of four measles virus strains. *Virology*, **78**, 463
6. Bellini, W.J., Trudgett, A. and McFarlin, D.E. (1979). Purification of measles virus with preservation of infectivity and antigenicity. *J. Gen. Virol.*, **43**, 633
7. McFarlin, D.E., Bellini, W.J., Mingioli, E.S., Behar, T.N. and Trudgett, A. (1980). Monospecific antibody to the haemagglutinin of measles virus. *J. Gen. Virol.*, **48**, 425
8. Bellini, W.J., McFarlin, D.E., Silver, G.D., Mingioli, E.S. and McFarland, H.F. (1982). Immune reactivity of the purified hemagglutinin of measles virus. *Infect. Immun.*, **32**, 1051
9. Gheuens, J., McFarlin, D.E., Rammohan, K.W. and Bellini, W.J. (1981). Idiotypes and biological activity of murine monoclonal antibodies against the hemagglutinin of measles virus. *Infect. Immun.*, **34**, 200
10. Jerne, N.K. (1974). Towards a network theory of the immune system. *Ann. Immunol.* (Inst. Pasteur), **125C**, 373

3
Studies on the intrathecal humoral immunity in multiple sclerosis

C. J. M. SINDIC, M. P. CHALON, C. L. CAMBIASO, E. C. LATERRE and
P. L. MASSON

INTRODUCTION

The most frequent immunological change which occurs in multiple sclerosis
(MS) is the oligoclonal pattern of IgG in electrophoresis of the concentrated
cerebrospinal fluid (CSF)[1-3]. This peculiar pattern is not seen at the electrophoresis of the paired serum. There are numerous studies supporting the
assumption that these oligoclonal IgG are locally produced in the central
nervous system of MS patients. In a recent study of 80 patients, we have
observed this restricted heterogeneity by agar gel electrophoresis in 61 cases
(76%) (Table 1). Several formulae have been proposed to estimate this local
biosynthesis, but the IgG index is the most commonly used[4]. The index takes
into account the influence of the serum concentration and the permeability of
the blood–CSF barrier. The latter factor is assessed by the gradient of albumin
between the two compartments. In our hands 66% of the cases had an
increased IgG index whereas 76% had an oligoclonal pattern. One key
question remains to know whether the local biosynthesis of IgG has a pathogenic significance. In addition to the study of IgG, we have investigated the
local production of other immunoglobulin (Ig) classes, namely IgM, IgA, IgE
and looked for the occurrence of immune complexes (IC) in the CSF.

Table 1 Changes in the CSF of MS patients

Oligoclonal pattern of IgG	61/80	(76%)		
High IgG index (>0.62)	53/80	(66%)		
High IgM index (>0.071)	26/80	(32%)		
with oligoclonal pattern of IgG			22/26	(85%)
with high IgG index			19/26	(73%)
High IgA index (>0.36)	12/45	(27%)		
High IgE index (>0.57)	0/71	(0%)		

MATERIALS AND METHODS

The levels of IgM, IgA and IgE were determined in the CSF by Particle Counting Immunoassay (PACIA). This automated technique is based on latex agglutination. Particles coated with antibodies are agglutinated by the antigen of interest[5-7]. The use of F(ab')$_2$ fragments rather than whole antibody prevents non-specific agglutination or inhibition of agglutination by proteins interacting with the Fc region of IgG[8]. Agglutination is measured by the counting of the residual unagglutinated particles in a conventional optical cell counter whose electronics have been modified to ignore aggregates.

For the assay of soluble IC, our method[9] is based on the inhibition by antigen–antibody complexes of the agglutinating activity of rheumatoid factors (RF) towards IgG-coated particles. Results are expressed in μg/ml equivalents of heat-aggregated human IgG (HAG). The IC were also measured in sera by a precipitating technique using polyethyleneglycol at the final concentration of 35 g/l and immunonephelometric determination of IgG and C4 in the precipitates.

RESULTS

IgE

With a limit of sensitivity of 0.2 IU/ml, IgE is not detected in CSF from non-neurological patients and infrequently in patients with MS: 13 cases out of 71 (18%). In these cases the levels of IgE in serum and CSF correlated significantly ($r = 0.78$; $n = 13$) and the mean IgE index was found to be 0.23 (SD $\pm$ 0.15). This value was not significantly different from the mean values observed in viral, pyogenic and cryptococcal meningitis ($\bar{x} = 0.33$; SD $\pm$ 0.08). However in tuberculous meningitis a high IgE index exceeding 0.57 occurred in most cases, suggesting a local biosynthesis of this immunoglobulin.

IgA

In a preliminary study, we have determined the IgA index in a group of non-neurological patients. The mean value, 0.22 (SD $\pm$ 0.07), was similar to that of IgE. This suggests that CSF contains essentially monomeric IgA. Values exceeding the upper reference limit were observed in 12 MS patients out of 45 (27%) (Table 1).

IgM

IgM is the first antibody to be produced in immune reactions. Therefore, its index could be particularly useful for the follow-up of the immune response. The mean IgM level in non-neurological patients was 97.5 μg/l and the mean IgM index, 0.021. The upper reference limit which was set up at 2 SD of log values above the mean, was found to be 0.071. In MS, the IgM index exceeded the reference limit in 26 cases out of 80 (32%).

Table 2 Relationships between very high IgM and IgG CSF indices and the clinical features of MS patients

	Number	Males	Females	Age of onset (±SD)		Interval between onset and sampling year (±SD)		Clinical state at the moment of sampling (number of patients)		
								Relapse	Remission	Slowly progressive course
Very high IgM index (>0.13)	11	7	4	29.5	(11.5)	5.1	(6.1)	8	2	1
Very high IgG index (>1.8)	8	1	7	27.5	(11.7)	10.7	(12.5)	7	0	1

12

The predominance of an Ig class during an immune response is dependent upon various factors such as age, sex and time after antigenic challenge. Therefore, we wondered how the IgM and IgG indices would be related. No correlation was observed between the two indices. Seven patients had a high IgM index with a normal IgG index and four of them with a normal pattern in agar gel electrophoresis. It should be noted that very high values of IgM index (> 0.13) were never associated with very high values of IgG index (> 1.8). Of the 11 patients with very high IgM index, seven were males, whereas of the 8 patients with very high IgG index, seven were females ($p = 0.035$ by Fisher's exact test) (Table 2). In addition to the influence of gender, other factors such as the age of onset, the interval between onset and sampling and the clinical state were considered. Of the 10 patients with a disease history exceeding 15 years, none had an IgM index exceeding the upper reference limit ($p<0.001$).

IC

The CSF of 21 non-neurological patients used as controls slightly inhibited the agglutinating activity of RF towards IgG-coated latex. This inhibition corresponded to a mean value of $2.8 \mu g/ml$ of HAG equivalents (SD ± 0.4). Values higher than 3.6 (mean $+ 2$ SD) which was considered as the upper reference limit were observed almost exclusively in herpetic encephalitis and pyogenic meningitis, but not in MS. In serum, results of the IC assay were in the normal range for the MS group. It should be noted that in herpetic encephalitis, the levels of CSF IC and the titres of anti-herpes antibody started to increase simultaneously about 12 days after onset. The levels of IC persisted at high values for 3–4 weeks and antibody titres for several months; no correlation was observed between the levels of IC in CSF and paired sera, and between the levels of IC in CSF and the IgG index.

Our negative results in sera of MS patients prompted us to perform a precipitation test using polyethyleneglycol and immunonephelometric determination of IgG and C4 in the precipitates. No significant differences were observed between the MS group, the group with minor neurosis and the group of patients with other neurological disorders. This latter group was made up of 13 patients with disc-prolapse, five with stroke, two with headache, two with seizure, seven with degenerative disorders of the nervous system and two with cervicarthrosis myelopathy. A significant correlation was found between the results obtained with the three tests (for PACIA vs. IgG in the precipitate, $r = 0.26$, $n = 90$, $p = 0.01$; for PACIA vs. C4 in the precipitate, $r = 0.35$, $p<0.001$, and between IgG and C4 in the precipitate, $r = 0.75$, $p<0.001$).

CONCLUSIONS

Our failure to detect soluble IC does not exclude the pathogenic role of IC in MS. Inflammation could be triggered by the deposits of IC which might be independent of circulating complexes. As in herpetic encephalitis, in MS the

IC could occur in the CSF for a very short time at the very beginning of the immune response and therefore be difficult to detect.

The local biosynthesis of Ig in the central nervous system of MS patients can be explained by polyclonal activation of specific immune response against either foreign or self antigens. In the first hypothesis the Ig production would be secondary to a proliferation of B lymphocytes under the mitogenic action of unknown endogenous or exogenous factors and would not play any pathogenic role in MS. The study of the IgG, IgA, IgM and IgE indices could give some insight into this still unresolved problem.

ACKNOWLEDGEMENTS

We are thankful to M. A. Crepin, M.P. van Antwerpen and J. L. Guarin for skilful technical assistance and to Mr M. Delory for competent editorial work. This work was supported by grants from the Fonds de la Recherche Scientifique Médicale (No 3.4529.79) and from the Groupe Belge d'Etude de la Sclérose en Plaques.

References

1. Lowenthal, A., Van Sande, M. and Karcher, D. (1960). *J. Neurochem.,* **6,** 31
2. Laterre, E. C. (1965). Les Protéines du LCR à l'état normal et pathologique. *Thèse.* Arscia, Bruxelles
3. Latterre, E. C., Callewaert, A., Heremans, J. F. and Sfaello, Z. (1970). *Neurology,* **20,** 982
4. Delpech, B. and Lichtblau, E. (1972). *Clin. Chim. Acta,* **37,** 15
5. Cambiaso, C. L., Leek, A. E., de Steenwinkel, F., Billen, J. and Masson, P. L. (1977). *J. Immunol. Methods,* **18,** 33
6. Sindic, C. J. M., Cambiaso, C. L., Depré, A., Laterre, E. C. and Masson, P. L. (1982). *J. Neurol. Sci.,* **55,** 339
7. Collet-Cassart, D., Mareschal, J. C., Sindic, C. J. M., Tomasi, J. P. and Masson, P. L. (1983). *Clin. Chem.* in press
8. Limet, J. N., Moussebois, C. H., Cambiaso, C. L., Vaerman, J. P. and Masson, P. L. (1979). *J. Immunol. Methods,* **28,** 25
9. Cambiaso, C. L., Riccomi, H., Sindic, C. J. M. and Masson, P. L. (1978). *J. Immunol. Methods,* **23,** 29

4
Antibody to viral antigens in multiple sclerosis demonstrated by ELISA method

M. CLANET, J. PUEL, F. BRETTE, M. ABBAL, A. BLANCHER
and A. RASCOL

Sera and CSFs of 47 patients with multiple sclerosis were assayed for IgG antibodies to measles, varicella zoster, rubella, cytomegalovirus, Herpes zoster 1 and 2, by ELISA technique: intrathecal antibody synthesis was calculated from sera and CSF titres and CSF albumin/serum albumin concentration ratio.

Intrathecal anti-measles antibody synthesis was observed in 59.5% of patients, anti-varicella zoster in 34%, anti-rubella in 29.7%, anti-Herpes HSV2 in 8.5%, HSV1 in 2.1%, anti-cytomegalovirus in 2.1%. Combined intrathecal synthesis was found in 21.3% of the cases to two viral antigens, in 17% to three viral antigens, in 4.2% to four viral antigens. High sera titres were frequently correlated with high CSF titres ($p < 0.001$).

Anti-measles and anti-rubella antibodies intrathecal synthesis was higher when patients were younger at the onset of disease ($p < 0.01$). Anti-measles intrathecal synthesis was higher in patients with remittent progressive types and severe disability scores ($p < 0.05$). Intrathecal synthesis of these several antiviral antibodies was not linked with the disease progression. Anti-measles, anti-varicella zoster, anti-rubella, anti-HSV1 intrathecal synthesis were strongly linked with IgG index ($p < 0.0001$), and with plasma call reaction in CSF. We did not find any correlation between sera and CSF titres, or antibody intrathecal synthesis and HLA antigens. These results and their relationships are discussed.

ACKNOWLEDGEMENTS

This investigation was supported by grants from the French Research association on MS (ARSEP).

5
Cerebrospinal fluid antibodies detect brain antigens

A. VANDENBARK, F. VAN ROMPAEY, D. NIJST, H. HEYLIGEN
and J. RAUS

ABSTRACT

Auto-immune destruction of central nervous system (CNS) antigens may contribute to the pathogenesis and prolonged clinical dysfunction in multiple sclerosis and other neurologic diseases. In an attempt to define relevant CNS auto-antigens, a sensitive assay (Enzyme Linked Immunosorbent Assay, ELISA) was developed, using as antigen, extracts of MS and control brains, and as antibody, cerebrospinal fluid (CSF). CSF from more than 80% of MS patients and less than 30% of control patients contained increased IgG anti-brain antibody levels. IgG_1 and IgG_3 were the predominant subclasses involved, but only IgG_3 demonstrated significantly more reactivity per μg antibody. Antibrain IgA and sometimes IgM levels were also elevated, but rarely IgD or IgE levels. Total reactivity to brain antigens rarely exceeded 0.1% of the antibody present. Total reactive antigen was extracted best with 1-butanol suggesting membrane association, and was extracted with similar efficiency from MS and control brains, from different areas of the same brain or from plaques or the corresponding periplaques from MS brains.

SUMMARY

Multiple sclerosis (MS) is characterized by increased auto-immune reactivity to brain antigens[1,2] which probably contributes to chronic demyelination, plaque formation, and motor dysfunction[3,4]. Of associated interest, the cerebrospinal fluid usually contains increased concentrations of intrathecally produced IgG[5] often resulting in oligoclonal bands[6]. To determine if this increased immuno-globulin production is directed against brain antigens, a sensitive enzyme linked immunosorbent assay (ELISA) was employed[7]. As antigen, crude 3 mol/l KCl extracts of brain were prepared and coated onto microtitre plates; the CSF antibody directed at the brain antigens was then detected using α-Ig class and subclass reagents. The results indicate that most MS patients and some other neurologic disease (OND) patients have elevated antibrain antibody levels.

METHODS

CSF samples, obtained from MS and OND patients from several clinics in Belgium and Copenhagen, Denmark, were centrifuged to remove cells, and were analyzed for oligoclonal bands and total IgG levels. Some CSFs were analyzed for circulating immune complexes[8].

Brain tissue, obtained at autopsy and frozen at $-80\,^{\circ}$C was extracted with 3 mol/l KCl[9], l-butanol[10], NaCl[11] or perchloric acid[12]. Myelin basic protein was prepared as described previously[13]. The ELISA test was carried out as described previously[1]. Reagents which detected Ig classes and subclasses were pretitrated to confirm specificity, and were often preabsorbed (see chapter P21 by Van Rompaey et al) on antibody of a different class to reduce non-specific background in the ELISA.

RESULTS

Preliminary experiments established optimal conditions for the ELISA test to detect antibrain and anti-myelin basic protein (MBP) IgG in neat CSFs. This reactivity was found to be dependent on the coating concentration of antigen and on the dilution of the CSF.

When antibrain IgG was evaluated in 64 MS patients and 171 OND patients, positive reactions were observed in 80% of the MS group and 30% of the OND group. The reactivity to MBP was lower in the MS group (70%) and higher in the OND group (45%). Within the OND group, patients with inflammatory or vascular disorders had a higher frequency of antibrain activity (43%) than patients with early neurologic symptoms (24%) or degenerative disorders (25%).

Analysis of oligoclonal bands (OCB), IgG levels and immune complexes indicated the following: patients with OCB had higher IgG levels and more antibrain IgG than patients without OCB. Individual comparisons confirmed a highly significant correlation of increasing antibrain IgG reactivity and increasing total IgG. All positive antibrain reactions exceeded the background reaction of normal human IgG tested at the same concentration. No correlation was observed between presence or levels of immune complexes and antibrain IgG activity.

Characterization of antibody

In further experiments IgG from MS and a pool of OND patients was separated over a Staph Protein A (SPA) column and tested for antibrain antibody activity. The SPA column eluate (IgG$_{1, 2}$, and $_4$ enriched fraction)

17

showed similar reactivity in MS and OND preparations (both above background IgG reactions), but the MS IgG_3 enriched fraction was significantly more reactive per μg IgG than the comparable OND preparation. The MS IgG_3 fraction was approximately 30 fold more reactive than the neat MS CSF, and 100 fold more reactive than the SPA column eluate. Direct analysis of IgG subclass reactivity to brain using α-subclass specific reagents confirmed the increased reactivity in the MS IgG_1 and IgG_3 subclasses. Similar experiments with Ig class specific reagents indicated that in addition to antibrain IgG, antibrain IgA and sometimes IgM was detectable in patients with elevated Ig levels. Increased antibrain IgD or IgE activity was not detected, however.

Characterization of antigen

In order to characterize the nature of the brain antigens which were recognized by CSF antibodies, several extraction methods were utilized. At comparable coating concentrations, the methods which extracted membrane associated antigens (1-butanol and KCl) had more reactivity than cytosol preparations (NaCl or PCA). To evaluate the distribution of the antigenic material, extracts from five areas of a normal brain, extracts from several MS and non-MS brains, and extracts from plaque and corresponding periplaque areas were compared. In general, the degree of myelination within the normal brain did not affect the antibrain reactivity. Similarly, unselected extracts from MS or non-MS brain produced comparable levels of antibrain reactivity, as did comparisons of plaque and periplaque extracts.

DISCUSSION

These data demonstrate clearly that patients with increased CSF IgG levels (including most MS patients and some OND patients with vascular and inflammatory diseases) have increased antibrain antibody activity. This antibody is of the IgG_1 and IgG_3 subclasses, usually includes IgA, and sometimes IgM and is probably directed at membrane associated antigens. Within the crude antigen mixtures, which are tested without further fractionation, no distinct activity can be associated with degree of myelination, patient source or plaque areas. Further fractionation by chromatofocusing, however, suggests that distinct antigenic differences can be detected in MS, Huntingtons and normal brain extracts (data presented in Chapter P10 by Heyligen et al).

The data presented above agree in general and extend the data of Ryberg[14] and Laurell and Link[15], and support the contention that most CSF auto-antibodies are produced in response to an initial tissue insult. As such, these antibodies may contribute to the chronic degenerative nature of MS; implication of auto-antibodies in the primary MS disease process (e.g. anti-acetylcholine receptor antibodies in myasthenia gravis) may require assays of greater sensitivity utilizing a restricted antigen repertoire (e.g. CNS neuroreceptor or neurotransmitter molecules).

ACKNOWLEDGEMENTS

The authors wish to thank A. Delsaer for typing the manuscript, and T. Van Galen for preparing the graphics for presentation at the 25th Anniversary Symposium of the Belgian Research Group for MS, Brussels, Belgium which this manuscript describes. This research supported by the Paul J. Cams Foundation of Belgium, the Wetenschappelijk Onderzoek MS Organization of Belgium and the United States Veterans Administration.

References

1. Knight, S.C. (1977). *Br. Med. Bull.*, **33**, 45
2. Iivanainen, M.V. (1981). *J. Neuroimmunol.*, **1**, 141
3. Caspary, E.A. (1977). *Br. Med. Bull.*, **33**, 50
4. Olsson, J.E., Link, H.R. and Müller, R. (1976). *J. Neurol. Sci.*, **27**, 233
5. Tourtelotte, W.W. and Ma, B.I. (1978). *Neurology*, **28**, 76
6. Kostulas, V.K. and Link, H. (1982). *J. Neurol. Sci.*, **54**, 117
7. Vandenbark, A.A., Van Rompaey, F., Heyligen, H., Nijst, D. and Raus, J. (1982). In Peeters, H. (ed.). *Protides of the Biological Fluids*, **30**, 231 (Oxford: Pergamon Press)
8. Stevens, W.J. and Bridts, C. (1981). *Immunol. Lett.*, **3**, 124
9. Meltzer, M.S., Leonard, E.J., Rapp, J.J. and Bersos, T. (1971). *J. Natl. Cancer Inst.*, **47**, 103
10. Le Grue, S.J., Kahan, B.D. and Pellis, N.R. (1980). *J. Natl. Cancer Inst.*, **65**, 191
11. Rastogi, S.C. and Clausen, J. (1980). *Clin. Chim. Acta*, **101**, 85
12. Comings, D.E. (1979). *Nature*, **277**, 2832
13. Diebler, G.E., Martenson, R.A. and Kies, M.W. (1972). *Prep. Biochem.*, **2**, 139
14. Ryberg, B. (1982). *J. Neurol. Sci.*, **54**, 239
15. Laurell, A.B. and Link, H. (1972). *Acta Neurol. Scand.*, **48**, 461

6
Immune complexes and the complement factors C4 and C3 in cerebrospinal fluid and serum from patients with multiple sclerosis

A. HELTBERG, H. JANS, I. ZEEBERG, J. HALKJAER KRISTENSEN,
N. E. RAUN and T. FOG

Multiple sclerosis (MS) seems associated with both the appearance of circulating immune complexes (CIC) and also, to a certain extent, the occurrence of immune complexes (IC) in cerebrospinal fluid (CSF). Furthermore, possible relationships between the occurrence of CIC, variations in the complement levels in serum and the activity of manifestations of the disease have been suggested.

Previous studies of the complement factors C4 and C3 in CSF from patients with MS seem to indicate a depressed level, but normal levels and elevated levels have also been described. As the complement system has a close functional relationship to IC it seems of importance to evaluate whether the occurrence of IC has any influence on the levels of some important complement factors.

In order to evaluate the possibility of an association between IC and the levels of C4 and C3 in CSF from patients with MS 32 patients with progressive and 'clinically definite' multiple sclerosis, according to the diagnostic criteria of Schumacher were studied. Before entering the study the patients were for at least 1 year monthly evaluated, according to an objective rating scale, measuring neurological deficit. Only patients, who according to these evaluations had a progressive course, entered the study.

The patients received information about the investigation, and all 32 patients accepted the drawing of blood samples, whereas 31 accepted the lumbar puncture. The clinical data are shown in Table 1.

The group of controls for the cerebrospinal fluid analyses constituted 61 persons, subjected to myelography for degenerative disorders of the spine and intervertebral discs. No patients with signs of tumours or regular inflam-

Table 1. *Patients* with multiple sclerosis

Total number	32
Sex:	18 men, 14 women
Age:	24–54 years (mean 36.6)
Duration of disease:	2–31 years (mean 10.3)
HLA-Dw2:	13 Dw2 + 19 Dw2
Course of disease:	remittant and progressive: 28
	progression from the start: 4

matory diseases in the nervous system were included in the control group. In the serum analyses the normal range was defined from groups of healthy persons.

Whole blood and cerebrospinal fluid samples were drawn simultaneously. Serum and 0.5% EDTA plasma were freshly frozen and stored at 80 °C. CSF samples were mixed with purified human albumin to a final concentration of 5% and were stored at 80 °C for not more than 3 days before analysis.

For detection of CIC all samples were double determined in the complement consumption test (CCT) and the polyethylene glycol precipitation test (PEGPT).

Presence of IC in a sample were considered if one of the two methods was found positive.

Quantitation of the complement components C4 and C3 in serum and identification of C4 and C3 activation products (C4 AP and C3 AP) in EDTA plasma were performed by means of rocket-immunoelectrophoresis. C4 and C3 in CSF were quantitated by means of rocket-immunoelectrophoresis. C4 AP and C3 AP in CSF were investigated by crossed immunoelectrophoresis.

In serum, CIC were found in 17 of the 32 sera (53%). in CSF IC were found in 9 of the 31 samples (29%). No correlation was found between the occurrence of IC in serum and in CSF. The levels of C4 and C3 in serum and CSF are shown in Table 2. A slightly elevated level of C4 was found in serum from MS patients, whereas the level of C4 in CSF from MS patients was significantly depressed when compared to controls.

C4 activation products and C3 activation products occurred simultaneously in plasma from 11 of the 32 patients (34%)*. C3 AP appeared alone in only one patient.

No C4 AP or C3 AP could be identified in the 31 CSF samples. As it appears from Table 3 a low level of C4 in CSF was significantly correlated to the presence of IC in CSF. No correlation could be found between the occurrence of IC in CSF and in serum, and no correlation could be established between the clinical type of disease, the occurrence of IC and the levels of complement in CSF or in serum.

In recent reports the frequencies of CIC and CSF-IC have been estimated to be 10%–77% and 10%–57%, respectively. Our observations are within these ranges. Also the observation of an independent appearance of IC in serum and CSF is supported by previous reports.

Although deposition of IC in the choroid plexus has been found in IC

---

*Nine patients with CIC and only two patients without CIC.

Table 2

	MS patients	Controls
Serum C4 %	126 (52–260) $p = 0.05$	112 (60–176)
Serum C3 %	114 (36–225)	104 (69–146)
CSF C4 mg/l	1.96 (0.90–3.32) $p < 0.01$	2.36 (1.19–3.88)
CSF C3 mg/l	2.64 (1.32–4.96)	2.64 (1.72–5.65)

Table 3

	IC present (n = 9)	IC absent (n = 22)
CSF C4 mg/l	1.34 (0.90–1.96) $p < 0.01$	2.11 (1.30–3.32)

related disease in animal models, there is no evidence for the IC in CSF to be a result of the occurrence of CIC. Previous studies have reported conflicting levels of C4 in CSF. Generally they have not taken the occurrence of IC in the CSF into consideration.

It has been suggested that CSF favours sustained binding of IC to complement receptors. Therefore, detectable IC in CSF should only be found when receptors are saturated, or when so much complement is consumed that solubilization mechanisms are compromised.

Some authors have demonstrated C3 AP in a small number of CSF samples from patients with MS, but our study has not been able to confirm this. Consequently, we have no evidence of complement activation and thereby evidence for an accelerated inflammatory reaction, but the simultaneous occurrence of IC in CSF and low CSF–C4 might be the result of receptor-binding of C4 and IC in complex.

We do not know the pathogenetic significance of the detectable IC in serum and CSF and their constituents are not known in detail, especially the antigenic part. We still have no indication of a reliable relation between IC, complement and the nature or the progress of the disease.

7
Characterization of circulating immunocomplexes in multiple sclerosis

J. CLAUSEN and M. UNGER

Circulating immunocomplexes were isolated from MS and control serum by precipitation at 3% w/v polyethylene glycol. The protein content of the precipitate was characterized by immuno- and polyacrylamide-SDS-electrophoresis. Furthermore, the DNA and RNA were isolated by hydroxyapatite chromatography after protein digestion and the total content of these constituents estimated. The native DNA fractions were characterized by their melting curves, their electrophoretic pattern after enzymic digestion and by hybridization experiments. Data will be presented elsewhere.

8
Immunoelectrophoretic characterization of immune complexes from CSF of multiple sclerosis patients

I. R. PEDERSEN and I. ZEEBERG

ABSTRACT

Immune complexes were isolated from the CSF of multiple sclerosis (MS) patients and non-neurological disease controls in order to examine if some of the antigens could be related to measles virus. The antigens were revealed by different immunoprecipitation methods by use of antibodies raised in rabbits against the immune complexes. The immune complexes used for immunization were isolated by crossed immunoelectrophoresis of the CSF against anti-human IgG. By this approach the rabbit anti-immune complex antibodies from both MS and control patients could be demonstrated to react with measles virus infected Vero cells, suggesting a persistent measles virus infection in the central nervous system.

INTRODUCTION

The present work deals with measles virus antigen in immune complexes isolated from MS patients. The presence of measles antigen in the CSF of MS patients could be expected for the following reasons. About 60% of MS patients have elevated measles antibodies in their CSF as compared to antibodies in the serum, and the measles antibodies are found in a much larger proportion of MS patients than are antibodies to other viruses[1,2]. Nearly 100% of adults have contracted measles, and approximately half of these have electroencephalographic changes during the acute phase of the disease, indicating that a measles infection involving the brain is a common event[3]. A direct proof of this notion is found in the fact that MS patients as well as non-MS patients harbour measles virus specific RNA in their brain cells as detected by *in situ* hybridization to measles cDNA[4]. Finally, about 49% of MS patients and 15% of normal persons have immune complexes in their CSF[5]. Thus, there is substantial evidence of the presence of measles antigen in the immune complexes isolated from the CSF of MS patients and perhaps also in the CSF of others.

METHODS AND RESULTS

Immune complexes from the CSF of MS patients and non-neurological controls were isolated and characterized by crossed immunoelectrophoresis of concentrated CSF against rabbit anti-human IgG serum as shown in Figure 1. A cathodic and an anodic precipitate were formed during the electrophoresis which could be seen with or without staining with Coomassie brilliant blue. The cathodic precipitate representing MS often increased in size, reflecting the fact that MS patients frequently have an increased CSF IgG level[6].

In order to characterize the antigenic part of immune complexes, antibodies were raised in rabbits against the cathodic and anodic precipitates obtained by crossed immunoelectrophoresis of CSF. The CSF material used was a pool of CSF from 12 patients with progressive MS and elevated CSF IgG, and from non-neurological disease patients used as controls. The precipitates used for the immunization were cut out of the electrophoresis gel while still wet and unstained, by use of a methodology for the production of monospecific measles antibodies as previously described[7]. The rabbits were given multiple injections and three rabbits were used for immunization with each precipitate. The rabbit anti-immune complex antibodies could be shown to react with measles infected Vero cells when different immunoprecipitation techniques were employed.

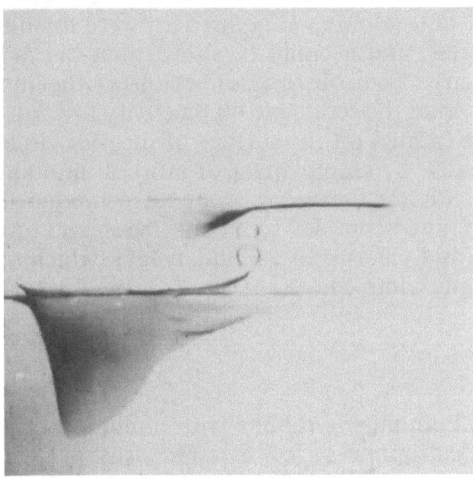

Figure 1 Crossed immunoelectrophoresis of CS from an MS patient. The wells in the centre were filled with CSF concentrated fifty times, from a patient with progressive MS. The components in the CSF were separated into a cathodic and an anodic part by first dimension electrophoresis. Next, second dimension electrophoresis was performed against rabbit anti-human IgG (Dako) $2\mu l/cm^2$ in the second dimension gel. This resulted in a lower cathodic and upper anodic precipitate representing isolated immune complexes.

In preliminary experiments, measles virus proteins labelled with ^{35}S-methionine were extracted from infected Vero cells, immunoprecipitated with rabbit anti-immune complex sera and analyzed by polyacrylamide gel electrophoresis. Four rabbit sera were obtained by immunization towards the cathodic and anodic MS and control immune complexes. These sera precipitated a measles protein with a molecular weight of about 60 kilodalton. Moreover, the rabbit sera representing the MS anodic immune complexes precipitated proteins from infected Vero cells with molecular weights of about 42, 100 and 200 kilodaltons. Of these, the 60 and 200 dalton proteins seemed to be specific for measles virus infected cells, as the other proteins could also be precipitated from non-infected Vero cells. The significance and identification of these Vero cell proteins remain to be shown. The precipitation pattern of measles virus infected Vero cells could also be seen with the application of a Western immune blotting technique.

The immunoreactivity of the four rabbit anti-immune complex sera was further tested by crossed immunoelectrophoresis of measles virus proteins. In this assay an extract of measles virus infected Vero cells was separated by electrophoresis in first dimension agarose gel. Second dimension electrophoresis was performed with rabbit anti-measles serum in the second dimension gel. The four rabbit anti-immune complex sera to be analyzed were placed separately in an intermediate gel between the first and second dimension gels. This technique has previously been used for the characterization of monospecific rabbit anti-measles antibodies[7]. All rabbit anti-immune complex sera reacted with measles virus nucleoprotein, although variable results were obtained in related assays, apparently due to the lower sensitivity of this technique as compared to the above mentioned techniques.

The four rabbit anti-immune complex sera were finally used in a measles plaque reduction test, and it could be shown that the different sera had no neutralizing capacity. This observation confirms the immunoprecipitation results which show that the sera have no reactivity towards the measles glycoproteins which are located on the surface of measles virus and measles virus infected cells. Finally, by employment of crossed immunoelectrophoresis of human serum proteins and the intermediate gel technique described above, the four rabbit anti-immune complex sera could be shown to react with complement factors C1q and C3 as well as human IgG, which are all known to be contained in immune complexes[8].

DISCUSSION

The advantage of immunizing rabbits with immunoprecipitates obtained by crossed immunoelectrophoresis of measles virus proteins is that even μg quantities of protein can be used for the production of antibodies[7]. By use of this technique, antibodies have been raised in rabbits against immune complexes which were isolated from the CSF of MS patients and non-neurological disease controls. The rabbit antibodies obtained could be shown to be reactive towards a measles protein with a molecular weight of about 60 kilodalton and which by crossed immunoelectrophoresis seemed to be identical with measles virus nucleoprotein. This reactivity was found with rabbit sera produced both against MS and control immune complexes. A parallel to this observation is the presence of measles virus nucleocapsid in the brain of SSPE patients[9,10]. Our findings suggest that a persistent infection in the central nervous system is not uncommon after contraction of measles. Whether a persistent measles infection is of primary importance for the development of MS remains to be shown. However, the measles infection can lead to demyelination of nerve sheaths in SSPE patients[9,10] and the closely related CDV virus can also cause demyelination, indicating that measles might play a major role in MS.

References

1. Norrby, E. (1977). Characterization of the virus antibody activity of oligoclonal IgG produced in the central nervous system of patients with multiple sclerosis. In ter Meulen, V. and Katz, V. (eds.). *Slow Virus Infections of the Central Nervous System*, p. 159 ff. (New York, Heidelberg, Berlin. Springer-Verlag)
2. Cook, S. D. and Dowling, P. C. (1980). Multiple sclerosis and viruses: An overview. *Neurology*, **302**, 80
3. Gibbs, F. A., Gibbs, E. L., Carpenter, P. R. and Spies, H. W. (1959). Electroencephalographic abnormality in 'uncomplicated' childhood diseases. *J.Am. Med. Assoc.*, **171**, 1050
4. Haase, A. T. and Ventura, P. (1981). Measles virus nucleotide sequences: Detection by hybridization *in situ*. *Science*, **212**, 672.
5. Tachovsky, T. G., Koprowski, H., Lisal, R. P., Theofilopoulos, R. P. and Dixon, F. J. (1976). Circulating immune complexes in multiple sclerosis and other neurological diseases. *Lancet*, **ii**, 997
6. Tourtellotte, W. W., Potvin, A. R., Fleming, J. O., Kolar, N. M., Levy, J., Syndulko, K. and Potvin, J. H. (1980). Multiple sclerosis: Measurement and validation of central nervous system IgG synthesis rate. *Neurology*, **30**, 240
7. Pedersen, I. R. (1983). Crossed immunoelectrophoresis of measles virus proteins. In Bjerrum, O. J. (ed.). *Electroimmunochemical analysis of membrane proteins*, pp. 409-418. (Amsterdam-Elsevier Science Publishers)
8. Theofilopoulos, A. N. and Dixon, F. J. (1980). Immune complexes in human disease. A review. *Am. J. Pathol.*, **100**, 531
9. Johnson, R. T. (1982). *Viral Infections of the Nervous System*, Chap. 10, pp. 237–270. (New York: Raven Press)
10. ter Meulen, V. and Carter, M. J. (1982). Morbillivirus persistent infections in animals and man. In Mahy, B. W. J., Minson, A. C. and Darby, G. K. (eds.). *Virus Persistence*, pp. 96–132, Symposium 33, The Society for General Microbiology. (Cambridge: Cambridge University Press)

9
Neurosurgery in the rehabilitation of hyperspasmodic and painful paraplegia in multiple sclerosis. Functional results in selective posterior rhizotomy

M. F. MILLET, C. BENETON, M. SINDOU, M. EYSSETTE and D. BOISSON

This study is about 22 MS patients, who became bedridden because of hyper-spasmodic paraplegia with irreducible triple flexion, associated with severe pain in 19 cases.

After the medical and physical therapy failed, the physiotherapist came to a therapeutic 'deadlock'. At this stage, he can have recourse to functional neurosurgical methods, like Selective Posterior Rhizotomy (SPR).

SPR consists of making a partial lateral incision on the posterior rootlets, on entering the spinal cord. It selectively interrupts the nociceptive fibres and myotatic fibres, while sparing most of the lemniscal fibres which are regrouped medially to reach the dorsal column.

The post-operative course, within the first 2 weeks, requires intensive care.

During the following 3 months, adapted nursing and kinesitherapy must be undertaken in specialized rehabilitation centres.

The risk of pressure sores remains the first patients' problem, over several months. Intensive kinesitherapy can be resumed because of pain relief, flexion spasms reduction, and abnormal postures correction, while a new neurological status appears.

All the 22 patients who were bedridden could recover a comfortable position in bed and wheelchair. Dressing and nursing have been ameliorated, as well as all daily life activities.

The results are then stable and long lasting with a follow-up period from 3 months to 10 years (more than 5 years in eight cases). They have allowed the patient to be reinstalled comfortably in a wheelchair and to resume a useful social life.

This paper was presented in this place due to the practicalities of the Symposium. It logically belongs in Section 3.

10
Immunological aspects of multiple sclerosis

J. MERTIN

INTRODUCTION

Multiple sclerosis (MS) and the immune system: to give a full review of this controversial field is an impossible task on an occasion such as this. I have decided, therefore, to centre my presentation on one aspect only, namely, the similarities between MS and one of its tentative animal models. This will provide a framework for the discussion of some of the more recent developments in MS research.

For some decades autoimmunity has been implicated in the aetiology and pathogenesis of multiple sclerosis. This theory has received its most convincing support so far from the similarities in clinical symptomatology and pathology between MS and an experimental autoimmune disease of the central nervous system (CNS), experimental allergic encephalomyelitis (EAE)[1,2]. The self-limiting disease process in conventional monophasic EAE contrasts distinctly with the chronicity of MS, and this has in the past cast doubt on the usefulness of EAE as a model for MS. This situation, however, has changed with the advent of chronic-relapsing EAE, which can be produced, under certain conditions, in guinea pigs, rats and mice[3-7]. Chronic-relapsing EAE resembles MS not only clinically and in the separation in space of the characteristic inflammatory and demyelinating lesions but also in their separation in time.

In EAE immunological tolerance against 'self' components of the CNS breaks down following injection of myelin, or of myelin basic protein (MBP), which have to be given in conjunction with an immunological adjuvant, usually Freund's complete adjuvant (FCA). In MS the antigen(s) responsible for the immunopathological process is(are) not known, nor do we have any definite clues yet as to the primary events initiating the disease. The most favoured theory at present is that autoimmunity in MS may result from a defect in immunoregulation, whereby the balance between intrinsic immune response-enhancing and suppressive mechanisms is disturbed. This would lead to autoaggressive reactions. The disturbance may have a genetic basis or may be acquired, for example, through a viral infection early in life involving nervous tissue and parts of the immune system.

SIMILARITIES BETWEEN CHRONIC-RELAPSING EAE AND MS

A summary of some of the most salient similarities between chronic-relapsing EAE and MS is given in Table 1.

Table 1 Some similarities between chronic-relapsing EAE and MS

Age	chronic-relapsing EAE: juvenile animals; MS: exposure to environmental factor before puberty
Clinical	characteristic clinical signs and clinical course (relapsing–remitting or progressive)
Pathological	perivascular infiltrations consisting of mononuclear cells; disseminated lesions of primary demyelination; gliosis, astrocytosis
Clinical/pathological	number, distribution and extent of lesions often correlate poorly with clinical illness
Genetical	genes of the major histocompatibility complex (MHC) and/or genes outside the MHC control susceptibility to the diseases
Immunological	intrathecal immunoglobulin production; restricted heterogeneity of the immunoglobulins in the CSF and in/around the lesions in the CNS (oligoclonal bands) sensitization of peripheral lymphocytes to MBP; direct cell-mediated cytotoxicity by peripheral blood lymphocytes against MBP and other myelin components; fluctuation of cell numbers in T cell subpopulations in relation to clinical attacks; suppression of disease activity by immunosuppressive treatment

Age

In order to produce chronic-relapsing EAE, sensitization with CNS-specific antigen has to be carried out in juvenile animals[3-7]. Age-dependancy is also a factor in MS, where the results of epidemiological studies have indicated that the patients were exposed to the aetiological environmental agent(s) before attaining puberty[8].

Clinical and pathological characteristics

The striking similarities in the clinical and pathological characteristics of chronic-relapsing EAE with those encountered in MS have been demonstrated convincingly by various authors[5,9]. This similarity also extends to the often poor correlation between pathological changes on the one hand and clinical signs on the other. In chronic-relapsing EAE of the strain 13 guinea pig, for example, Suckling *et al*[10] have observed that '... those animals with macroscopically visible plaques showed the most severe perivascular and meningeal changes, although these changes were not necessarily indicative of clinical illness'. Until recently there has been some agreement that in MS the number, distribution and extent of inflammatory and demyelinating lesions correlate closely with the clinical status of the patients. However, we have become increasingly aware of the possibility that this may not necessarily be so. Apart from the occasional discovery of so-called 'silent MS' in post mortem examinations[11] there are other observations supporting the view that clinical relapses, their frequency and severity are not indicative of the activity of the disease process *per se*. For example, pathological changes in the visual evoked potentials (VEP) can be detected in a high percentage of patients with 'spinal MS' who have never shown symptoms indicating involvement of parts of the CNS above the foramen magnum[12]. Furthermore, studies using computer tomography and, more recently, nuclear magnetic resonance (NMR) tomography have revealed discrepancies between clinically-diagnosed lesions and the actual site, number and extent of lesions detected with these methods. Thus, Young *et al*[13] have demonstrated a disturbingly high number of lesions, detected by the NMR method, in patients with relatively mild clinical disease. Some of the patients had distinct brainstem lesions but did not show any clinical signs indicative of lesions in this region. These observations suggest that typifying subgroups of MS patients for the purpose of stratification of therapeutic trials or for immunological research according to clinically-diagnosed lesions or the clinical course of the disease may be unwarranted. To be provocative: the relapsing–remitting clinical course shown by the majority of MS patients, especially during the earlier stages of the disease, is an epiphenomenon and does not reflect the true nature of a progressive disease process. Therefore, the preoccupation of many investigators in searching for changes in parameters which are closely linked to the changes in clinical illness may well be a fallacy, leading merely to the description of secondary phenomena. This we have to bear in mind when discussing some of the findings in EAE and MS research.

Genetic factors influencing susceptibility to EAE and MS

Acute monophasic EAE can only be induced reproducibly in guinea-pigs, rats and mice if certain inbred strains are used for the experiments. Susceptibility to chronic-relapsing EAE is further restricted since it can only be produced – in a regular fashion – in guinea-pigs of the strain 13, in Lewis rats and in SJL mice. This clearly indicates genetic control of susceptibility, and indeed various studies have shown that susceptibility is closely associated with genes linked to the major histocompatibility complex (MHC)[14-16]. Recent data on EAE in mice have indicated control of susceptibility also by genes outside the major histo-compatibility complex[17].

In MS genetic population and family studies have shown an association of the disease with the human major histocompatibility complex, the HLA system[18]. A preponderance of the HLA antigens A3, B7, Dw2 and DR2 has been found in North European and American MS patients of Caucasian race.

Different associations were detected for Mediterranean, African and Japanese populations. An 'MS susceptibility gene' appears to be closely linked to DR genes, but is of low penetrance and only leads to MS when combined with an environmental factor[19]. Also genes outside the HLA complex may influence susceptibility to MS. Important candidates are genes coding for immuno-globulin G allotypes (Gm). Interacting with HLA, Gm genes seem to influence the incidence of chronic active hepatitis in man[20] and Graves' disease[21]. An increased frequency of the Gm 1, 17, 21, 26 haplotype has been described in patients with MS[22].

The results of population studies have indicated an increase of this Gm haplotype in the northern areas of Europe[23], and this would fit in well with the known North–South gradient of the prevalence of MS.

Apart from contributing to the aetiology of MS, HLA-linked factors may also influence the rate of progression of the disease and the effectiveness of treatment[24,25]. Correlation between the beneficial effect of immunosuppressive treatment with HLA DR2 has been reported by Hommes et al[26] and Madigand et al[27]. In a recently completed double-blind controlled trial we have found a significant reduction in the rate of acute clinical exacerbations in HLA A3-positive patients treated with immunosuppression when compared with placebo-treated A3-positive patients[28]. If such observations could be confirmed in extended studies then one day it may be possible to identify sub-groups of MS patients for whom the benefits of certain treatments would be more predictable than they are today.

THE IMMUNOLOGY OF CHRONIC-RELAPSING EAE AND MS

Before discussing the immunology of chronic-relapsing EAE and MS, let me first mention some of the more recent advances in the field of immunology in general (Figure 1)[29].

The immune system

Both cell-mediated immune responses (mediated by T lymphocytes) and humoral responses (mediated by B lymphocytes) can precipitate clinical hyper-sensitivity reactions, resulting in immunological inflammation and tissue damage. In recent years, we have witnessed considerable progress in the under-standing of the function of the immune system. It has become evident that T lymphocytes are essentially required for immune recognition and the genera-tion of immune responses. Antigens are recognized by T cells only when presented to them on the surface of cells expressing 'self'[30]. In such antigen-presenting cells (APC) surface molecules signalling 'self' are controlled by the MHC. Cytotoxic T cells (T_C) recognize antigens associated with class I products of the major histocompatibility complex (HLA A and B, in man) whereas T-helper cells (T_H) and T cells producing delayed hypersensitivity reactions (T_{DTH}) require class II MHC products (HLA D), the immune response-associated (Ia) histocompatibility antigens for recognition.

The best known APC are macrophages and monocytes, but current

32

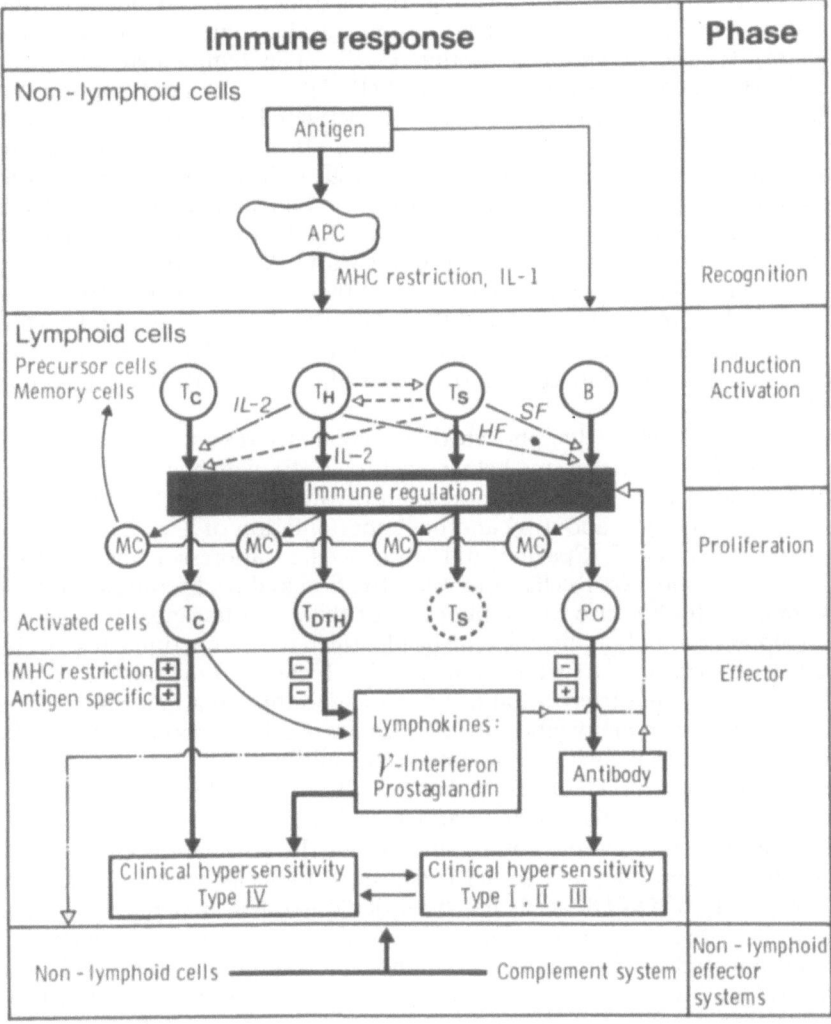

Mertin and Fierz, 1982

Figure 1 Schematic representation of immune responses leading to clinical hypersensitivity reactions[29]. APC = antigen-presenting cell; MHC = major histocompatibility complex; IL-1 = interleukin 1; IL-2 = interleukin 2; T_C = cytotoxic T-cell; T_H = helper T-cell; T_S = suppressor T-cell; T_{DTH} = T-cell mediating delayed type hypersensitivity; B = B-cell; PC = plasma cell; MC = memory cell; HF = helper factor(s); SF = suppressor factor(s)

evidence suggests that dendritic cells may be of even greater importance for MHC-restricted antigen recognition[31]. The group of dendritic cells comprises the Langerhans cells of the skin, dendritic cells in the lymphoid organs, veiled cells in the afferent lymph[32] and possibly also microglial cells in the CNS. It is assumed that these cells derive from a common stem cell in the bone marrow and migrate to their respective tissues.

Activated APC, besides providing the specific 'self' signal allowing recognition, also produce and release a non-specific soluble factor which is mandatory for the activation of resting T cells. This lymphocyte activating factor (LAF) has been termed interleukin 1 (IL-1)[33]. IL-1 is a polypeptide and acts as an inducer of T cell maturation. Once activated T_H cells produce T cell growth factors (TCGF), termed interleukin 2 (IL-2)[34]. IL-2 is required to promote and maintain the proliferation of T cells following their stimulation. IL-2 has already proved to be invaluable for the establishment of specific T cell lines in culture. For example, with the help of T cell growth factor, clones of myelin basic protein-specific T cells from rats with EAE have been propagated as continuous cell lines[35]. These cells retained their EAE-inducing activity for up to 8 months after establishment of the cultures. When given in numbers too low to transfer the disease to the recipient animals these cells had a protective effect against EAE as induced by inoculation of the rats with CNS antigen in FCA[36].

In contrast to T cells, B lymphocytes can respond to free antigen, but usually depend on help conveyed by helper factors (HF) which are released by specifically activated T_H cells. Suppression of the activity of B cells, on the other hand, is brought about by another subpopulation of T cells, namely T suppressor (T_S) cells[37]. Specific and non-specific suppressor factors (SF) produced by suppressor T cells suppress activation and proliferation not only of B lymphocytes but also of lymphocytes of the T cell lineage.

Subpopulations of lymphocytes can be identified using functional tests or by detection of specific cell surface markers. With the introduction of monoclonal antibodies characterization of lymphocyte subpopulations has become routine procedure in many laboratories. Human T cell subpopulations can be identified, for example, with monoclonal OKT antibodies[38]. These allow us to distinguish between T_H (= OKT4$^+$) and T_S (= OKT8$^+$) cells, but not between T_H and T_{DTH} cells, nor between T_S and T_C cells.

There is still considerable controversy about the correlation between cell marker on the one side, and actual function of the cells on the other. Suppressor activity of OKT8$^+$ cells has been demonstrated *in vitro*, but little is known about the *in vivo* function of such cells. Moreover, the concept of immunosuppression by discrete lymphocyte subpopulations has been challenged by investigators such as Knight *et al*[39,40] who could demonstrate suppression in lymphocyte cultures as a function of normal cell growth dynamics. Another factor limiting the interpretation of changes in the numbers of peripheral lymphocytes is the fact that the blood represents only a small part of the lymphoid system: changes herein do not necessarily indicate alterations within the extravascular compartments of the lymphoid system. Furthermore, lymphocytes specifically involved in disease processes comprise only a small fraction of the total number of cells of the different lymphocyte subpopulations, and global changes in the subpopulations may not reflect changes in the number of specific cells. Today, this field is dominated by what some authors have called 'a recent conceptual epidemic'[41]. There is widespread speculation on the role of non-specific suppressor cells in diseases. This is, in my view, somewhat premature: as long as basic immunological research has not been able to define the *in vivo* role of cells which after stimulation with mitogen cause suppression in tissue cultures, clinical investigators should not rely on the activity of such cells in their patients.

Interleukins, helper and suppressor factors and other lymphokines, together with antibodies, anti-antibodies, antigen–antibody complexes, and various intercellular mediator substances produced by lymphoid and non-lymphoid cells such as interferons, prostaglandins, leukotrienes and hormones, all contribute to an intricate network of regulatory circuits summarized in Figure 1 as 'immunoregulation'. The mechanisms of immunoregulation are poorly understood, and this limits the possibilities for modifying immune function for therapeutic purposes. For example, in treatment with cytotoxic drugs or antilymphocyte globulin, immunosuppression is essentially produced by reduction in the numbers of potentially harmful lymphocytes, without discrimination, however, for functionally different lymphocyte subpopulations. A first step towards a more specific immunosuppressive treatment has been the discovery of cyclosporin A (CyA). This fungal metabolite is not cytotoxic but has been found to interfere with the production and release of IL-2 by activated T_H cells as well as with the action of IL-2 on IL-2-dependent cells[42,43]. There is no effect of CyA on suppressor activity. A double blind trial to test this new substance in the treatment of MS is presently being carried out in London, England.

Humoral immune responses in EAE and MS

EAE is a cell-mediated autoimmune disease which can be transferred from afflicted animals to 'naïve' recipients of the same genetic background (in adoptive transfer) with the help of T cells, but not with antibodies or B cells. Nevertheless, sensitization with components of the central nervous system also causes humoral immune reactions which may contribute considerably to the disease process. In animals with EAE, as well as in patients with MS, there is a local production of immunoglobulin (Ig) in the central nervous system combined with increased concentrations of immunoglobulin in the cerebrospinal fluid (CSF). In both circumstances the immunoglobulin is of restricted heterogeneity[44,45] which results in the occurrence of oligoclonal bands in agar gel electrophoreses or after separation by isoelectric focussing. Studies in guinea-pigs with chronic-relapsing EAE have revealed that the majority of the oligoclonal antibodies are directed against components of the mycobacterium of the adjuvant[46] and not against components of the central nervous system. This is somewhat similar to MS, where it was hoped in the past that the discovery of oligoclonal antibodies would lead to the identification of an MS-specific antigen. This hope, however, has been greatly frustrated by findings showing that these antibodies are directed against a variety of bacterial and viral antigens with no specific relationship to the disease. It would appear that these 'nonsense antibodies' – as some authors have called them[47] – are produced by B lymphocytes and plasma cells trapped within lesions and in the cerebrospinal fluid, and activated by non-specific stimuli. Nevertheless, some of these antibodies could still be crossreacting with components of the central nervous system or the blood–brain barrier, and so contribute to the disease process.

Cell-mediated immunity in EAE and MS

In EAE sensitization of peripheral blood lymphocytes to components of the CNS, such as MBP, can be detected readily using various *in vitro* assay techniques. The evidence for similar findings in MS is still equivocal.

Cytolytic activity directed against MBP has been detected after incubation of spleen cells from MBP sensitized guinea-pigs with target cells which were coated with basic protein[48]. Adapting this method to human peripheral lymphocytes Frick[49] has demonstrated marked cytolytic activity by lymphocytes from MS patients directed not only against MBP but also against cells coated with encephalitogenic peptide, cerebrosides and gangliosides. The author concluded that 'cytotoxicity against the encephalitogenic peptide can be considered as a pathogenic factor for the demyelinization process in MS'. Independent confirmation supporting this speculation has yet to be published. There is, on the other hand, also the question whether the activity of cytotoxic T cells as detected *in vitro* has any relevance for their *in vivo* action. It has been shown that for adoptive transfer of EAE in mice and rats only those T cells are required which carry the surface characteristics of T helper lymphocytes[50,51]. Moreover, little is known about the occurrence and distribution of products of the major histocompatibility complex on the various cell types of the nervous system. So far, only Ia molecules have been detected on glial cells[52,53], and this again would favour the T_H cell as a candidate for the initiation of immunologic inflammation in the central nervous system. The abundance or relative lack of Ia molecules on cells of the nervous tissues may be one of the factors determining susceptibility to EAE in different animal strains. It will be important to find out whether cells bearing Ia molecules are evenly distributed throughout the central nervous system, or whether there may be regions which are predominantly populated by such cells. Should the latter be the case then this could have some relevance in explaining those sites in the central nervous system known to be preferentially afflicted by the demyelinating processes in EAE and MS.

Suppressor cells

Various methods have been used to detect changes in suppressor activity, or in the actual number of cells carrying suppressor cell markers, in the peripheral blood of animals with EAE and in patients with MS. Recent investigations using monoclonal antibodies for the identification of lymphocyte subpopulations have confirmed earlier studies showing a decrease in the numbers of suppressor cells in relation to clinical attacks in chronic-relapsing EAE[54] and in MS[55]. It has been speculated that such changes may be causally connected with clinical exacerbations of the disease process. However, changes in the number of specific cells in the peripheral blood can be detected in many conditions, including some unrelated to immunological events, e.g. after open heart surgery or after physical exertion. Moreover, Arnason and co-workers have recently suggested that during clinical attacks suppressor cells may not be physically removed from the circulation of MS patients but lose the surface markers identifying them as such[56]. With this in mind, and considering the frequent disparity (mentioned earlier in this review) between clinical illness and pathology, one may suspect that these changes in the numbers of identifiable cells may be secondary phenomena, and thus be without specific relevance to the basic pathology of the disease.

Immunosuppressive treatment

EAE can be readily suppressed by tolerization of the animals with MBP or encephalitogenic peptide in non-immunogenic preparations[57], or by immuno-suppression with cytotoxic drugs[58], antilymphocyte globulin[59], essential fatty acids[60], and CyA[61]. The results of attempts to suppress progression of the disease process in MS patients using the same substances, have so far been less convincing[62]. Nevertheless, most of the many uncontrolled and the few controlled trials of immunosuppressive treatment reported in the literature have shown some degree of amelioration, and this should be sufficiently encouraging for continued efforts in this direction. The pragmatic approach, with strictly controlled clinical trials of immunological treatment, may in the end prove to be as valuable as that of basic research in solving the problem of multiple sclerosis.

References

1. Alvord, E. C., Shaw, C. M., Hruby, S. and Kies, M. W. (1965). *Ann. N.Y. Acad. Sci.,* **122**, 333
2. Paterson, P. Y. (1977). In Talal, N. (ed.). *Autoimmunity, Genetics, Immunologic, Virologic and Clinical Aspects,* pp. 643–692 (New York: Academic Press)
3. Raine, C. S. and Stone, S. H. (1977). *N.Y. State J. Med.,* **77**, 1693
4. Wisniewski, H. M. and Keith, A. B. (1977). *Ann. Neurol.,* **1**, 144
5. Lassmann, H. and Wisniewski, H. M. (1979). *Archs. Neurol.,* **36**, 490
6. McFarlin, D. E., Blank, S. E. and Kibler, R. F. (1974). *J. Immunol.,* **113**, 712
7. McFarlin, D. and Waksman, B. (1982). *Immunology Today,* **3**, 321
8. Kurtzke, J. F. (1983). In Hallpike, J. F., Adams, C. W. M. and Tourtelotte, W. W. (eds.). *Multiple Sclerosis. Pathology, Diagnosis and Management,* pp. 47–95 (London: Chapman and Hall)
9. Raine, C. S. (1983). In Hallpike, J. F., Adams, C. W. M. and Tourtelotte, W. W. (eds.). *Multiple Sclerosis. Pathology, Diagnosis and Management,* pp. 413–460 (London: Chapman and Hall)
10. Suckling, A. J., Wilson, N. R., Kirby, J. A. and Rumsby, M. G. (1983). *Neuropath. Appl. Neurobiol.* (in press)
11. Mackay, R. P. and Hirano, A. (1967). *Archs. Neurol.,* **17**, 588
12. Halliday, A. M. (1978). In Matthews, W. B. and Glaser, G. H. (eds.). *Recent Advances in Clinical Neurology,* pp. 47–74 (Edinburgh: Churchill Livingstone)
13. Young, I. R., Hall, A. S., Pallis, C. A., Legg, N. J., Bydder, G. M. and Steiner, R. E. (1981). *Lancet,* **2**, 1063
14. Williams, R. M. and Moore, M. J. (1973). *J. Exp. Med.,* **138**, 775
15. Kies, M. W., Driscoll, B. F., Lisak, R. P. and Alvord, E. C. (1975). *J. Immunol.,* **115**, 75
16. Bernard, C. C. A. (1977). *J. Immunogenet.,* **3**, 263
17. Montgomery, I. N. and Rauch, H. C. (1982). *J. Immunol.,* **128**, 412
18. Jersild, C., Dupont, B., Fog, T., Plate, P. and Svejgaard, A. (1975). *Transplant. Rev.,* **22**, 148
19. Ho, H-Z., Tiwari, J. L., Haile, R. W., Terasaki, P. I. and Mortion, N. E. (1982). *Immunogenetics,* **15**, 509
20. Whittingham, S. J., Matthews, J. D., Schanfield, M. S., Tait, B. D. and Mackay, I. R. (1981). *Clin. Exp. Immunol.,* **43**, 80
21. Uno, H., Sasazuki, T., Tamai, H. and Matsumoto, H. (1981). *Nature,* **292**, 768

22. Pandey, J. P., Goust, J-M, Salier, J-P and Fudenberg, H. H. (1981). *J. Clin. Invest.*, **67**, 1797
23. Steinberg, A. G. and Cook, C. E. (1981). *The Distribution of the Human Ig allotypes*, (Oxford: Oxford University Press)
24. Mertin, J. (1978). *Med. Klin.*, **73**, 1752
25. Mertin, J., Harding, B., Knight, S. C. and Hall, P. J. (1979). In Miescher, P. A., Bolis, L., Gorini, S., Lambo, T. A., Nossal, G. J. V. and Torrigani, G. (eds.). *The Menarini Series on Immunopathology*, Vol. 2. pp. 873–885 (Basel, Stuttgart: Schwabe)
26. Hommes, O. R., Lamers, K. J. B. and Reekers, P. (1980). In Bauer, H., Ritter, H. and Poser, I. (eds.). *Progress in MS – Research*, pp. 396–400. (Berlin, Heidelberg, New York: Springer)
27. Madigand, M., Oger, J. J-F, Gauchet, R., Sabouraud, O. and Genetet, B. (1982). *J. Neurol. Sci.*, **53**, 519
28. Mertin, J., Rudge, P., Kremer, M., Healey, M. J. R., Knight, S. C., Compston, A., Batchelor, J. R., Thompson, E. J., Halliday, A. M., Denman, M. and Medawar, P. B. (1982). *Lancet*, **2**, 351
29. Mertin, J. and Fierz, W. (1982). *Proceedings of the Workshop on Immunosuppressive Treatment in MS*, Nijmegen, (in press)
30. Zinkernagel, R. M. and Doherty, P. C. (1979). *Adv. Immunol.*, **27**, 51
31. Nussenzweig, M. C. and Steinman, R. M. (1982). *Immunology Today*, **3**, 65
32. Knight, S. C., Balfour, B. M., O'Brien, J., Buttifant, L., Sumerska, T. and Clarke, J. (1982). *Eur. J. Immunol.*, **12**, 1057
33. Watson, J. D. (1982). *Transplantation*, **31**, 313
34. Morgan, D. A., Ruscetti, F. W. and Gallo, R. (1976). *Science*, **193**, 1007
35. Benn-Nun, A., Wekerle, H. and Cohen, I. R. (1981). *Eur. J. Immunol.*, **11**, 195
36. Ben-Nun, A., Wekerle, H. and Cohen, I. R. (1981). *Nature*, **292**, 60
37. Germain, R. N. and Benacerraf, B. (1981). *Scand. J. Immunol.*, **13**, 1
38. Reinherz, E. L. and Schlossmann, S. F. (1980). *Cell*, **19**, 821
39. Knight, S. C., Harding, B., Burman, S., O'Brien, J. and Farrant, J. (1979). In Kaplan, J. (ed.). *The Molecular Basis of Immune Cell Function*, pp. 181–192, (Amsterdam: Elsevier: North Holland)
40. Knight, S. C., (1982). *J. Immunol. Meth.*, **50**, R51
41. Goodwin, J. S. and Williams, R. C. Jr. (1979). *J. Clin. Lab. Immunol.*, **2**, 89
42. Larsson, E. L. (1980). *J. Immunol.*, **124**, 2828
43. Green, C. J. (1981). *Diagnostic Histopath.*, **4**, 157
44. Whitacre, C. C., Mattson, D. H., Paterson, P. Y., Roos, R. P., Peterson, D. J. and Arnason, B. G. W. (1981). *Neurochem. Res.*, **6**, 87
45. Thompson, E. J. (1977). *Br. Med. Bull.*, **33**, 28
46. Glynn, P., Weedon, D., Edwards, J., Suckling, A. J. and Cuzner, M. L. (1982). *J. Neurol. Sci.*, **57**, 369
47. Mattson, D. H., Roos, R. P. and Arnason, B. G. W. (1980). *Nature*, **287**, 335
48. Eggers, A. E. and Hibbard, C. A. (1981). *J. Neurol. Sci.*, **49**, 109
49. Frick, E. (1982). *J. Neurol. Sci.*, **57**, 55
50. Pettinelli, C. B. and McFarlin, D. E. (1981). *J. Immunol.*, **127**, 1420
51. Holda, J. H. and Swanborg, R. H. (1982). *Eur. J. Immunol.*, **12**, 453
52. Ting, J. P. Y., Shigekawa, B. L., Linthicum, D. S., Weiner, C. P. and Frelinger, J. A. (1981). *Proc. Natl. Acad. Sci. (USA)*, **78**, 3170
53. Carrel, S., de Tribolet, N. and Gross, N. (1982). *Eur. J. Immunol.*, **12**, 354
54. Traugott, U., Stone, S. H. and Raine, C. S. (1979). *J. Neurol. Sci.*, **41**, 17
55. Reinherz, E. L., Weiner, H. L., Hauser, S. L., Cohen, J. A., Distaso, J. A. and Schlossman, S. F. (1980). *N. Engl. J. Med.*, **303**, 125
56. Arnason, B. W. G., Oger, J. J-F., Antel, J. P. and Szuchet, S. (1982). *Neuroscience*, **7**, 59
57. Levine, S., Sowinski, R. and Kies, M. W. (1972). *Proc. Soc. Exp. Biol. Med.*, **139**, 506
58. Paterson, P. Y. (1971). *J. Immunol.*, **106**, 1473
59. Leibowitz, S., Lessof, M. H. and Kennedy, L. A. (1968). *Clin. Exp. Immunol.*, **3**, 753
60. Mertin, J. and Stackpoole, A. (1981). *Cell. Immunol.*, **62**, 393
61. Bolton, C., Allsopp, G. and Cuzner, M. L. (1982). *Clin. Exp. Immunol.*, **47**, 127
62. Mertin, J. (1982). *Clinics Immunol. Allergy*, **2**, 385

11
Myelin basic protein and its antibodies in the cerebrospinal fluid in experimental allergic encephalomyelitis, multiple sclerosis and other diseases

E. C. ALVORD, Jr., S. HRUBY, C. M. SHAW and J. SLIMP

Myelin basic protein (BP) has been extensively studied not only as the cause of experimental allergic encephalomyelitis (EAE) but also, when released into the cerebrospinal fluid (CSF), as an indicator of activity of demyelinating diseases, especially multiple sclerosis (MS). Gutstein and Cohen[1] reported that EAE differed from MS in having antibodies to BP, but not BP itself, in the CSF. Our studies, however, have revealed no essential differences between EAE in monkeys and MS and other CNS diseases in humans. High concentrations of BP occur early, especially if no anti-BP antibodies are also present. Lower concentrations of BP follow and may be associated with the presence of anti-BP antibodies. In EAE these antibodies come from the relatively strong peripheral sensitization to BP and enter the CSF through a damaged blood–brain barrier, in MS they come from the relatively weak immunologic stimulation probably evoked by previous attacks of the disease. Proteolytic enzymes[2] also enter the CSF and produce peptide fragments of BP, whose differing antigenic compositions permit antibodies to some fragments to coexist with other fragments antigenically unrelated but detected as 'BP' *in vitro*. Since oligoclonal immunoglobulins (IgG) occur more often in MS than in other diseases, one can expect to find BP, anti-BP antibodies and oligoclonal IgG more often in MS, but even the combination is not specific for MS. Consideration of the temporal and immunochemical relationships as well as of the differential diagnosis provides a basis for the understanding of the significance of BP, its antibodies and other immunoglobulins in the CSF.

ACKNOWLEDGEMENT

Supported by NMSS grant RG-805-E-20

References

1. Gutstein, H. S. and Cohen, S. R. (1978). *Science*, **199**, 301
2. Alvord, E. C. Jr., Hruby, S. and Sires, L. R. (1979). *Ann. Neurol.*, **6**, 474

12
Identification of myelin basic protein (MBP) as an antigenic component of circulating immune complexes (CIC) in MS patients

M. K. DASGUPTA, T. A. McPHERSON, I. CATZ, K. G. WARREN
and J. B. DOSSETOR

INTRODUCTION

Multiple sclerosis (MS) remains a disease of unknown aetiology. Auto-immunity is postulated, involving an antigen of myelin or oligodendrocytes (glial cells responsible for production and maintenance of myelin in CNS) or alternatively some form of viral or other infective process[1]. This auto-immunity hypothesis is supported by evidence from experimental allergic encephalitis (EAE), a useful, but not exactly similar experimental model of MS[2,3]. Many clinical investigators have sought to implicate myelin basic protein (MBP), the causative antigen in EAE, in the pathogenesis of MS. To this end:

(1) MBP has been identified and quantitated in the cerebrospinal fluid (CSF) of patients with active demyelination, including MS[4-6];
(2) antibodies to MBP have been identified in patients with MS[7], and
(3) aspects of cellular immunity to MBP have been identified in MS patients[8,9].

Several laboratories have shown that CIC occur in serum of patients with multiple sclerosis (MS) though no specific antigen was reported[10-17]. We reported data on the prevalence of CIC in 254 MS patients, using the Raji cell radioimmunoassay (Raji-RIA), and have shown a relationship to disease activity[18]. In this report we present further observations on the character of the antigenic component of CIC in MS. We find MBP to be an antigenic component in some CIC isolated from sera of patients with MS.

PATIENTS AND MATERIALS

Serum

Eighteen serum samples were obtained from 15 MS patients. Disease control sera were collected from three patients with virus encephalitis, two patients with Guillain–Barré syndrome, four patients with active systemic lupus erythematosus, two patients with subacute bacterial endocarditis, and one patient with myasthenia gravis. Neurological diagnosis was made by one of us (KGW) according to criteria previously reported[18]. Serum samples, for prospective studies, were collected and stored at −70 °C. They were analysed without the knowledge of clinical condition of the serum donor.

METHODS

Raji-RIA for CIC

Serum samples were analysed for CIC by Raji-cell radioimmunossay (Raji-RIA) as originally described by Theofilopoulos et al[19] except that 8–10 normal sera were included with each sera and mean and standard deviations (SD) determined for each day's assay. Results were expressed as SD units above the normal mean for each day. Values 2 SD above the mean were abnormal[20].

Characterization of MBP containing complexes bound to Raji cells

Acid elution of Raji cell adsorbed immune complexes

Complexes present in MS sera were eluted by isotonic citrate buffer at pH 2.8–3.0 after adsorption to Raji cells by following the method described by Theofilopoulos et al[21]. Briefly, 40×10^6 Raji cells were incubated at 37 °C for 45 minutes with 200 μl of test serum and were washed three times. Washed Raji cells were then incubated for 7 minutes in freshly prepared isotonic citrate buffer (containing 1% BSA) at pH 2.8–3.0. Cells were then centrifuged at 500 g for 7 minutes and supernates were collected, coded and passed on for further characterization by gel electrophoresis.

SDS polyacrylamide gel electrophoresis (PAGE) of Raji acid eluates

The preparative procedure for SDS-PAGE was that of Carson et al[22]. 10 μl of sample were mixed with 50 μl 1% SDS and 40 μl of 0.01 mol/l phosphate buffer, boiled for 90 s, with 10 μl of BME and 10 μl of glycerol and bromphenol blue were added. The sample was underlayered on 10% polyacrylamide gels which were run at 8 mA per gel for about 4 hours at room temperature. After electrophoresis, gels were removed from the tubes, stained overnight in 0.1% Coomassie blue. Excess stain was removed by diffusion using several changes of 10% acetic acid.

After destaining, gels were sliced into 3 mm slices. Each slice was macerated and protein extracted by incubation in 1.5 ml T_3 buffer (0.2 mol/l Tris, 1%

Triton X100, 0.1% Trasylol, pH 7.2). 1 hour at 37 °C and overnight at room temperature. Duplicate 0.5 ml aliquots were subjected to analysis for MBP by competitive inhibition radioimmunoassay (RIA).

Radioimmunoassay (RIA) for myelin basic protein (MBP)

Details have already been described by us[23]. Antibody to human MBP was raised in female New Zealand white rabbits as described by Thomas *et al*[24] and by J. N. Whitaker[25]; MBP was isolated from human brain by the method of Diebler *et al*[26] and iodinated by the chloramine-T method[23]; a fresh preparation of ^{125}I-MBP being prepared at least every 4 weeks.

Eluate from each gel slice was incubated with 0.3 ml normal rabbit serum, 0.1 ml concentrated T_3 buffer and antibody to BP to a final dilution of 1:1500. After incubation for 18 h at 4 °C, ^{125}I-BP was added (0.2 ng – 25 000 cpm) and incubation continued overnight at 4 °C, being terminated by the addition of 0.5 ml of 16 g/100 ml silica gel. Results were expressed as percentage bound to antibody or as percentage inhibition (% bound in the sample minus % bound in the non-specific binding tube).

Silica gel RIA can detect down to 1 ng of MBP/ml of CSF. Specificity is checked by including different quantities of lysozymes, histones and EAE nonapeptide (Beckman). Negligible cross-reactivity was detected. MBP or its fragments were detected, according to their molecular weights, in three different peaks:

(1) Peak I = 'MBP' – molecular wt 18 000,
(2) Peak II = 'fragments of MBP' – molecular wt <18 000 and
(3) Peak III = 'high molecular wt MBP' – molecular wt approximately 50 000, also referred to as 'Big BP'[22].

Total inhibition, as well as inhibition associated with each of three particular locations on the gels, was computed, with the total inhibition from a particular gel expressed as nanograms of MBP equivalent per ml.

Preparation of in vitro MBP–anti-MBP complexes

A constant amount of antibody (rabbit antisera to MBP at 1/150 dilution) was added to increasing amounts of ^{125}I-MBP until the zone of equivalence was identified (40 ng/ml of MBP); complexes were thus formed between anti-MBP and various doses of unlabelled MBP. These were added to NHS for 30 min at 37 °C, and the mixtures were then added to the Raji cells for adsorption and elution studies.

Statistical analysis

Correlation coefficient by linear regression was used to determine the relation between MBP and CIC in serum.

RESULTS

Detailed results of the presence of CIC and MBP in eluates from Raji cells, using sera from MS and control populations, are given in Table 1 and 2. Quantitative MBP is expressed in ng/ml of MBP equivalents; inhibition by

Table 1 Results of Raji cell acid elution of MBP from circulating immune complexes (CIC) and Raji-RIA for CIC–MS patients

Disease status	Sample no	MBP components (ng/ml) I	II	III	MBP-equivalents† (ng/ml)*	CIC† (SD units)
Relapse	1	0	19	14	33	8.6
	2	14	9	1	24	4.7
	3	1	0	3	4	6.4
	4	1	0	0	1	4.4
	5	0	1	0	1	5.1
	6	0	1	0	1	0.1
	7	0	0	0	0	8.5
Progressive	8	2	0	4	6	1.8
	9	0	3	0	3	3.8
	10	0	0	1	1	0.8
	11	0	0	0	0	4.4
Remission	12	1	2	1	4	2.4
	13	0	0	0	0	6.0
	14	0	0	0	0	0
	15	21	0	0	21	3.8
Stable	16	1	0	2	3	0.3
	17	0	0	0	0	3.7
	18	0	0	0	0	0

†No statistical significance was found when MBP-equivalents as a group were compared to CIC as a group (Pearson's correlation coefficient: $r = 0.38$; $r^2 = 0.15$; $p > 0.05$)
*MBP results > 1ng/ml represent·values above 2 SD of the mean baseline observations

Table 2 Results of MBP acid eluted from CIC and Raji-RIA for CIC: Control groups

	MBP equivalents (ng/ml)	Raji-RIA for CIC SD
Neurologic controls		
(1) Herpes virus encephalitis	9	0 –
(2) Herpes virus encephalitis	0	1.6 –
(3) Guillain–Barré syndrome	0	0.6 –
(4) Guillain–Barré syndrome	0	1.1 –
(5) Viral encephalitis	0	0.1 –
(6) Myasthenia gravis	0	8.1 +
Non-neurologic controls		
(1) SLE (active disease)	0	7.7 +
(2) SLE (active disease)	0	27.6 +
(3) SLE (active disease)	0	5.2 +
(4) SLE (active disease)	0	8.8 +
(5) Subacute bacterial endocarditis (SBE)	0	24.8 +
(6) Subacute bacterial endocarditis (SBE)	0	7.4 +

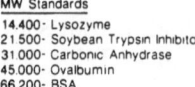

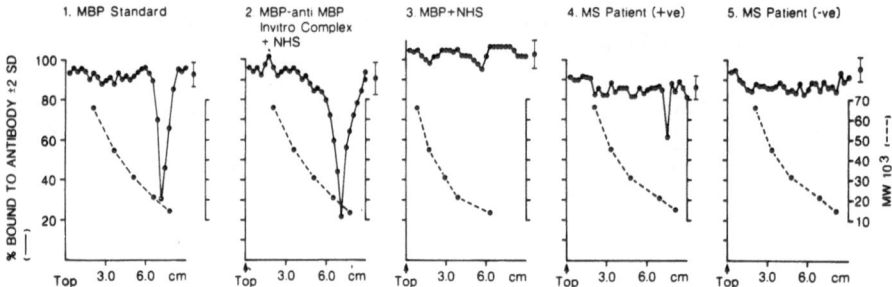

Figure 1 Shows result of sodium dodecyl sulphate-polyacrylamide gel electrophoresis (SDS-PAGE) and RIA for myelin basic protein (MBP) (see methods) from Raji cell acid eluates on MS sera, controls and MBP standard solution. MBP eluted from each gel strip is shown as solid line (•——•) in relation to left ordinate; the molecular weight (MW) standards simultaneously run, are shown as interrupted line (•---•) in relation to right ordinate. Different MW markers used are identified at the top of the Figure. Positions of each gel peak in relation to MW markers are shown in the abscissa. Solution of MBP standard (75 ng/ml in T_3 buffer) is run straight in the SDS-PAGE system and results are shown in Gel #1. MBP/anti-MBP *in vitro* complex (in 3:1 antigen/antibody ratio) added to NHS and equivalent amount free MBP (120 ng/ml) added to NHS are absorbed and acid eluted on Raji cells (Gel #2 and 3). SDS-PAGE and RIA for MBP of these two gels show clear peak of MBP in the complexed form of MBP (88 ng/ml, Gel #2) and none in the free form (Gel #3). Two representative samples of MS sera, one positive and another negative for MBP, are shown in Gel #4 and 5. In the positive sample (Gel #4) only peak I is observed, but in other samples different peaks of MBP were also noted and details are given in Table 1.

more than 2 SD below the mean baseline is given by any concentration in excess of 1 ng/ml of MBP equivalent. Thus values in excess of 1 ng/ml are considered positive for MBP. Using this criterion, as shown in Table 1, 12 of 18 samples from MS patients were positive for CIC; of these six were also positive for MBP. Two of the CIC-negative sera were also positive for MBP containing more than 1 ng/ml of MBP-equivalent. Six samples, clearly positive for CIC, had 1 or less than 1 ng of MBP-equivalent in the eluate. One eluate from a serum of a patient with viral encephalitis showed 9 ng/ml of MBP-equivalent (component I = 3 ng/ml, and component III = 6 ng/ml); all other 11 non-MS samples, 7 of which had very high levels of CIC (8.1, 7.7, 27.6, 5.2, 8.8, 24.8 and 7.4 SD units) had no detectable MBP-equivalents (Table 2). To ensure specificity, a variety of controls were treated exactly as described for the MS serum samples. An *in vitro* prepared solution of MBP/anti-MBP immune complexes in 3:1 antigen–antibody ratio (Figure 1) was shown to contain 88 ng/ml of MBP in Raji eluate, whereas the same quantity of MBP in normal human serum (NHS) with T_3 buffer was negative for MBP (Figure 1). MBP in isotonic acid citrate buffer applied directly to the SDA-PAGE system, as a positive control, showed marked evidence of MBP activity after elution from the polyacrylamide gel when tested by RIA.

In Table 1, CIC results by Raji-RIA do not correlate well with positive evidence of MBP in eluates from Raji cells ($r = 0.38, p > 0.05$). This could be due to differential sensitivity of the two assay conditions (gel electrophoresis of eluates versus Raji-RIA for CIC) or, alternatively, all IgG-complexes detected by Raji assay in sera from MS patients may not contain MBP. A third possibility is that free MBP (and not complexed MBP) could bind to Raji cells, i.e. non-specific binding of free MBP to Raji cells. To eliminate this possibility, we added different amounts of free MBP to Raji cells (2–200 ng/ml) *without addition of normal human serum (NHS);* no MBP was found in acid eluates from these cells. Further, we added *free* MBP and *artificial* MBP/anti-MBP complexes *to NHS*, exposed these mixtures to Raji cells and then performed acid elution. Antigen–antibody ratios varied from antibody excess to 12 times antigen excess (see methods). Binding of *free MBP in NHS* to Raji cells was negligible up to 120 ng/ml (Figure 1, gel 3) and was only appreciable when 160 ng/ml or more was added. In contrast, MBP present in artificial complexes with about 3:1 antigen–antibody ratio *in NHS* gave striking MBP elution from Raji cells (see Figure 1, gel 2). Additionally, at no time did we find detectable free MBP (by RIA) in the serum samples from MS patients shown in Table 1. We, therefore, concluded that the detection of MBP in acid eluates from Raji cells exposed to MS sera (when later studied by SDS-PAGE RIA) could not be due simply to the presence of free MBP in MS serum.

DISCUSSION

CIC are known to be present in serum and CSF from MS patients[10-17]. In a recent study of 254 MS patients, we found a correlation between CIC and disease activity[18]. This study shows that MBP and/or a component of serum which is antigenically cross-reactive with MBP is detectable in the CIC in serum of some MS patients. Not all MS patients' sera contain CIC, not all CIC from MS serum samples contain MBP or MBP-equivalents, and MBP (measured by binding inhibition as MBP-equivalents) can sometimes be eluted from Raji cells after incubation with serum which is not positive by Raji-RIA for conventional CIC. This latter observation may be due to differential sensitivity of SDS-PAGE elution technique and Raji-assay or that not all CIC on Raji cells contain IgG. We have evidence that it is not due to free MBP being absorbed to Raji cells as all of the serum samples shown in Table 1 were negative for free MBP when reacted directly in RIA. Also, the range of MBP concentrations found in Raji-acid eluates (0–33 ng/ml) is well below the minimum range for binding of free MBP to Raji cells *in vitro* (> 120 ng/ml). Thus, it is clear that MS serum can contain CIC which may contain MBP. What is not yet clear is whether such MBP-containing complexes play a role in the development or evolution of MS.

ACKNOWLEDGEMENTS

This research is supported in part by the following agencies: Medical Research Council (Canada), Multiple Sclerosis Society (Canada), The Friends of MS Research, Edmonton, the Association of Canadian Travellers of Edmonton, Kidney Foundation of Canada and the Alberta Heritage Foundation for Medical Research (AHFMR). Dr M. K. D. is a scholar of the AHFMR.

References

1. Paterson, P. Y. (1977). In Talal, N. (ed.). *Autoimmunity: Genetic, Immunologic, Virologic and Clinical Aspects*, pp. 643–692. (New York: Academic Press)
2. Gutstein, H. S. and Cohen, S. R. (1978). *Science*, **199**, 301
3. McFarlin, D. E., Hsu, S. C. L., Slamenda, S. B., Chou, F. C. H. and Kibler, R. F. (1975). *J. Exp. Med.*, **141**, 72
4. McPherson, T. A., Gilpin, A. and Seland, T. P. (1972). *Can. Med. Assoc. J.*, **107**, 856
5. Cohen, S. R., Herndon, R. M. and McKhann, G. M. (1976). *N. Engl. J. Med.*, **295**, 1455
6. Whitaker, J. N. (1977). *Neurology* (Minneapolis), **27**, 911
7. Panitch, H. S., Hafler, D. A. and Johnson, K. P. (1980). In Bauer, H. J., Poser, S. R. and Ritter, G. (eds.) *Progress in Multiple Sclerosis Research*, pp. 98–105. (Berlin, Heidelberg, New York: Springer-Verlag)
8. Kallen, B., Nilsson, O. and Thelin, C. (1977). *Acta Neurol. Scand.*, **55**, 33
9. Lisak, R. P. and Zweiman, B. (1977). *N. Engl. J. Med.*, **297**, 850
10. Deicher, H., Schwabedissen, H. M., Liman, W., Baruth, B., Patzold, U. and Haller, P. (1980). In Bauer, H. G., Poser, S. and Ritter, G. (eds.). *Progress in Multiple Sclerosis Research*, pp. 200–206. (Berlin: Springer-Verlag)
11. Goust, J. M., Chenais, F., Carnes, J. E., Hames, C. G., Fudenbergh, H. H. and Hogan, H. L. (1978). *Neurology*, **28**, 421
12. Jacques, C., Davous, P. and Baumann, N. (1977). *Lancet*, **2**, 408
13. Jans, H., Jersild, C., Taaning, E., Dybkjaer, E., Fog, T. and Heltberg, A. (1980). In Bauer, H. G., Poser, S. and Ritter, G. (eds.). *Progress in Multiple Sclerosis Research*, pp. 195–199. (Berlin: Springer-Verlag)
14. Schocket, A. L., Carr, R. I. and Hardtke, M. A. (1980). *Clin. Immunol. Immunopathol.*, **17**, 477
15. Tachovsky, T. G., Lisak, R. P., Koprowski, H., Theofilopoulos, A. N. and Dixon, F. J. (1976). *Lancet*, **2**, 997
16. Trouillas, P., Vincent, C. and Revillard, J. V. (1980). *J. Clin. Lab. Immunol.*, **4**, 77
17. Noronha, A. B. C., Antel, J. P., Roos, R. P. and Medof, E. M. (1981). *Neurology (NY)*, **31**, 1402
18. Dasgupta, M. K., Warren, K. G., Johny, K. V. and Dossetor, J. B. (1982). *Neurology (NY)*, **32**, 1000
19. Theofilopoulos, A. N., Wilson, C. B. and Dixon, F. J. (1976). *J. Clin. Invest.*, **57**, 169
20. Johny, K. V., Dasgupta, M. K., Nakashima, S. and Dossetor, J. B. (1981). *J. Immunol. Methods*, **40**, 61
21. Theofilopoulos, A. N., Eisenberg, R. A. and Dixon, F. J. (1978). *J. Clin. Invest.*, **61**, 1570
22. Carson, J. H., Barbarese, E., Braun, P. E. and McPherson, T. A. (1978). *Proc. Natl. Acad. Sci. USA*, **75**, 1976
23. Hsiung, H. M., Wu, J. and McPherson, T. A. (1978). *Clin. Biochem.*, **11**, 54
24. Thomas, D. G. T., Palfreyman, J. W. and Ratcliffe, J. G. (1978). *Lancet*, **i**, 113
25. Whitaker, J. N. (1975). *J. Immunol.*, **114**, 823
26. Diebler, G. E., Martenson, R. C. and Kies, M. (1972). *Prep. Biochem.*, **2**, 139

13
Sensitization of cerebrospinal fluid and peripheral blood lymphocytes to brain glycolipids in multiple sclerosis

ANNA CZLONKOWSKA and Z. RZEPECKI

SUMMARY

The sensitization of cerebrospinal fluid (CSF) and peripheral blood lymphocytes (PB) to galactocerebroside and gangliside in multiple sclerosis (MS) was studied by use of the antigen active E rosette assay.

In CSF the majority of patients suffering from MS and almost 40% of those with other neurological disease (OND) showed a sensitization to both glycolipids. In PB sensitization was also observed in the lymphocytes from healthy persons. In MS in the course of relapse, sensitization was greater in CSF and PB than during the chronic progressive stage.

The results suggest that the sensitization to glycolipids in CSF is a result of the breakdown of tolerance to self-produced antigens, but that in PB it may also be caused by a cross-reactivity with environmental factors.

It is very probable that the observed delayed type of hypersensitivity to glycolipids is an epiphenomenon associated with white matter destruction and cross reactivity with commonly distributed antigens.

INTRODUCTION

There is much evidence that in the pathogenesis of multiple sclerosis (MS) autoimmune phenomena play an important role, and that this disease results from abnormalities in immunoregulation[1]. However, it is not, as yet, clear at which white matter component the autoimmune process is directed. Myelin basic protein (MBP) is regarded as a most important antigen involved in the autoimmune reaction of the central nervous system (CNS). Other potential targets of an autoimmune reaction (either humoral or cellular) against CNS white matter include myelin-associated glycoprotein, myelin ganglioside, galactocerebroside and antigens located on the surface of oligidendrocytes.

Glycolipids are important contributors to the antigenicity of the mammalian cell surface. In the brain, major glycolipids are the galacto-cerebroside and ganglioside. Galactocerebroside is a myelin lipid, whether ganglioside is present in the neuron as well as other neural elements. They are powerful haptens and combine readily with immunogenic carriers to induce formation of antibodies[2,3]. Antibodies to glycolipids are able to produce certain pathological changes in the peripheral and central nervous system such as allergic neuritis[4,5], demyelination upon intraneural injection[6], epileptic discharges[7] or behavioural disturbances[8].

There is less evidence that cerebral glycolipids are able to induce a delayed type of hypersensitivity. Certain authorities maintain, however, that these haptens are unable to initiate cell-mediated immunity[9,10]. However, Nagai et al[4] injecting ganglioside into experimental animals were able to demonstrate blastoid cell transformation *in vitro* upon incubation of lymphocytes with myelin containing ganglioside antigen.

In human pathology, antibodies to galactocerebroside and ganglioside have been demonstrated in peripheral blood (PB) of patients suffering from MS or other neurological disease (OND)[11,12]. Recently it has been found that lymphocytes from the PB of MS patients and patients suffering from other types of autoimmune diseases are sensitized to brain glycolipids[13-15]. Antibodies to glycolipids have been detected in the cerebrospinal fluid (CSF) only sporadically[16]. Nothing is known about the sensitization of CSF lymphocytes to the lipid components of myelin. The aim of the present work was to examine CSF and PB lymphocyte sensitization to galactocerebroside and ganglioside in MS.

MATERIALS

The following groups were included in the study:

(1) Fifty patients with MS, aged 13–66 years, a median age of 34 years. Clinical criteria of the diagnosis were according to Rose et al[17] and Cendrowski[18].

Upon clinical criteria patients were divided into three groups:
(a) clinically definite – 38 persons,
(b) clinically probable – 5 patients and
(c) clinically possible – 7 persons.

The patients were also divided into two groups according to the activity of the disease process:
(i) patients in relapse – 31 persons. An exacerbation was defined as the sudden appearance of new symptoms and signs or the sudden reappearance or worsening of previous findings, in each case in excess of 4 days in duration[19].
(ii) 19 patients with progressive symptoms of at least 2 years in duration in the absence of any sudden changes.

(2) Sixteen patients with other neurological diseases (OND), aged 16–67 years, median age 38 years. Four of these suffered from Parkinson's

disease, 2 from epilepsy, 2 from cerebrovascular disease, 1 from Huntington's disease, 1 from habit spasm, 1 from tumour of the brain stem, 1 from paresis n. VI, 1 from mental retardation, 1 from alcoholic polyneuropathy, 1 from leucodystrophy and 1 from myelosis funicularis.

(3) Thirteen subjects served as a healthy control group, aged 20–42 years, median age 28 years. All of these displayed neuroses and revealed no abnormalities upon neurological examination.

MS and OND patients had not been treated with ACTH, corticosteroids or immunomodulatory drugs in the 3 months preceding this study.

METHODS

The antigen-active rosette forming cells assay (Ag-ARFC) of Felsburg and Edelman[20] was used. For CSF study an 8–10 ml sample was taken by lumbar puncture. The sample was divided into three equal parts and put into separate tubes. Cells were centrifuged at $300\,g$, the supernatant was removed and the cells resuspended in 0.1 ml TC 199 medium. The cell concentration was 1–$2 \times 10^3/0.1$ ml. To one sample $10\,\mu l$ of 0.9% NaCl was added and to others $10\,\mu l$ of saline containing glycolipids. Samples were incubated at room temperature for 15 min after which 0.1 ml of 0.2% sheep red blood cells in TC 199 medium containing 10% calf serum and 5% of human AB serum were added. The mixture was immediately centrifuged at $50\,g$ for 3 min. About half of the supernatant was taken off and the pellet was gently resuspended, and a smear was made on a glass slide.

The preparation was fixed in 95% ethanol and stained with Giemsa. At least 10^2 lymphocytes were counted, and the % of rosette forming lymphocytes more than 3 red cells attached was calculated. For PB the method described by Offner et al[13] was used. Details of the method used in our laboratory are provided elsewhere[21].

As antigens bovine cerebroside (Sigma type IV) and ganglioside (Sigma type III) were used. Cerebrosides were dissolved in ethanol and gangliosides in saline. Further dilutions were made in saline[13].

In the case of CSF the assay was performed with one concentration of lipids 5 pg/0.1 ml of lymphocyte culture. For PB two concentrations were used, 1 and 5 pg/0.1 ml of lymphocyte culture.

The results are given as the percentage of active rosette forming cells (ARFC) and the percentage of ARFC after stimulation with antigen (Ag-ARFC). From these values the antigen sensitization index Ag-SI, i.e. Ag-ARFC:ARFC ratio was calculated. The subject was regarded as positively reacting with the antigen when the Ag-SI was in excess of 1.15.

The Students t-test for unpaired and paired variables, the Wilcoxon rank test and χ^2 test were used for statistical calculations.

RESULTS

Glycolipids in relation to clinical status

The sensitization to glycolipids in MS in relation to the clinical status of the disease is shown in Table 1 and Figure 1.

Table 1 Sensitization of CSF and PB lymphocytes to glycolipids in MS patients, persons with other neurological diseases and a healthy control group. Results as antigen sensitization index (mean ±SD)

| | CSF | | PB | | | |
	Cerebroside 5pg	Ganglioside 5pg	Cerebroside 1pg	Cerebroside 5pg	Ganglioside 1pg	Ganglioside 5pg
MS definite (n = 38)	1.50[a,b] ±0.27[c]	1.34[a,b] ±0.26[c]	1.34[a] ±0.47	1.30[a,b] ±0.23	1.14[a] ±0.13	1.19[a] ±0.15
MS probable (n = 5)	1.38[a,b] ±0.18	1.46[a,b] ±0.24	1.61[a] ±0.52	1.47[a,b] ±0.21	1.27[a] ±0.22	1.27[a] ±0.19
MS possible (n = 7)	1.41[a,b] ±0.13	1.39[a,b] ±0.15	1.40[a,b] ±0.32	1.26[a,b] ±0.16	1.25[a] ±0.17	1.37[a] ±0.35
OND (n = 16)	1.14 ±0.16	1.15 ±0.31	1.19 ±0.13	1.09 ±0.13	1.10 ±0.29	1.12 ±0.23
Control (n = 13)	1.00 ±0.12	1.02 ±0.09	1.01 ±0.10	1.03 ±0.11	0.98 ±0.11	1.06 ±0.13

a = $p < 0.05$ vs. control group
b = $p < 0.05$ vs. OND group
c = $p < 0.05$ CSF vs. PB (in the same concentration)

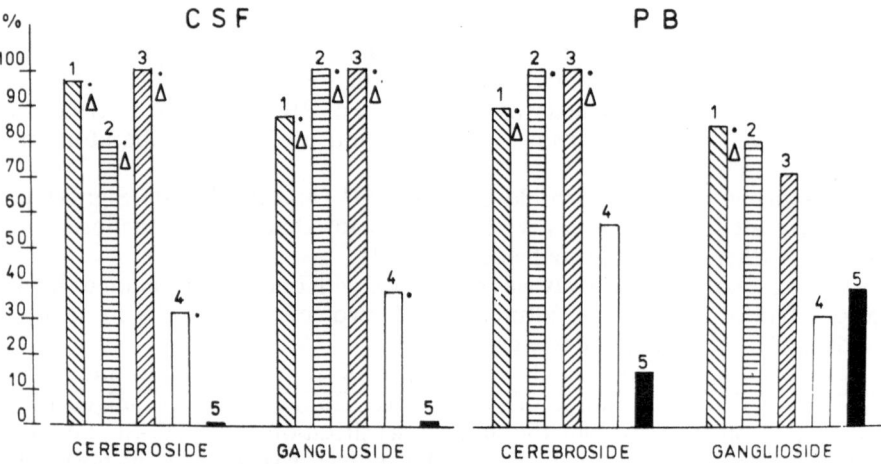

Figure 1 Frequency of lymphocyte sensitization to glycolipids in CSF and PB in the various groups. Results as % of persons having AG-SI higher than 1.15.

1 - MS definite (n = 38); 2 - MS probable (n = 5); 3 - MS possible (n = 7); 4 - OND (n = 16); 5 - healthy control (n = 13).
   • $p < 0.05$ vs. a healthy control group.
   Δ $p < 0.05$ vs. OND group.

CSF

In all MS groups, Ag-SI was significantly higher when each of the glycolipids was used as compared to the OND and control group. The frequency of the positive reactions (with a Ag-SI higher than 1.15) was similar for both lipids in all MS groups and higher than in the OND and control group.

In the control group, no individual had Ag-SI values higher than 1.15 when cerebroside and ganglioside were used as antigens. In the OND group, 5 of 16 patients (31.25%) responded to cerebroside and 6 of 16 (37.35%) to ganglioside.

PB

In all MS groups Ag-SI was higher (at least at one lipid concentration) than in the control group and OND group when cerebroside was used as the antigen. When ganglioside was used as the antigen Ag-SI was higher than in the control group but did not differ from that in the OND group.

The frequency of positive reactions to both lipids was similar in all MS groups, but higher than in the OND and control groups. In the OND group 9 of 16 patients (56.25%) had a positive Ag-SI to cerebroside and 5 of 16 (31.25%) to ganglioside. In the OND group the highest values of Ag-SI were to cerebroside and ganglioside respectively, in case of leucodystrophy (1.21 and 1.68), tumour of the brain stem (1.20 and 1.80), myelosis funicularis (1.33 and 1.14), epilepsy (1.34 and 1.08), Parkinson's disease (1.30 and 1.25). In the control group 2 persons of 13 (15.38%) displayed positive reaction to cerebroside and 5 of 13 (38.4%) to ganglioside. The control and OND groups did not differ significantly in the frequency of positive Ag-SI for each of the lipids.

In the clinically definite MS group when cerebroside was used as the antigen in a concentration of 5 pg, Ag-SI was significantly higher than in PB. In other MS groups there was no difference between CSF and PB in Ag-SI.

Sensitization to glycolipids in MS patients according to the activity of the disease (Table 2)

CSF

When cerebroside was used as the antigen no difference in Ag-SI was observed between patients in the relapse and in the chronic progressive stage of the disease. When ganglioside was used as antigen Ag-SI was higher in the relapse than in the chronic progressive stage.

In the chronic progressive stage, Ag-SI was higher when cerebroside as compared to ganglioside was used as antigen.

PB

In the relapse group with cerebroside in a dose of 5 pg and for ganglioside in both concentrations Ag-SI was higher than in the chronic progressive stage.

51

Table 2 Sensitization of CSF and PB lymphocytes in MS patients in different stages of the disease. Results as antigen sensitization index (mean ± SD)

	CSF		PB			
	Cerebroside 5pg	Ganglioside 5pg	Cerebroside 1pg	Cerebroside 5pg	Ganglioside 1pg	Ganglioside 5pg
MS relapse (n = 31)	1.45 ± 0.20	1.41[a] ± 0.25	1.44[b] ± 0.35	1.37[a] ± 0.21	1.24[a] ± 0.17	1.30[a] ± 0.27
MS chronic progressive (n = 19)	1.43[b,c] ± 0.25	1.28[c] ± 0.15	1.35 ± 0.74	1.24 ± 0.19	1.08 ± 0.14	1.13 ± 0.16

a = $p < 0.05$ vs. progressive stage
b = $p < 0.05$ vs. ganglioside in the same group
c = $p < 0.05$ CSF vs. PB (in the same concentration of glycolipids)

Only in the active stage when cerebroside was used in a dose of 1 pg Ag-SI was higher than when ganglioside was used in an equivalent concentration.

In relapse there was no difference in Ag-SI between CSF and PB for each glycolipid. In the chronic progressive stage, Ag-SI was higher in CSF than in PB when both lipids were used as the antigens.

DISCUSSION

In the present work to study the sensitization of lymphocytes to glycolipids the antigen active E rosette test was used. This test has been shown to correlate with delayed type of hypersensitivity[20,22].

Lymphocytes from the PB in 80% of clinically definite MS patients were sensitized to cerebroside and in 85% to ganglioside. Although the number of persons showing sensitization to glycolipids in the MS group was higher, many patients with OND and persons from the healthy control group also displayed a positive reaction to glyclopids. The response to stimulation by galacto-cerebroside was stronger in MS patients than in the OND group, but that to ganglioside was similar in MS compared to the OND group.

Our results are not in complete agreement with those obtained by others[13-15]. By using the same method these authors found only a sporadic reactivity of PB lymphocytes with glycolipids in patients with OND, and never among healthy persons. However, most of their patients with rheumatoid arthritis responded to glycolipids[12]. Frieck and Stickl[15] have found antibodies reacting with galactocerebroside and ganglioside in more than 50% patients with various neurological disease, syphilis and in many with rheumatoid arthritis, but never in the sera of normal controls. Each of the above mentioned studies is in line with present results, that patients with MS manifest a high incidence of sensitization to cerebroside and ganglioside.

Hirsch and Parks[23] detected an antibody to digalactodiglyceride in 43% of normal subjects. The presence of the immune reaction in PB to brain glycolipids in MS, rheumatoid arthritis, OND and occasionally in the healthy person indicate that this phenomenon is not unique to MS, and does not just reflect a breakdown of the tolerance to own antigens. Glycolipids are widely distributed in the plant and animal kingdom, and are present as surface components in not only mammalian cells but also in bacteria and viruses. In many micro-organisms they are closely associated with substances possessing powerful immunogenic and adjuvant properties. These are circumstances favourable to the formation of the cross-reacting immune response.

In the CSF in contrary to PB we could not observe any sensitization of lymphocytes in normal probands. The incidence of sensitization in MS patients was greater than in OND, but in the OND group reached nearly 40%. In MS in relapse, and in the chronic progressive stage sensitization to cerebroside was similar but the response to ganglioside was greater in relapse.

It can be postulated that the immunological reaction with cerebrcside and ganglioside in the CSF reflects primarily a local failure to maintain the tolerance to self-generated glycolipids. In contrast to PB, cross-reactivity with environmental micro-organisms in CSF appears improbable. In other cases from the OND group and MS, viral infection of the nervous system was not apparent.

Glycolipids in the brain are relatively inaccessible to immunocompetent cells and bound to autologous protein. Breakdown of tolerance may occur as a result of damage to nerve tissue and the consequent facilitation of access to immunocompetent cells. Sensitization of glycolipids in PB and CSF is greater in relapse than in the chronic progressive stage. In relapse, no difference in the severity of reaction between CSF and PB is evident, but in the chronic progressive stage the immune response in CSF is greater than in PB. This finding may support the view that sensitization in CSF results from a destruction of CNS tissue. During relapse there is a greater presence of antigen in the CSF, and secondly also in PB, owing to the blood–brain barrier destruction. This may cause a higher sensitization of PB lymphocytes. In the chronic progressive stage, there is similarly a degradation of brain tissue but the barrier is not disturbed. Active sensitization in CSF may still occur but the supply of antigen to the PB is diminished. In CSF of MS patients an increased level of glycolipids is observed[24,25].

At present it is impossible to resolve the question as to whether the observed delayed type of hypersensitivity to glycolipids in CSF and in PB plays any role in the pathogenesis of MS. It is very probable that it is only an epiphenomenon associated with white matter destruction and cross-reactivity with environmental factors.

ACKNOWLEDGEMENTS

The authors would like to thank Dr H. Offner for providing galacto-cerebroside and ganglioside.

This work was supported by grant No D-12 from the Ministry of Health.

References

1. Weiner, H. L. and Hauser, S. L. (1982). Neuroimmunology I: Immunoregulation in neurological disease. *Ann. Neurol.*, **11**, 437

2. Rapport, M. N. and Graf, L. (1969). Immunochemical reactions of lipids. *Progr. Allergy,* **13,** 273

3. Czlonkowska, A. and Leibowitz, S. (1974). The effect of homologous and heterologous carriers on the immunogenicity of the galacto-cerebroside hapten. *Immunology,* **27,** 117

4. Nagai, Y., Momoi, T., Saito, M., Mitsuzawa, E. and Ontani, S. (1976). Ganglioside syndrome, a new autoimmune neurologic disorder, experimentally induced with brain ganglioside. *Neurosci. Lett.,* **2,** 107

5. Saida, T., Saida, K., Dorfman, S. H., Silberberg, D. H., Sumner, A. J., Manning, M. G., Lisak, R. P. and Brown, M. J. (1979). Experimental allergic neuritis induced by sensitization with galactocerebroside. *Science,* **204,** 1103

6. Saida, K., Saida, T., Brown, M. J. and Silberg, D. H. (1979). *In vivo* demyelination induced by intraneural injection of antigalactocerebroside serum: a morphology study. *Am. J. Pathol.,* **95,** 99

7. Karpiak, S. E., Mahadik, S. P., Graf, L. and Rapport, M. M. (1981). An immunological model of epilepsy; seizures induced by antibodies to G_{M1} ganglioside. *Epilepsia,* **22,** 189

8. Rick, J. T., Gregson, A., Adinolfi, M. and Leibowitz, S. (1981). The behaviour of immature and mature rats exposed prenatally to anti-ganglioside antibodies. *J. Neuroimmunol.,* **1,** 413

9. Niedieck, B. (1975). On the glycolipid hapten of myelin. *Progr. Allergy.,* **18,** 353

10. Leibowitz, S. (1980). Glycolipid haptens in disease of the nervous system. In Boese, A. (ed.). *Search for the cause of multiple sclerosis and other chronic diseases of the central nervous system.* pp. 117-126. (Weinheim: Verlag Chemie)

11. Arnon, R., Crisp, E., Kelley, R., Ellison, G. W., Myers, L. W. and Tourtellotte, W. W. (1980). Anti-ganglioside antibodies in multiple sclerosis. *J. Neurol. Sci.,* **46,** 179

12. Frick, E. and Stickl, H. (1982). Specificity of antibody-dependent lymphocyte cytotoxicity against cerebral tissue constituents in multiple sclerosis. *Acta Neurol. Scand.,* **65,** 30

13. Offner, H. and Konat, G. (1980). Stimulation of active E-rosette forming lymphocytes from multiple sclerosis patients by gangliosides and cerebrosides. *J. Neurol. Sci.,* **46,** 101

14. Offner, H., Konat, G. and Sela, B. (1981). Multi-sialo brain gangliosides are powerful stimulators of active-rosetting lymphocytes from multiple sclerosis patients. *J. Neurol. Sci.,* **52,** 279

15. Offner, H., Pedersen, K. and Konat, G. (1981). Lymphocyte stimulation by gangliosides, cerebrosides and basic protein in juvenile rheumatoid arthritis. *J. Clin. Lab. Immunol.,* **6,** 35

16. Ryberg, B. (1978). Multiple specificities of antibrain antibodies in multiple sclerosis and chronic myelopathy. *J. Neurol. Sci.,* **38,** 357

17. Rose, A. S., Ellison, G. W., Myers, L. W. and Tourtellotte, W. W. (1976). Criteria for the clinical diagnosis of multiple sclerosis. *Neurology,* **26,** 20

18. Cendrowski, W. (1980). Criteria of clinical diagnosis of multiple sclerosis. *Neurol. Neurochir. Pol.,* **14,** 445

19. McAlpine, D., Lumsden, C. E. and Acheson, E. D. (1965). *Multiple sclerosis: a reappraisal.* (Edinburgh: Livingstone)

20. Felsburg, J. P. and Edelman, R. (1977). The active E rosette test: a sensitive *in vitro* correlate for human delayed-type hypersensitivity. *J. Immunol.,* **118,** 62

21. Czlonkowska, A., Póltorak, M., Cendrowski, W. and Korlak, J. (1982). Sensitization of cerebrospinal fluid and peripheral blood lymphocytes to myelin basic protein in multiple sclerosis. *Acta Neurol. Scand.,* **66,** 121

22. Hashim, G. A. (1978). Myelin basic protein: structure, function and antigenic determinants. *Immunol. Rev.,* **39,** 60

23. Hirsch, H. E. and Parks, M. E. (1976). Serological reactions against glycolipid sensitized liposomes in multiple sclerosis. *Nature,* **264,** 785

24. Tourtellotte, W. W. and Haerer, A. F. (1969). Lipids in cerebrospinal fluid. Part 12 (In multiple sclerosis and retrobulbar neuritis). *Arch. Neurol.,* (Chicago), **20,** 605

25. Nagai, Y., Kanfer, J. J. and Tourtellotte, W. W. (1973). Preliminary observations of gangliosides of normal and multiple sclerosis cerebrospinal fluid. *Neurology* (Minneap.), **23,** 945

14

Interferon production and natural killer (NK) activity in multiple sclerosis

G. VERVLIET, H. CLAEYS, H. VAN HAVER, H. CARTON, C. VERMYLEN and A. BILLIAU

The purpose of the present study was to compare the ability of peripheral blood leukocytes (PBLs) of MS patients and of normal donors to respond to well-characterized inducers of HuIFN-α and HuIFN-γ. Both the production of interferons and the enhancement of NK activity were used as parameters of the response. A possible association of the responses with the DR2 HLA phenotype was examined by stratification of both patients and donors in DR2 + and DR2 −. The results of this study will be published *in extenso* elsewhere (*J. Neurol. Sci.*, (1983), **60**, 137–150).

Fifty-four MS patients and 29 normal blood donors were included in the study. All patients had clinically manifest MS. Twenty-six were female, 28 were male patients. Twelve patients had a chronic progressive disease course from the onset (CP), 42 had a remitting relapsing course or a remitting relapsing course followed by chronic progression (RR). All were in the stable phase of the disease, the last relapse having occurred more than 3 months earlier. The patients all had disability scores between 1 and 7 as evaluated by the Kurtzke Disability Status Scale. The control subjects were healthy blood donors (mean age, 30 years; range 20–40 years).

Mononuclear cells were separated from heparinized blood by density gradient centrifugation (Ficoll Isopaque, Pharmacia, Uppsala, Sweden). After three washes with Dulbecco's phosphate buffered saline (PBS) the cells were resuspended in Hepes-buffered RPMI-1640 medium supplemented with 10% fetal calf serum (Flow Laboratories, Irvine, Scotland) and 1% glutamine. One ml aliquots of the cell suspension (3×10^6 cells/ml) were incubated in the presence of Sendai virus (10^2 EID$_{50}$/cell); Concanavalin A ($10 \mu g$/ml) or a HuIFN-α preparation ($3 \log_{10}$ units/ml). The culture supernatant fluids were harvested at 18 h by centrifugation ($500 g$, 10 min). The supernatants from Sendai virus-induced cell cultures were dialyzed at pH 2.0 for 48 h before interferon assay. All samples were stored at $-20\,^{\circ}$C until further assay.

As can be seen from Table 1, all cultures, whether from MS patients or

Table 1 Interferon production by PBLs of MS patients and normal donors after *in vitro* stimulation by Sendai virus or ConA

	Stimulation with Sendai virus			Stimulation with ConA		
		Responders[a]			Responders[a]	
Donor group	Total number	n	Average titre ($\log_{10}$ U/ml)	Total number	n	Average titre ($\log_{10}$ U/ml)
MS patients	48	48	3.4 (0.06)[b]	54	20	2.8 (0.18)
Controls	29	29	3.5 (0.07)	27	23	2.8 (0.17)

a = Interferon titre$\geqslant 1.5 \log_{10}$ U/ml
b = Mean (SE)

normal blood donors, produced interferon in response to Sendai virus. Moreover, the same mean interferon titre was reached by both groups of cultures. In contrast, when Concanavalin A (ConA) was used as the inducer, only 37% of the cultures from MS patients produced detectable interferon, as opposed to 85% of the cultures prepared from normal blood donors (probability of results under null-hypothesis by χ^2-analysis <0.005). However, the mean titre reached by responding cultures of MS patients was the same as that reached by cultures of normal donors.

The interferons were characterized by the use of potent and specific antisera. PBL cultures derived from both MS patients and blood donors produced HuIFN-α in response to Sendai virus and HuIFN-γ in response to ConA (data not shown).

The rates of interferon responsiveness to ConA stimulation among the PBL cultures of MS patients were not correlated with age, sex, type of disease or disease duration (data not shown). In contrast, the response rates did show some correlation with severity of disease. In the groups of patients with indices 1-4, the response rate was about 50%. Lower response rates, down to zero, were noted in cultures from patients with indices 5, 6 and 7. The association between interferon response and disability index was found to be statistically significant ($p<0.005$) in a χ^2-test performed on patients grouped in two categories: index $\leqslant 4$ and index $\geqslant 5$. The mean and median progression rate of the 20 patients in the group that produced HuIFN-γ in response to ConA was significantly lower than in the group of 34 non-responders (Table 2). This is remarkable since the mean disease duration was very similar in both groups. After a mean duration of 7.1 years the responding group had attained a mean

Table 2 ConA-stimulated interferon response rates among PBL cultures of 54 MS patients by disease progression rate

		Disease progression rate[a]		
	Number	Median	Mean[b]	± SE
Responders	20	0.41	0.49	0.09
Non-responders	34	0.63	0.81	0.12

a = Expressed as disability index divided by number of years disease duration
b = Significance tests:
   Mann–Whitney: U = 204; $p < 0.05$
   Student's *t*-test: $t = 2.16$; $p < 0.05$

Table 3 Analysis by DR2 – phenotype of the average ConA-induced interferon yields in PBLs from MS patients and normal donors[a]

	MS patients			Controls		
Phenotype	Total number examined[b]	Responders	Average IFN titre ($\log_{10}$ U/ml)	Total number examined	Responders	Average IFN titre ($\log_{10}$ U/ml)
DR2 +	18	4 (22%)	2.4 (0.4)[c]	8	7 (88%)	2.5 (0.3)
DR2 –	25	12 (48%)	2.8 (0.2)	13	10 (77%)	3.0 (0.3)

a = p values for χ^2-tests are given in the text
b = Total number differs from those in Table 1, because samples for HLA determination were not available for all donors
c = Mean (SE)

disability score of 2.55. In the group of non-responders a mean disability score of 4.11 was reached after 7.4 years.

Stratification of MS patients and controls as a function of DR2 + phenotype (Table 3) revealed that in both subgroups the percentage of responders was lower for the MS patients. However, the difference was less pronounced (statistically not significant: $p<0.1$) in the DR2 – group than in the DR2 + group ($p<0.005$). This suggests that, on the population level, the presence of the DR2 + haplotype contributes to the non-responsiveness of MS patients but cannot completely explain it. The interferon responsiveness of normal donors was certainly not reduced by DR2 +, again indicating that belonging to the DR2 + category by itself cannot explain non-responsiveness of MS patients. However, in the MS patients the presence of the DR2 + phenotype seemed to further reduce the already diminished responsiveness.

Spontaneous NK activity varied widely in both PBL cultures from normal donors and MS patients, and mean values were not different between the two groups. Stimulation by Sendai virus, ConA and HuIFN-α resulted in significant increases of the NK activity, and these increments were of similar size in PBL cultures of normal donors and MS patients.

However, when the results of the NK activity were further analyzed in function of the ConA-induced HuIFN-γ production, or in function of the DR2 + typing, potentially significant differences became apparent. The

Table 4 NK activities of PBLs of MS patients and normal donors by DR2 + and DR2 – HLA phenotypes

Donor group		Total number examined	NK activity (expressed as LU_{50}) Spontaneous[a]	After incubation with HuIFN-α	After stimulation with ConA
DR2 +	MS patients	18	3.6 (0.73)[b]	8.9 (1.69)	7.8 (1.62)
	Controls	8	5.0 (1.1)	10.9 (2.8)	10.7 (1.44)
DR2 –	MS patients	25	7.0 (1.18)	14.5 (1.82)	12.6 (1.56)
	Controls	12	5.6 (0.30)	12.5 (2.2)	11.4 (1.52)

a = PBLs cultured in plain medium with serum
b = Mean (SE)

average NK activity after ConA stimulation for the HuIFN-γ-producing MS-PBLs was 12.4 (SE 1.90; $n = 20$) as compared to a value of 9.5 (SE 1.13; $n = 34$) for the non-producing cultures. Table 4 shows the analysis of NK activities in function of the DR2 phenotype. Within the MS patient group both spontaneous and stimulated NK activities were lower in cultures from patients who were DR2+ than from those who were DR2− (statistically significant as analyzed by Student's t-test: $p < 0.025$). PBL cultures of normal donors did not display this DR2-dependent difference in NK activities. The effectiveness of stimulation by ConA and leukocyte interferon was the same in all groups: treatment with HuIFN-α provoked a 2.0–2.5-fold increase in NK activity and ConA caused a 1.8–2.2-fold increase.

In conclusion, at the population level, there seems to be an association between the occurrence of certain, as yet undefined MS pathogenic factors, defective responsiveness to mitogens (as measured by HuIFN-γ production and NK cell activities), and presence of HLA DR2-controlled antigens.

The true nature of this association is not clear at present. Neither is it evident whether HuIFN-γ and NK cell activity are intervening variables in this association, or simple epiphenomena.

ACKNOWLEDGMENTS

Support for this study was received from the Belgian Foundations for Scientific Research on Multiple Sclerosis: WOMS and BSMS.

15
α-Albumin in cerebrospinal fluid of patients with multiple sclerosis and other neurological diseases – comparison with other brain specific proteins

R. CROLS, M. NOPPE, and A. LOWENTHAL

ABSTRACT

α-Albumin (an astrocyte specific protein) was determined in cerebrospinal fluid (CSF) of 142 patients without CNS disease, 79 multiple sclerosis patients and 1060 patients with other neurological diseases. In control and other neurological diseases, the CSF α-albumin (GFA) level was comparable with that of other brain specific proteins. However in MS, CSF α-albumin was within the normal range even during exacerbations, contrasting with the CSF levels of MBP and S100, which were correlated with the disease activity. This difference could be of diagnostic value if confirmed in further studies.

INTRODUCTION

During recent years, several central nervous system (CNS) specific proteins have been described: protein 14-3-2 is a neuron specific enolase (NSE), myelin basic protein (MBP) is specific for CNS myelin and the proteins α-albumin (immunologically identical to glial fibrillary acidic protein (GFA)[1,2]) and S100 are two different markers for astroglial cells. It seems logical that their level in cerebrospinal fluid (CSF) correlates with pathological changes in the CNS. For instance, an increase of MBP in CSF has been shown in patients during multiple sclerosis (MS) exacerbations[3-7]. We performed a large scale study on CSF α-albumin[8,9]. In the present paper we compare the results of our study with publications on other brain specific proteins demonstrated in CSF of several neurological diseases, with special emphasis on MS.

RESULTS

The normal value for CSF α-albumin was determined with a two-site immuno-radiometric assay[10] in 142 CSF samples of patients without CNS disease (disc herniation, peripheral ophthalmological or otovestibular disease and non-organic psychiatric diseases). The mean value was 3.2 ng/ml and the standard deviation 3.1 ng/ml. Values above the mean + 2 SD or 9.4 ng/ml were considered pathological.

Table 1 Mean CSF α-albumin levels in some neurological diseases

Diagnosis	Number of cases	CSF α-albumin (ng/ml) Mean	Range
Encephalitis	14	120.2	1–636
Astrocytic tumours	12	43.3	2–151
Syringomyelia	10	42.5	0–259
Bacterial meningitis	13	19.0	1– 74
Acute cerebrovascular disease	82	16.1	0–342
Alzheimer's disease	46	8.4	0– 74
Controls	142	3.3	0– 23

In Table 1 several neurological diseases were classified in decreasing order of pathological values. High values were found in most cases of encephalitis, astrocytic tumours, syringomyelia and bacterial meningitis and less in acute cerebrovascular disease. Slightly elevated values were found in patients with chronic cerebrovascular disease and Alzheimer's disease. Pathological values were rarely found in aseptic meningitis, amyotrophic lateral sclerosis (ALS), Parkinson's disease and MS. Even in patients with definite MS (stable or active) the incidence of pathological CSF α-albumin values did not increase (Table 2).

Table 2 CSF α-albumin in MS

MS	Number of cases	CSF α-albumin (ng/ml) Mean	Range	% Pathological cases (> 9.4 ng/ml)
Probable	37	9.7	0–242	8.1%
Definite stable	33	3.6	0– 15	9.9%
Definite active	9	3.1	0– 11	11.1%
All	79	6.4	0–242	8.9%

DISCUSSION

In Table 3 the CSF levels of the CNS specific proteins (α-albumin, MBP, NSE and S100) are compared in control subjects and in several CNS diseases. All four proteins are increased in the CSF of brain tumours[5,6,8,9,11,12]. α-Albumin, MBP and S100 are increased in encephalitis,[5,8,9,12,13]. α-Albumin, NSE and S100 are increased in congenital malformations[8,9,11]. Patients without CNS

Table 3 Brain specific proteins in CSF

Disease	α-albumin	MBP	NSE	S100
Controls	−	−	−	−
Brain tumours	+ +	+ +	+ +	+ +
Encephalitis	+ +	+ +	n.d.	+ +
Congenital malformations	+ +	n.d.	+ +	+ +
Active MS	−	+ +	n.d.	+ +
Stable MS	−	+	n.d.	+

+ + increased in most cases
　+ increased in some cases
　− rarely increased
n.d. not determined

disease have normal CSF levels for all four CNS specific proteins[3,5,7-9,11,12,14].

There thus seems to be a parallelism between the CSF levels of these four CNS specific proteins, all being increased or normal depending on the pathological condition. There is only one exception. In MS, the levels of MBP and S100 correlate with the disease activity, being more increased in active than in stable MS[3-6,12,15]. In addition, an increase of total CSF enolase activity (neuron-specific or non-neuron-specific) has been shown in active MS[16]. This contrasts strongly with α-albumin, which lies within the normal range in MS patients, even during acute bouts[9]. Only a few increased values were reported in a previous study[17].

This result is unexpected because there is a clear astrocytic reaction in MS: GFA (immunologically identical to α-albumin[1,2]) was isolated out of MS plaques, containing many reactive astrocytes[18]; an increase of S100 protein was demonstrated in the CSF of active MS[12,15]; increased serum levels of auto-antibodies against α-albumin and S100 were shown in MS[19]. The reason why α-albumin is not increased in MS is unclear. It could be due to local factors, inhibiting the transition from the structural non-hydrosoluble to the free hydrosoluble form or inhibiting the release of α-albumin into the CSF.

Since the presence of MBP or the absence of α-albumin in CSF is not specific by itself, they cannot be used individually as a diagnostic test in MS bouts. However, the combination of both seems to be specific for MS and could be of clinical value, if confirmed in prospective studies.

References

1. Gheuens, J., Lowenthal, A., Karcher, D. and Noppe, M. (1978). Similarities between the nervous tissue proteins α-albumin and glial fibrillary acidic protein. In Schoffeniels, E., Franck, G., Hertz, L. and Tower, D. B. (eds.). *Dynamic Properties of Glial Cells*, pp. 257–266. (Oxford: Pergamon Press)
2. Gheuens, J., Karcher, D., Noppe, M. and Lowenthal, A. (1979). Comparison of brain specific protein α-albumin and GFA (glial fibrillary acidic protein). *Acta Neurol. Belg.*, **79**, 314
3. Biber, A., Engler, D., Dommash, D. and Hempel, K. (1981). Myelin basic protein in cerebrospinal fluid of patients with multiple sclerosis and other neurological diseases. *J. Neurol.*, **225**, 231
4. Cohen, S. R., Herndon, R. M. and McKhann, G. M. (1976). Radioimmunoassay of myelin basic protein in spinal fluid: an index of active demyelination. *N. Engl. J. Med.*, **295**, 1455

5. Cohen, S. R., Brooks, B. R., Herndon, R. M. and McKhann, G. M. (1980). A diagnostic index of active demyelination: myelin basic protein in cerebrospinal fluid. *Ann. Neurol.*, **8**, 25

6. Matthieu, J. M. and Bürgisser, P. (1983). Radioimmunological determination of myelin basic protein in the CSF of neurological patients. In Peeters, H. (ed.). *Protides of the Biological Fluids: Proceedings of the 30th Colloquium 1982*, pp. 223–226. (Oxford: Pergamon Press)

7. Whitaker, J. N., Lisak, R. P., Basher, R. M., Fitch, O. H., Seyer, J. M., Krance, R., Lawrence, J. A., Ch'ien, L. T. and O'Sullivan, P. (1980). Immunoreactive myelin basic protein in the cerebrospinal fluid in neurological disorders. *Ann. Neurol.*, **7**, 58

8. Crols, R., Noppe, M., Tasnier, A., Lowenthal, A. and Karcher, D. (1983). Determination of α-albumin in cerebrospinal fluid. In Peeters, H. (ed.). *Protides of the Biological Fluids: Proceedings of the 30th Colloquium 1982*, pp. 209–212. (Oxford: Pergamon Press)

9. Crols, R., Noppe, M., Caers, J. and Lowenthal, A. α-Albumin (GFA) as a marker of astrocytic involvement in human cerebrospinal fluid. *Neurochem. Pathol.* (in press)

10. Noppe, M., Lowenthal, A., Karcher, D. and Gheuens, J. (1979). A two-site immunoradiometric assay for the determination of α-albumin. *J. Immunol. Methods*, **27**, 75

11. Kato, K., Nakajima, T., Ishiguro, Y. and Matsutani, T. (1982). Sensitive enzyme immunoassay for S-100 protein: determination in human cerebrospinal fluid. *Biomed. Res.*, **3**, 24

12. Michetti, F., Massaro, A., Russo, G. and Rigon, G. (1980). The S-100 antigen in cerebrospinal fluid as a possible index of cell injury in the nervous tissue. *J. Neurol. Sci.*, **44**, 259

13. Jacque, C., Delasalle, A., Rancurel, G., Raoul, M., Lesourd, B. and Legrand, J. C. (1982). Myelin basic protein in CSF and blood. Relationship between its presence and the occurrence of a destructive process in the brains of encephalitic patients. *Arch. Neurol.*, **39**, 557

14. Scarna, H., Steinberg, R., Delafosse, B., Debilly, G., Mandrand, B., Keller, A. and Pujol, J. F. (1983). Neuron-specific enolase (NSE) in biological fluids: a marker of neuronal lesions. In Peeters, H. (ed.). *Protides of the Biological Fluids: Proceedings of the 30th Colloquium 1982*, pp. 55–60. (Oxford: Pergamon Press)

15. Michetti, F. and Massaro, A. (1983). Studies on the S-100 antigen in cerebrospinal fluid of neurological patients. In Peeters, H. (ed.). *Protides of the Biological Fluids: Proceedings of the 30th Colloquium, 1982*, pp. 205–208. (Oxford: Pergamon Press)

16. Royds, J. A., Timperly, W. R. and Taylor, C. B. (1981). Levels of enolase and other enzymes in the cerebrospinal fluid as indices of pathological change. *J. Neurol., Neurosurg. Psych.*, **44**, 1129

17. Lowenthal, A., Noppe, M., Gheuens, J. and Karcher, D. (1978). α-Albumin (glial fibrillary acidic protein) in normal and pathological human brain and cerebrospinal fluid. *J. Neurol.*, **219**, 87

18. Eng, L. F., Vanderhaeghen, J. J., Bignami, A. and Gerstl, B. (1971). An acidic protein isolated from fibrous astrocytes. *Brain Res.*, **28**, 351

19. Melse, J., Noppe, M., Crols, R., Gheuens, J. and Lowenthal, A. (1983). Autoantibodies to brain specific proteins in human serum from normal and several pathological conditions. *Acta Neurol. Belg.*, **83**, 17

16
The Transferrin–Tau ratio of the CSF

B. TAVOLATO, P. GALLO and C. De ZANCHE

INTRODUCTION

Transferrin (Tr) is a major serum protein with a MW of 90000 and a serum concentration of 200–320 mg/100 ml (about 4 per cent of the total serum proteins). Each molecule of Tr can bind two atoms of trivalent iron (Fe^{3+}). Normally only 30 per cent of the total iron binding capacity of the Tr is saturated.

Several genetic variants of Tr have been described in different racial groups. The major Tr (phenotype C) is however present in almost all the racial groups. With standard electrophoresis (EF) Tr migrates in the β-1 area, separating in two bands. With isoelectricfocusing Tr shows an isoelectric point at about pH 5.9, separating in several bands[1,2].

The concentration of Tr in the CSF is higher than might be expected from the MW and the hydrodynamic radius of the protein[3]. The concentrations reported in normal CSF are around 15 mg/l (with minor variations according to the different methods of measurement employed), and represent about 8 per cent of the total CSF proteins[4,5]. No modifications of the CSF Tr concentration are described in specific neurological diseases, except when the total protein concentration is increased.

It is known from Bucher et al[6] that Tr of the CSF is divided by electrophoretic methods in two fractions: the major one is more anodic and corresponds to the serum Tr, while the minor one, more cathodic (migrating in the β-2 zone) corresponds to the so called Tau fraction[7-9]. The Tau fraction is immunologically identical to Tr and differs from Tr only because it lacks four molecules of sialic acid[10] The Tau fraction still has the capacity to bind iron, and has been sometimes observed as a double fraction in degenerative diseases of the CNS[10,11].

In the present study, the proteins of the β-zone were studied with electroimmunofixation on cellulose acetate strips. A densitometric method to evaluate the relative per cent of Tr/Tau proteins was devised, and the Tr/Tau ratio was estimated in different neurological diseases.

63

MATERIALS AND METHODS

We studied 124 CSF from 'normal' subjects and from patients with different neurological diseases. Five ml of CSF were concentrated 25–30 times using a Minicon B-15 chamber (Amicon). The amount of concentrated CSF used for EF was calculated from the amount of total protein (TP) in the concentrated CSF. The amount of TP necessary for immunofixation was found to be one half of the amount used for EF.

The EF was carried out on cellulose acetate strips (Cellogel RS – Chemetron, Milano) using a Tris-glycine buffer (pH 9.5). The migration lasted $4\frac{1}{2}$ hrs at 240 V: This 'long migration' allowed a good separation of the β-zone bands.

After EF the strips were cut in half along the longitudinal axis. One half was used for immunofixation with anti-Tr antiserum (100 μl of the antiserum were uniformly distributed on a glass plate and the half strip was carefully placed on the antiserum for 15 minutes). After immunofixation the strip was washed three times for 20 minutes each in PBS. The standard EF strip and the immunofixation strip were stained with Coomassie BB 250 R and destained as usual.

For the densitometric measurement of the Tr and Tau fractions an automatic densitometer ('Cellomatic 2') was used. The densitometer provided the profile of the β-zone and the relative per cent of the Tr and Tau fractions. On the basis of these data we calculated the Tr/Tau ratio.

RESULTS

Immunofixation studies of the CSF β-zone

On standard EF with Cellogel RS three or four bands were visible in the β-zone in 'normal' and most of the pathological CSF. After immunofixation with anti-Tr antiserum four bands were regularly precipitated (Figure 1). The pattern of these bands was highly reproducible. The two more anodic bands corresponded to the serum Tr, while the two more cathodic bands corresponded to the Tau fractions. The major Tr was always more anodic than the minor one; while for the Tau fraction the major was more cathodic than the minor one. The minor Tau was not always visible with standard EF, but it became clearly visible after immunofixation (due to the enhancing effect of the immunoprecipitation reaction).

After EF of the sera no Tau fraction could be immunoprecipitated with the anti-Tr antiserum (Figure 1).

In pathological conditions bands not related to Tr proteins were sometimes visible between the Tr and Tau bands. In one case a huge band due to IgA was identified. The patient was affected by amyotrophic lateral sclerosis with IgA paraproteinaemia (serum IgA 1400 mg/100 ml) and the CSF IgA band was similar to the serum band. In two cases affected by Guillain–Barré syndrome the extra bands in the β-zone were precipitated with the anti-C3c and anti-C4 antisera. In two patients affected by subarachnoid haemorrhage with 'xanthochromic' CSF two extra bands were present between the Tr and Tau bands. In these cases the extra bands were precipitated by the anti-Tr antiserum.

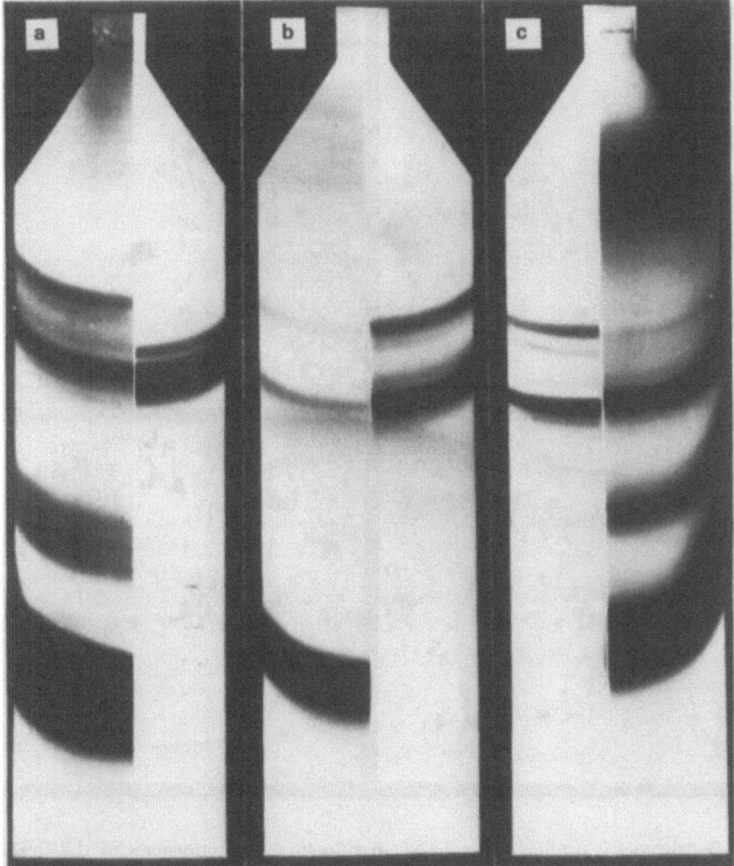

Figure 1 (a) Electrophoresis of serum: immunofixation with anti-Transferrin antiserum on the right half of the strip. Only two bands of Transferrin are precipitated. (b): Electrophoresis of CSF: immunofixation with anti-Transferrin antiserum on the right half of the strip. Four bands are precipitated; the two more cathodic bands are due to the Tau fraction. (c): Immunofixation on the left half of the strip. The minor Tau fraction is clearly separated.

Such bands were considered as Tr of serum origin, partially deprived of sialic acid and with an EF mobility intermediate between Tr and Tau. These cases are indicative of a direct enzymatic degradation of Tr (of serum origin) to Tau protein inside the CNS.

Quantitative studies of the Tr/Tau ratio

The β-zone could be easily scanned with a standard densitometer. The Tr and Tau peaks could always be separated and measured. The two Tr subfractions and the two Tau subfractions were often very close or not visible (the latter condition was however noted only for the minor Tau fraction). Therefore, the

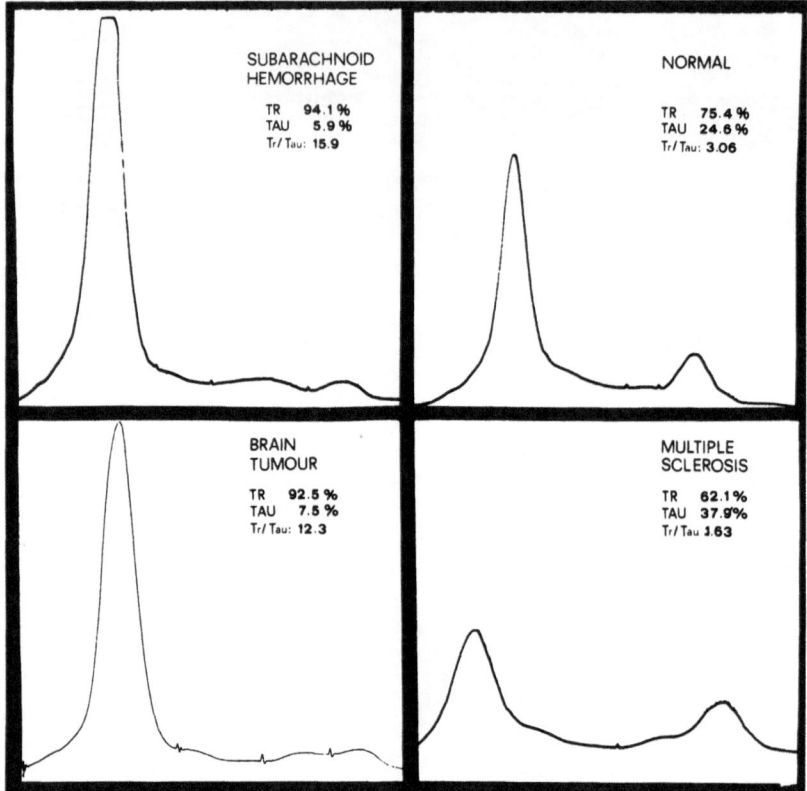

Figure 2 Densitometric profiles of the β-zone in different CSF. In normal CSF the Tau fraction is about 25% of the total. In a subarachnoid haemorrhage (or in a brain tumour) a marked percentage increase of the Transferrin is observed (influx of Transferrin through a damaged blood–brain barrier). In MS a relative increase of the percent of the Tau fraction can be observed (myelin damage with liberation of neuraminidase, without blood–brain barrier damage?)

data were expressed as relative per cent of total Tr and total Tau. The Tr/Tau ratio was also calculated (Figure 2).

In the cases in which extra bands were visible the percentages due to these bands were subtracted and the Tr and Tau percentages were recalculated without the extra bands.

In 'normal' CSF the per cent of Tr and Tau fractions and the Tr/Tau ratio proved to be rather constant with small variations (mean 2.77 ± 0.61).

In pathological conditions instead, large variations of the Tr/Tau ratio were observed (Figure 2). As predicted the increase of the ratio is not disease specific, but it mainly reflects the damage of the blood–brain barrier and correlates with the total proteins of the CSF (Table 1).

From Figure 3 it can be observed that 14 cases (all from pathological CSF) had a normal total protein level and a Tr/Tau ratio higher than normal. Vice

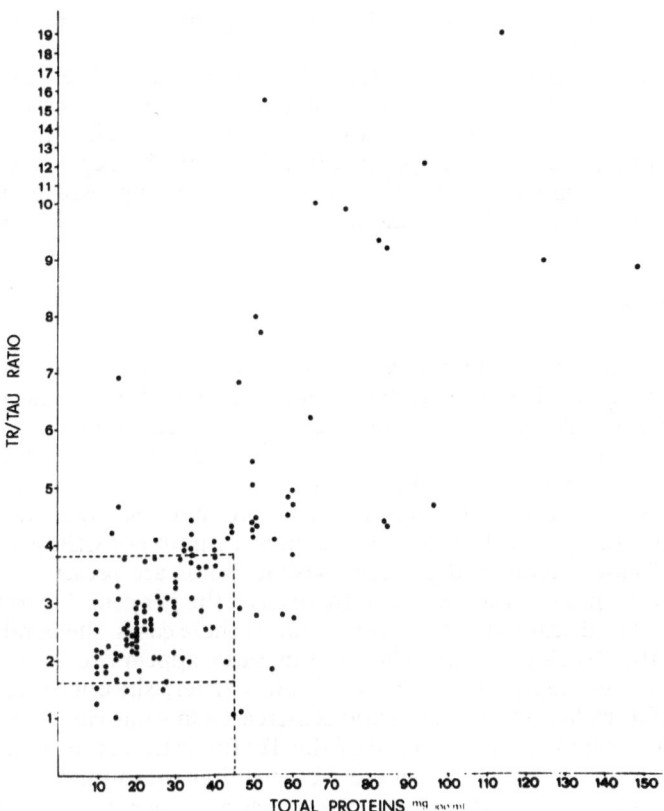

THE TRANSFERRIN-TAU RATIO OF THE CSF

Figure 3 Correlation between total protein and Transferrin/Tau ratio ($r^2 = 0.48$). The dotted lines enclose the normal values

Table 1 Transferrin per cent, Tau per cent and Tr/Tau ratio in 124 CSF. Significantly increased Tr/Tau ratio in some neurological disease groups (*$p < 0.001$, **$p < 0.01$)

	No CSFs	Transferrin Per Cent	Tau Per Cent	Tr/Tau Ratio	Total proteins mg/100ml
Multiple sclerosis	56	72.80	26.20	2.81 ± 1.01	30.64
Alzheimer disease	10	78.75	21.25	4.20 ± 2.13	30.64
Brain tumours	7	82.61	17.39	6.02 ± 3.74**	49.16
Meningitis	6	83.20	16.80	5.37 ± 2.10*	59.00
Amyotrophic lateral sclerosis	6	72.70	27.30	2.67 ± 0.24	22.6
Guillain-barré syndrome	8	84.90	15.10	6.10 ± 2.43*	80.75
Subarachnoid haemorrhage	4	92.75	7.25	13.83 ± 4.50*	98.23
Optic neuritis	4	68.60	31.40	2.21 ± 0.46	27.00
Polyneuropathies	3	70.90	29.10	2.87 ± 1.16	22.00
Various	10	73.07	26.93	2.71 ± 1.55	35.06
'Normals'	10	72.90	27.10	2.77 ± 0.61	21.75

versa only seven CSF were found with a normal ratio and a total protein level higher than normal.

In seven cases a ratio lower than normal (<1.6) was also observed. Most of such cases have a low total protein content (only in one case CSF TP > 45 mg/100 ml). Again these cases were not disease specific (five MS, one polyneuropathy, one subacute paraneoplastic cerebellar degeneration), but the cases were all from patients with chronic demyelinating diseases, probably without any blood–brain barrier damage.

DISCUSSION

The increase of the Tr in the CSF from patients with damage of the blood–brain barrier has already been reported (it is part of the so called 'transudative profile')[9]. However our quantitative densitometric method of estimation of the Tr/Tau ratio offers a simple and economic tool which can be easily added to standard CSF EF.

The presence of other proteins in the β-zone not related to the Tr/Tau system, is not relevant with the use of a standard amount of CSF protein. In a minority of cases (about 6–8 per cent) visible bands are present in the area between the Tr and the Tau bands. In these cases the per cent due to the extra bands should be discarded, although in some of these cases, the bands are still related to the Tr/Tau system. The Tr/Tau ratio appears to be a valuable indicator of the integrity of the blood–brain barrier, since its variability in normal CSF is rather limited. The ratio is increased in some cases with normal TP content. Therefore, the increase of the Tr/Tau ratio can be considered a more efficient marker of the blood–brain barrier than the estimation of the TP, which is influenced by several factors (i.e. selective increase of γ-globulins, without blood–brain barrier damage).

From our data the increase ($0.01 < p < 0.005$) of the Tr/Tau ratio in cases of Alzheimer's disease is of particular interest. However, this group of patients also differs from the other groups in the mean age of the patients. Therefore, the increase of the ratio in Alzheimer's disease may also be an age-related phenomenon (the increase of CSF albumin and TP with age is well known)[12].

A decrease of the Tr/Tau ratio was observed only in seven CSF. Most (four of these cases) had a low TP content (<20 mg/100 ml), and only one case was over 45 mg/100 ml. All the cases with Tr/Tau ratio lower than normal were from patients with demyelinating diseases (five were from MS). Since it is known that neuraminidase is localised in myelin sheaths[13] it is probable that the decrease of the Tr/Tau ratio is due to recent demyelinating activity with liberation of neuraminidase in the CSF. However, this phenomenon was observed in a minority of the cases of MS. It is known that a relative damage of the blood–brain barrier exists in MS[14]. Therefore, MS can influence the Tr/Tau ratio in both directions, and the final result will depend on the dynamic equilibrium between demyelinating activity (with neuraminidase liberation in CSF) and blood–brain barrier damage (with influx of Tr from serum).

References

1. Hovanessian, G. and Awden, L. (1976). 'Gel isoelectricfocusing of human serum Transferrin. *Eur. J. Biochem.*, **68**, 333
2. Makey, D. G. and Seal, V. S. (1976). The detection of four molecular forms of human Transferrin during the iron binding process. *Biochem. Biophys. Acta*, **453**, 250
3. Felgenhauer, K. (1974). Protein size and CSF composition. *Klin. Wochenschr.*, **52**, 1158
4. Goodmann, M. and Vulpe, M. (1961). A quantitative immunochemical method for determining serum and CSF proteins. *World. Neurol.* **2**, 589–601
5. Schuller, E., Tompe, L., Lefevre, M. and Moreno, P. (1970). Electroimmunodiffusion des proteines du liquide céphalorachidien: dosage de la préalbumine, de l'Alpha 1-anti-trypsine, de l'Alpha 2-Haptoglobine, de l'Alpha-Macroglobuline et de la Transferrine. *Clin. Chim. Acta.*, **30**, 73
6. Butcher, T., Matzelt, D. and Pette, D. (1952). Papierelektrophorese von Liquor Cerebrospinalis. *Klin. Wochenschr.*, **30**, 325
7. Pette, D. and Stupp, I. (1960). Die Tau-Fraktion in Liquor Cerebrospinalis. *Klin. Wochenschr.*, **38**, 109
8. Lowenthal, A. (1964). *Agar Gel Electrophoresis in Neurology*, p. 55 (Amsterdam, New York, London: Elsevier)
9. Latterre, E. Chr. (1964). *Les Protéines du LCS à l'État Normal et Pathologique* (Bruxelles: ARSCIA)
10. Parker, C. and Bearn, A. (1967). Studies on the Transferrin of adult serum, cord serum and CSF. *J. Exp. Med.*, **115**, 83
11. Rocchelli, B., Roloni, M., Delodovici, M., Mazzarello, P. and Losi, V. (1979). The CSF Tau-Transferrin Isoelectricfocusing study on 674 neurological patients. *Ital. J. Neurol. Sci.*, **4**, 251
12. Eeg-Olofsson, O., Link, H. and Wigertz, A. (1981). Concentrations of CSF proteins as a measure of blood brain barrier function and synthesis of IgG within the CNS in 'normal' subjects from the age of 6 months to 3 years. *Acta Paediatr. Scand.*, **70**, 167
13. Tettamanti, G., Venerando, B., Preti, A., Lombardo, A. and Zambotti, V. (1974). Brain Neuraminidases. In *Glycolipids, glycoproteins, alpha mucopolysaccharides of the nervous system*. Adv. Exp. Med. Bio., **25**, 161
14. Lumsden, C. E. (1972). The clinical pathology of multiple sclerosis. In McAlpine, D., Lumsden, C. E. and Acheson, E. D. (eds.). *Multiple Sclerosis*, p.311 (Edinburgh & London: Churchill Livingstone)

17
Auto-antibodies to brain specific proteins

M. NOPPE, J. MELSE, R. CROLS, J. GHEUENS
and A. LOWENTHAL

INTRODUCTION

Destruction of cells in the brain can release specific markers from these cells. Some of these markers are immunogenic. We studied the auto-antibody immune response against glial fibrillary acidic protein (GFA)[1], S100[2] and myelin basic protein (MBP)[3], known to be markers for astroglial cells and myelin, respectively.

This study was designed to clarify whether the determination of auto-antibodies has a practical diagnostic value.

METHODS

A solid phase immunoassay was used[4]. Cellulose CNBr coupled antigen is incubated with the patient's serum. After a first incubation, the immuno-adsorbant is washed, and radiolabelled *Staphylococcus* protein A is added. After 1 hour, the immuno-adsorbant is washed and the bound radioactivity is measured.

Affinity purified radiolabelled anti-human IgG gives similar results as using *Staphylococcus* protein A; so does isolated γ-globulin.

IgG binds aspecifically to MBP[5,6], we, therefore, bring all sera to the same level of total IgG (12mg/100ml).

In order to compare results obtained in different experiments, we express the results as the per cent radioactivity bound in comparison to a reference serum.

RESULTS

A first group of 190 sera of patients from the neurological department were screened and showed that patients with MS, polyneuropathy, astroglial tumours and dementia had significantly elevated levels of auto-antibodies against the three antigens under study. As a control group we took 21 blood donors.

No difference was found between sex, total protein, total IgG and the levels of the auto-antibodies. The highest levels of auto-antibodies were found in rheumatoid patients.

For further study we used sera of patients with MS, polyneuropathy, astroglial tumours and senile and presenile dementia. A summary of the results is given in Table 1.

Table 1

	N	Anti-GFA (% ref)	Anti-S100 (% ref)	Anti-MBP (% ref)
Polyneuropathy	40	88.0 ± 44.5	49.5 ± 25.1	86.6 ± 50.9
Astroglial tumours	15	58.5 ± 31.8	41.6 ± 26.7	60.6 ± 23.5
MS	47	98.8 ± 34.7	50.6 ± 22.7	76.1 ± 22.6
Dementia	30	77.9 ± 40.9	41.2 ± 15,9	67.4 ± 18.6
Control	21	41.8 ± 10.2	34.9 ± 12.4	47.1 ± 12.5

Results are given as mean ± SD

In 32 patients we compared the levels of auto-antibodies in serum and CSF. No correlations between serum and CSF values were found for anti-S100 and anti-GFA. For anti-MBP we found a correlation coefficient of 0.817.

CONCLUSION

Using this solid phase immunoassay, we were able to demonstrate auto-antibodies against S100, GFA and MBP in neurological patients as well as in blood donors. Very high levels are seen in rheumatoid patients.

Significant levels are seen in MS, polyneuropathy, senile and presenile dementia and astroglial tumours. There are no significant differences between these groups. CSF levels do not correlate with serum levels except for anti-MBP.

References

1. Eng, L. F., Vanderhaeghen, J. J., Bignami, A. and Gerstl, B. (1971). An acidic protein isolated from fibrous astrocytes. *Brain Res.*, **28**, 351
2. Moore, B. W., Perez, V. J. and Gehring, M. (1968). Assay and regional distribution of a soluble protein characteristic of the nervous system. *J. Neurochem.*, **15**, 75
3. Eylar, E. H., Salk, J., Beveridge, G. C. and Brown, L. V. (1969). Experimental allergic encephalomyelitis basic protein from bovine myelin. *Arch. Biochem.*, **132**, 34
4. Melse, J., Noppe, M., Crols, R., Gheuens, J. and Lowenthal, A. (1983). Autoantibodies to brain specific proteins in human serum from normal and several pathological conditions. *Acta Neurol. Belg.*, **83**, 17
5. Aarli, J. A., Aparicio, S. R. and Lumsden, C. E. (1975). Binding of normal human IgG to myelin sheets, glia and neurons. *J. Immunol.*, **28**, 171
6. McPherson, T. A., Marchalonis, J. J. and Lennon, V. (1970). Binding of encephalitogenic basic protein by serum α-globulins. *J. Immunol.*, **19**, 929

18
The effect of monoclonal anti-T cell antibodies on the clinical course of experimental allergic encephalomyelitis in rats

C. J. J. BRINKMAN, H. J. ter LAAK and O. R. HOMMES

Much evidence exists regarding the role of T lymphocytes in the pathogenesis of multiple sclerosis (MS). By means of monoclonal anti-T cell antibodies, abnormalities and fluctuations in T cell subsets depending on disease activity have been found in the blood of MS patients[1]. Furthermore, it has been demonstrated that cells in the cerebrospinal fluid[2,3] and perivascular infiltrates[4-6] of the central nervous system of MS patients predominantly consist of T lymphocytes. The majority of these T cells showed the characteristics of helper/inducer T lymphocytes[4,5]. Moreover, it was demonstrated in our laboratory that part of the T lymphocytes in the cerebrospinal fluid[2] and in the perivascular cuffs were Ia$^+$, i.e. were in an activated state[7].

In view of our intention to treat MS patients with monoclonal anti-T cell antibodies, we primarily investigated the influence of this type of immunosuppression on the induction and the clinical course of experimental allergic encephalomyelitis (EAE).

EAE was induced in male Lewis rats by subcutaneous injection of whole guinea-pig spinal cord emulsified with Freund's complete adjuvant in the hind footpads[8]. The animals were observed and weighed daily. The clinical symptoms of EAE were scored[9] from 0 to 8.

Prophylactic immunosuppression

Monoclonal anti-rat-T cell antibodies (Sera Laboratories, Sussex, Great Britain) were dissolved in phosphate buffered saline (PBS). Between day 0 (day of immunization) and day 15, the rats received eight injections, each of 20 μg monoclonal antibodies, subcutaneously on the back. The monoclonal antibodies used were W3/13, W3/25 and OX8 labelling, respectively, all rat T lymphocytes, rat T helper lymphocytes and rat T non-helper lymphocytes. Rats treated with diluted mouse serum in a parallel fashion were used as controls. Surviving rats were killed at day 26.

Therapeutic immunosuppression

Twelve rats were used in this experiment. All rats were immunized as described. As soon as tail flaccidity appeared, five rats received a total dose of 230µg W3/13 (anti-rat total T cell antibodies), dissolved in PBS, subcutaneously on the back during the 3 consecutive days. Mouse serum, injected in a similar fashion, was used as control in the other seven rats. Surviving rats were killed at day 40.

Table 1 shows that prophylactic treatment of rats with monoclonal antibodies to all peripheral T lymphocytes (W3/13) significantly ($p < 0.001$) reduced the clinical signs of EAE compared to rats which received mouse serum (controls). Similar results were obtained with animals treated with monoclonal antibodies to T helper cells (W3/25) mixed with monoclonal antibodies to T non-helper cells (OX8) as compared to the control animals ($p < 0.0001$). Animals treated with either W3/25 or OX8 developed EAE with comparable clinical intensity ($p > 0.1$) as the control rats. The duration of EAE was reduced significantly ($p < 0.01$) in all groups treated with monoclonal antibodies as compared to the mouse serum treated animals. Treatment of rats with monoclonal antibodies to all T lymphocytes (W3/13) after the onset of the first clinical symptoms of EAE (tail flaccidity) resulted in a less fatal course of the disease compared to the control group (Table 2). This difference was on the borderline of significancy ($p = 0.06$).

Table 1 Influence of various monoclonal anti-T lymphocyte antibodies on the development of clinical EAE in Lewis rats

Injected material	No of rats	Mean clinical severity (grade 0–8)	Mean disease duration (days)	No of animals which died from EAE
Mouse serum (controls)	16	5.5	6.9	5
W3/13 (anti-T total antibodies)	11	1.9*	3.7*	0
W3/25 (anti-T helper antibodies)	11	4.4	5.5*	4
OX8 (anti-T non-helper antibodies)	8	4.5	4.9*	2
W3/25 + OX8**	12	1.5*	3.2*	0

*Significantly different from control group ($p < 0.01$, Mann-Whitney U test)
**Each rat received 13 µg W3/25 mixed with 7 µg OX8 per injection

These results demonstrate that prophylactic elimination of peripheral T lymphocytes by monoclonal anti-T cell antibodies diminished or prevented the clinical signs of EAE. This decline in clinical EAE was only successful when monoclonal antibodies to all T lymphocytes or a mixture of monoclonal antibodies to T helper cells and monoclonal antibodies to T non-helper cells were used. Monoclonal antibodies to T cell subsets, injected separately, were not effective in decreasing the clinical severity of EAE although the disease

Table 2 Effect of monoclonal anti-T cell antibodies injected from the onset of clinical EAE on the course of EAE in Lewis rats compared with control serum

| Injected material | Clinical severity of EAE | | | | | | | | | |
---	0	1	2	3	4	5	6	7	8	p*
Anti-T total antibodies		1	1		1		1		1	0.06
Mouse serum (controls)				1			1		5	

*Two sided p-value exact test

duration was shortened. Histologically, the differences between the animal groups were less obvious and these will be discussed in a future paper[8]. Furthermore, it was shown that treatment of rats with EAE with monoclonal anti-T cell antibodies from the onset of clinical symptoms resulted in a better prognosis of the disease.

Considering the abnormalities in T lymphocytes and T lymphocyte subsets in the various tissues of MS patients and the observed similarities between MS and EAE, specific elimination of T lymphocytes by monoclonal anti-T cell antibodies in MS patients might be beneficial for the course of this demyelinating disease.

References

1. Reinherz, E.L., Weiner, H.L., Hauser, S.L., Cohen, J.A., Distaso, J.A. and Schlossman, S.F. (1980). Loss of suppressor T cells in active multiple sclerosis. Analysis with monoclonal antibodies. *N. Engl. J. Med., 303,* 125
2. Brinkman, C.J.J., Nillesen, W.M. and Hommes, O.R. (1983). T cell subpopulations in blood and cerebrospinal fluid of multiple sclerosis patients: effect of cyclophosphamide. *Clin. Immunol. Immunopath.* (in press).
3. Panitch, H.S. and Francis, G.T. (1982). T-lymphocyte subsets in cerebrospinal fluid in multiple sclerosis. *N. Engl. J. Med.,* **307,** 560
4. Brinkman, C.J.J., ter Laak, H.J., Hommes, O.R., Poppema, S. and Delmotte, P. (1982). T-lymphocyte subpopulations in multiple sclerosis lesions. *N. Engl. J. Med.,* **307,** 1644
5. Nyland, H., Matre, R., Mørk, S., Bjerke, J.R. and Naess, A. (1982). T-lymphocyte subpopulations in multiple sclerosis lesions. *N. Engl. J. Med.,* **307,** 1643
6. Traugott, U., Reinherz, E.L. and Raine, C.S. (1983). Multiple sclerosis: Distribution of T cell subsets within active chronic lesions. *Science,* **219,** 308
7. Reinherz, E.L., Kung, P.C., Pesando, J.M., Ritz, J., Goldstein, G. and Schlossman, S.F. (1979). Ia determinants on human T-cell subsets defined by monoclonal antibody. Activation stimuli required for expression. *J. Exp. Med.,* **150,** 1472
8. Brinkman, C.J.J., ter Laak, H.J. and Hommes, O.R. (1983). Suppression of experimental allergic encephalomyelitis in Lewis rats by monoclonal anti T cell antibodies. *Eur. J. Immunol.,* submitted
9. Mertin, J. and Stackpoole, A. (1978). Suppression by essential fatty acids of experimental allergic encephalomyelitis is abolished by indomethacin. *Prostaglandin and Medicine,* **1,** 283

19
Changes of polymorphonuclear neutral proteinase activity in multiple sclerosis patients before and after plasma exchanges

B. M. GUARNIERI, L. AMADUCCI, F. CAMBI, R. CAPPARELLI, C. ARFAIOLI, G. AVANZI and C. FRANCO

There is much evidence that multiple sclerosis (MS) is a neurological disease autoimmune in nature.

Since 1966[1] and 1968[2] it was hypothesized that proteolytic enzymes could play an important role in demyelination, and that peptides derived from proteolysis of myelin basic protein (MBP) could be encephalitogenic. Later, several authors studied various aspects of the role of proteolytic enzymes in demyelination occurring in MS and experimental allergic encephalomyelitis (EAE)[3-15].

Classical histological observations indicate a strict correlation between perivascular cuffing and demyelination in MS plaques as well as in EAE lesions[16,17]: such observations led many researchers to consider lymphocytes and macrophages the main source of proteolytic enzymes[13,18,19]. The electron microscope too showed that demyelination occurs before phagocytosis which highly enhances acid protease level[20,21]: so the enzymes early involved in demyelination seem to be neutral proteinases mainly derived from stimulated macrophages[18]. Rastogi and Clausen[22] found that neutral proteinase activity of MS peripheral polymorphonuclear (PMN) leukocytes increases when PMN cells are incubated with MS-specific brain antigens, a mixture of antigens prepared from MS brains[23,24]. Starting from data by Cuzner et al[19,25] we assayed PMN neutral proteinase activity in MS, in other neurological diseases and in normal subjects. According to previous data we found a significant increase of PMN neutral activity in active[26] MS compared to inactive[26] MS and neurological and normal controls: we also found lower values in patients with inactive MS when compared to normal subjects[27].

Our further data confirm such findings (Tables 1 and 2). We have been working to understand the role of this phenomenon, and if it is specific or not

Table 1 PMN neutral proteinase activity in 'definite' multiple sclerosis and other controls

Subjects	Number of subjects	Age	PMN neutral proteinase activity (μmoles mg protein^{-1} hour^{-1})
(1) Multiple sclerosis active*	36	20–57	1.670 ± 0.200[a]
(2) Multiple sclerosis inactive**	39	20–58	1.100 ± 0.160
(3) Normal controls	19	20–45	1.220 ± 0.160
(4) Neurological controls	43	20–64	1.200 ± 0.190

[a] The differences for group (1) versus groups (2), (3) and (4) are significant ($p<0.01$)
* Acute relapse and progressive disease[26]
** Stable for at least 6 months before sampling[26]

Table 2 PMN neutral proteinase activity in 'definite' multiple sclerosis *inactive* and normal controls

Subjects	Number of subjects	Age	PMN neutral proteinase activity (μmoles mg protein^{-1} hour^{-1})
(1) Multiple sclerosis inactive**	39	20.58	1.100 ± 0.160[a]
(2) Normal controls	19	20–45	1.220 ± 0.160

[a] The differences for group (1) versus group (2) are significant ($p<0.05$)
** Stable for at least 6 months before sampling[26]

for MS. In fact, we found a significant increase in such enzyme activity in the initial phases of subacute sclerosing panencephalitis (SSPE), intracranial neoplasm and recent craniocerebral trauma. On the other hand, we did not find the same increase in myasthenia gravis, dermatomyositis, amyotrophic lateral sclerosis, chronic neuropathies and Duchenne muscular dystrophy[27]. These data lead us to consider such an enzymatic increase as an effect of demyelination, in accordance with previous findings by Cuzner et al.[19]

Among leukocytes, PMN cells are the richest in neutral proteinases (i.e. elastase, collagenase, cathepsin G[28,29]). PMN functions, however, are influenced by antigens, antibodies and immune-complexes[30-32]. PMN cells are not considered as key cells in the immune system, but the study of their neutral proteinase gives us new tools to understand some aspects of the complex pathophysiological mechanism of the immune regulation in MS, and also an interesting peripheral marker of the activity of the disease. We assayed PMN neutral proteinase activity in MS patients before and after a cycle of plasma-exchanges in comparison with other MS subjects under different therapies.

METHODS

Patients

The sample population consisted of 35 patients with definite MS, 18 females and 17 males, aged between 21 and 57 years. Patients were subdivided as having active or inactive[26] MS (12 active and 23 inactive).

No patients received corticosteroids or other immunosuppressive agents during the month before the enzyme assay. No patients had neutrophilic leukocytosis and intercurrent infectious diseases.

Initially, three patients received six plasmapheresis (900 ml each) only. Later, 17 patients received six plasma-exchanges, three patients received four: each change consisted of 2000 ml. The last group received two plasma-exchanges a week plus azathioprine (150 mg per day) according to a specific protocol. Four patients with active MS received dexamethasone i.m. (16 mg for the first, 8 mg for the second and 4 mg for the third week). One case of active and one case of inactive MS were treated with azathioprine only (75 mg per day).

PMN neutral proteinase activity was assayed before the beginning of each therapy and after a period of therapy not longer than one month. In six drug-free patients with inactive MS, two enzyme assays were performed with an interval of one month, in order to see spontaneous changes occurring in the disease.

Isolation of PMN cells

Each sample of 20 ml of whole blood was collected into heparinized tubes and layered onto Ficoll Hypaque gradient. Leukocytes were separated from the plasma layer after clumped erythrocytes had passed into the Ficoll phase. PMN cells were further separated, always on a Ficoll gradient. The PMN pellet was suspended in a known volume of phosphate saline buffer[33,34].

Enzyme assay

Total proteins in the PMN lysate were assayed by the Lowry method[35]. Neutral proteinase activity was assayed in a pH range 7.4–7.6 using haemoglobin as a substrate[19].

RESULTS

Among patients who underwent a cycle of plasma-exchanges (2000 ml each plus azathioprine), seven patients with active MS showed a significant decrease of PMN neutral proteinase activity after such therapy (Table 3). On the other hand 13 patients with inactive MS showed a significant increase in such enzyme activity (Table 4). Similarly, three patients with inactive MS who received only plasmapheresis of 900 ml each, showed an increase in PMN neutral proteinase activity and patient S.P. experienced a relapse during plasmapheresis (Table 5). In six drug-free patients with inactive MS we found varying values of PMN neutral proteinase activity during the period of observation (Table 6).

In four patients with active MS, treated with dexamethasone, we found a decrease of PMN neutral proteinase activity after a cycle of therapy: such a decrease was not significant (Table 7). Two patients (one with inactive, the

Table 3 Analysis of PMN neutral proteinase activity in patients with *active** MS who underwent plasma exchanges (2000 ml each)

Patients	Sex	Age	PMN neutral proteinase activity (μmoles mg protein^{-1} hour^{-1}) before	after
L.E.	M	36	1.436	1.384
G.G.	F	45	1.587	1.581
B.F.	M	45	1.835	0.872
M.E.	F	45	2.046	1.269
B.B.	F	35	1.960	1.331
P.E.	F	57	1.686	1.548
S.M.	F	42	1.768	1.126
		Mean ± SD	1.760 ± 0.210	1.302 ± 0.250†

* Acute relapse and progressive disease[26]
† $p < 0.05$

Table 4 Analysis of PMN neutral proteinase activity in patients with *inactive** MS who underwent plasma exchanges (2000 ml each)

Patients	Sex	Age	PMN neutral proteinase activity (μmoles mg protein^{-1} hour^{-1}) before	after
B.V.	F	42	1.260	1.502
S.T.	F	57	1.278	1.356
M.F.	F	28	1.023	1.368
F.F.	M	33	1.066	1.397
V.F.	F	44	1.105	1.530
G.A.	F	55	1.600	1.630
G.I.	F	35	1.332	1.777
C.M.	F	50	1.109	1.448
M.A.	F	45	0.890	0.994
M.S.	F	44	1.131	1.233
B.M.	M	27	1.534	1.588
B.C.	M	21	1.276	2.027
B.P.	M	54	1.320	1.412
		Mean ± SD	1.225 ± 0.200	1.482 ± 0.252†

* Stable for at least 6 months before sampling[26]
† $p < 0.01$

Table 5 Analysis of PMN neutral proteinase activity in patients with *inactive** MS who underwent a cycle of plasmapheresis (900 ml each)

Patients	Sex	Age	PMN neutral proteinase activity (μmoles mg protein^{-1} hour^{-1}) before	after
M.F.	M	24	0.916	1.416
S.P.	M	34	1.075	1.553
P.F.	F	41	1.214	1.434
		Mean ± SD	1.068 ± 0.149	1.468 ± 0.074†

* Stable for at least 6 months before sampling[26]
† $p < 0.05$

Table 6 Analysis of PMN neutral proteinase activity in drug-free patients with *inactive** MS·
(1 month observation)

Patients	Sex	Age	PMN neutral proteinase activity (μmoles mg protein^{-1} hour^{-1})	
			before	after
G.F.	F	44	1.128	1.210
L.G.	M	43	1.017	1.067
M.S.	M	24	0.620	1.016
E.S.	M	32	1.266	0.833
S.F.	M	34	1.018	0.861
Z.G.	F	28	0.800	0.797
		Mean ± SD	0.975 ± 0.232	0.964 ± 0.161†

* Stable for at least 6 months before sampling[26]
† Not significant

Table 7 Analysis of PMN neutral proteinase activity in patients with *active** MS treated with
dexamethasone (1 month observation)

Patients	Sex	Age	PMN neutral proteinase activity (μmoles mg protein^{-1} hour^{-1})	
			before	after
B.O.	M	54	1.681	1.320
P.C.	M	32	1.823	1.250
M.R.	M	36	1.474	1.268
M.A.	F	29	1.324	1.342
		Mean ± SD	1.576 ± 0.221	1.295 ± 0.043†

* Acute relapse and progressive disease[26]
† Not significant

Table 8 Analysis of PMN neutral proteinase activity in two patients with MS (one inactive and
one active) treated with azathioprine (1 month observation)

Patients	Clinical phase	Sex	Age	PMN neutral proteinase activity (μmoles mg protein^{-1} hour^{-1})	
				before	after
P.R.	Inactive	M	21	1.084	0.500
P.G.	Active	M	32	1.562	1.355

other with active MS) treated with azathioprine only both showed a decrease in
PMN neutral proteinase activity (Table 8).

DISCUSSION

In active MS we could consider the increase of PMN neutral proteinase activity
as an effect of the presence, in serum, of neuroantigens, antibodies and
immune-complexes: considering this we could use such enzyme activity to
monitor the clinical phases of MS.

As our data show, various therapies influence such enzyme activity, so we could use such an enzyme assay to investigate the efficacy of various therapies and their eventual effects on some immunoregulatory mechanisms. There are data about peripheral mechanisms of immune-unresponsiveness (antigen blockade, antibody feedback, suppressor cells[36]) in MS and EAE.

Some researchers affirmed that the reactivity of T cells that recognize determinants on MBP may be partly attenuated by circulating fragments of autologous MBP. Such MBP serum fragments (MBP-SF) were detected using a radioimmune assay in suckling rats[37], in adult normal rats and in Lewis rats at the time of the manifestations of EAE[38,39]. Concentrations of these MBP-SF progressively declined, correlating inversely with the age-related increasing ability of Lewis rats to develop EAE[40]. Recently, Paterson et al[41] detected endogenous MBP-SF and anti-MBP antibodies in human sera: their findings give additional support to the hypothesis that circulating MBP factors may function as neuro-autotolerogens that reduce expansion of MBP reactive lymphoid cell clones having potential injurious effect on central nervous system tissue.

So, in addition to a possible role in the pathogenesis, circulating antibodies may be implicated in the regulation of EAE and MS.

In MS, plasma-exchanges interfere with such circulating neuro-antigens, antibodies and complexes; in such a way plasma-exchanges might determine different effects on PMN neutral proteinase activity in the inactive compared to the active phases of the disease. Our studies need to examine a larger number of patients, and to verify in animal models the findings suggested by our data on human populations.

References

1. Nakao, A. W., Davis, W. J. and Einstein, E. R. (1966). Basic protein from the acidic extract of bovine spinal cord, Part 1 (isolation and characterization). *Biochim. Biophys. Acta*, **130**, 163

2. Chao, L. P. and Einstein, E. R. (1968). Isolation and characterization of an active fragment from enzymatic degradation of encephalitogenic protein. *J. Biol. Chem.*, **243**, 6050

3. Adams, C. W. M., Hallpike, J. F. and Bayliss, O. B. (1971). Histochemistry of myelin. XIII. Digestion of basic protein outside acute plaques of multiple sclerosis. *J. Neurochem.*, **18**, 1479

4. Einstein, E. R., Cseytey, J., Dalal, K. B., Adams, C. W. M., Bayliss, O. B. and Hallpike, J. F. (1972). Proteolytic activity and basic protein loss in and around multiple sclerosis plaques. Combined biochemical and histochemical observations. *J. Neurochem.*, **19**, 653

5. Einstein, E. R., Dalal, K. B. and Csejtey, S. (1970). Increased protease activity and changes in basic protein and lipids in multiple sclerosis plaques. *J. Neurol. Sci.*, **11**, 109

6. Govindarajan, K. R., Rauch, H. C., Clausen, J. and Einstein, E. R. (1974). Changes in cathepsins B–1 and D, neutral proteinase and 2', 3' cyclic nucleotide-3'-phosphohydrolase activities in monkey brain with experimental allergic encephalomyelitis. *J. Neurol. Sci.*, **23**, 295

7. Hallpike, J. F. and Adams, C. W. M. (1969). Proteolysis and myelin breakdown: a review of recent histochemical and biochemical studies. *Histochem. J.*, **1**, 559

8. Hallpike, J. F., Adams, C. W. M. and Bayliss, O. B. (1970). Histochemistry of myelin, part 8 (proteolytic activity in and around MS plaques). *Histochem. J.*, **2**, 199

9. Hirsch, H. E. and Parks, M. E. (1979). A thiol proteinase highly elevated in and around the plaques of multiple sclerosis. *J. Neurochem.*, **32**, 505

10. Rauch, H. C., Einstein, E. R. and Cseytey, J. (1973). Enzymatic degradation of myelin

basic protein in central nervous system lesions of monkeys with experimental allergic encephalomyelitis. *Neurobiology*, **3**, 195

11. Riekkinen, P.J., Rinne, U.K., Aristila, A.V. and Frey, V. (1970). Enzymic changes in the white matter of multiple sclerosis brains. In *6th International Congress of Neuropathology*, pp. 490–491. (Paris: Masson)

12. Sato, S., Quarles, R.H. and Brady, R.O. (1982). Susceptibility of the myelin associated glycoprotein and basic protein to a neutral protease in highly purified myelin from human and rat brain. *J. Neurochem.*, **39**, 97

13. Smith, M.E. (1979). Neutral protease activity in lymphocytes of Lewis rats with acute experimental allergic encephalomyelitis. *Neurochem. Res.*, **4**, 689

14. Smith, M.E. and Amaducci, L. (1982). Observations on the effects of protease inhibitors on the suppression of experimental allergic encephalomyelitis. *Neurochem. Res.*, **7**, 541

15. Wood, J.G., Davison, R.M.C. and Hauser, H. (1974). Effect of proteolytic attack on the structure of myelin membrane. *J. Neurochem.*, **22**, 637

16. Allen, I.V., Glover, G., McKeown, S.R. and McCormick, D. (1979). The cellular origin of lysosomal enzymes in the plaque in multiple sclerosis. Part 2 (A histochemical study with combined demonstration of myelin and acid phosphatase). *Neuropathol. Appl. Neurobiol.*, **5**, 197

17. Alsopp, G., Roters, S. and Turk, J.L. (1980). Characterization of infiltrating cells in the central nervous system of experimental allergic encephalomyelitis in the guinea pig. In Davison, A.N. and Cuzner, M.L. (eds.). *The suppression of experimental allergic encephalomyelitis and multiple sclerosis*, pp. 31–43. (London: Academic Press)

18. Cammer, W., Bloom. B.R., Norton, W.T. and Gordon, S. (1978). Degradation of basic protein in myelin by neutral proteases secreted by stimulated macrophages: a possible mechanism of inflammatory demyelination. *Proc. Natl. Acad. Sci., USA*, **75**, 1554

19. Cuzner, M.L., McDonald, W.I., Rudge, P., Smith, M., Borshell, N. and Davison, A.N. (1975). Leucocyte proteinase activity and acute multiple sclerosis. *J. Neurol. Sci.*, **26**, 107

20. Lampert, P.W. and Carpenter, S. (1965). Electron microscope studies on the vascular permeability and the mechanism of demyelination in EAE. *J. Neuropathol. Exp. Neurol.*, **24**, 11

21. Lampert, P. (1967). Electron microscopic studies on ordinary and hyperacute experimental allergic encephalomyelitis. *Acta Neuropathol.*, **9**, 99

22. Rastogi, S.C. and Clausen, J. (1980). Loss of lysosomal neutral proteinase from leucocytes induced by the action of multiple sclerosis specific brain antigens. *Clin. Exp. Immunol.*, **42**, 50

23. Rastogi, S.C., Clausen, J., Offner, H., Konat, Gi. and Fog, T. (1979). Partial purification of multiple sclerosis specific brain antigens. *Acta Neurol. Scand.*, **59**, 281

24. Rastogi, S.C. and Clausen, J. (1980). A simple method for the isolation of multiple sclerosis specific brain antigens. *Clin. Chim. Acta*, **101**, 85

25. Cuzner, M.L., Davison, A.N. and Rudge, P. (1978). Proteolytic enzyme activity of blood leucocytes and cerebrospinal fluid in multiple sclerosis. *Ann. Neurol.*, **4**, 337

26. Reinherz, E.L., Weiner, H.L., Hauser, S.L., Cohen, J.A., Distaso, J.A. and Schlossman, S.F. (1980). Loss of suppressor T cells in active multiple sclerosis. *N. Engl. J. Med.*, **303**, 125

27. Amaducci, L., Massacesi, L. and Guarnieri, B.M. (1982). Proteases, protease inhibitors and immune-mediated diseases of the nervous system. *Acts of the first International Congress on Neuroimmunology*, Stresa, 27th September–1st October (in press).

28. Janoff, A. (1972). Neutrophil proteases in inflammation. *Ann. Rev. Med.*, **23**, 177

29. Starkey, P.M. (1977). Elastase and cathepsin G; the serine proteinases of human neutrophil leucocytes and spleen. In Barret, A. (ed.). *Proteases in mammalian cells tissues*, p. 57. (Amsterdam: Elsevier, North Holland)

30. Ragsdale, C.G. and Arend, W.P. (1979). Neutral protease secretion by human monocytes. *J. Exp. Med.*, **149**, 954

31. Messner, R.P. and Jelinek, J. (1970). Receptors for human γG.globulin on human neutrophils. *J. Clin. Invest.*, **49**, 2165

32. Quie, P.G., Messner, R.P. and Williams, R.C. Jr. (1968). Phagocytosis in subacute bacterial endocarditis: localization of the primary opsonic site to Fc fragment. *J. Exp. Med.*, **128**, 553

33. Boyum, A. (1964). Separation of white blood cells. *Nature*, **204**, 793
34. Boyum, A. (1968). Isolation of leucocytes from human blood. Further observation. *Scand. J. Clin. Lab. Invest.*, **21**, (suppl.) 31
35. Lowry, O. H., Rosebrough, N. J., Farr, A. L. and Randall, R. J. (1951). Protein measurement with the folin phenol reagent. *J. Biol. Chem.*, **193**, 265
36. Weigle, W. O. (1981). Analysis of autoimmunity through experimental models of thyroiditis and allergic encephalomyelitis. *Adv. Immunol.*, **30**, 159
37. Day, E. D., Varitek, V. A., Fujinami, R. S. and Paterson, P. Y. (1978). MBP-SF, a prominent serum factor in suckling Lewis rats that additively inhibits the primary binding of myelin basic protein (MBP) to syngenic anti-MBP antibodies. *Immunochemistry*, **15**, 1
38. Day, E. D., Varitek, V. A. and Paterson, P. Y. (1978). Myelin basic protein serum factors (MBP-SF) in adult Lewis rats: a method for detection and evidence that MBP-SF influence the appearance of antibody to MBP in animals developing experimental allergic encephalomyelitis, *Immunochemistry*, **15**, 437
39. Paterson, P. Y., Fujinami, R. S., Day, E. D., Varitek, V. A., Pescovitz, M. D., Kelly, J. and Lorand, L. (1977). Immunologic determinants of experimental neurologic autoimmune disease and approaches to the multiple sclerosis problem. *Trans. Am. Clin. Climat. Assoc.*, **89**, 109
40. Fujinami, R. S., Paterson, P. Y., Day, E. D. and Varitek, V. A. (1978). Myelin basic protein factor (MBP-SF): an endogenous neuroantigen influencing development of experimental allergic encephalomyelitis in Lewis rats. *J. Exp. Med.*, **148**, 1716
41. Paterson, P. Y., Day, E. D., Whitacre, C. C., Berenberg, R. A. and Harter, D. H. (1981). Endogenous myelin basic protein-serum factors (MBP-SF$_s$) and anti-MBP antibodies in humans. Occurrence in sera in clinically well subjects and patients with multiple sclerosis. *J. Neurol. Sci.*, **52**, 37

20
Acid phosphatase activity of cerebrospinal fluid cells in multiple sclerosis and related neurological disorders

J. DE REUCK, W. DE COSTER and H. VANDER EECKEN

ABSTRACT

Cerebrospinal fluid cells, obtained from 140 lumbar punctures and stained, after centrifugation, for demonstration of acid phosphatase activity, are compared in various neurological disorders. In multiple sclerosis, Guillain–Barré syndrome and subacute sclerosing panencephalitis the enzyme activity is absent or discreté. In cases of recent leptomeningeal haemorrhage and bacterial meningitis mono-histiocytic cells, and to a lesser degree granulocytes, show a strong acid phosphatase staining.

The histochemical demonstration of acid phosphatase activity appears not useful in the diagnosis of inflammatory demyelinating disorders, but the increased activity reflects a severe blood–brain barrier destruction in various neurological diseases.

INTRODUCTION

In multiple sclerosis it has been postulated that the release of lysosomal enzyme activity is responsible for the initial attack on the myelin sheath. In the active demyelinating plaque an increase is found in a wide spectrum of lysosomal hydrolases, while in established chronic lesions the largest increase is in the activity of acid phosphatase[1]. Elevated values of lysozyme are also found in the cerebrospinal fluid of patients with multiple sclerosis[2]. The histochemical demonstration of acid phosphatase activity is now widely used as an approach to show the lysosomal character of hydrolytic enzymes in cells[3]. In cerebrospinal fluid cells an increased activity of lysosomal enzymes is thought to be characteristic of mono-histiocytic proliferation[4,5].

The purpose of the present study is to analyse if an increased acid phosphatase activity can be demonstrated in cerebrospinal fluid cells of patients, suffering from multiple sclerosis and related neurological diseases, and if this method can be a useful diagnostic tool.

MATERIAL AND METHODS

Cerebrospinal fluid cells were obtained from 140 lumbar punctures. A Shandon cytocentrifuge was used at a rotation speed of 800 rpm and 2 microscope slides of each 2 ml fluid were obtained. One slide was stained by the May–Grünwald–Giemsa method[6] and the other by the Gömori method[7] for demonstration of acid phosphatase.

The results of 11 samples of patients with proven multiple sclerosis, six with Guillain–Barré syndrome and two with subacute sclerosing panencephalitis were compared with those found in toxic and metabolic encephalopathies (13), in cerebral infarcts (37), in bacterial and viral meningitis (36), in leptomeningeal haemorrhage (21) and after a traumatic tap (13). The criteria for recognition of the cells were those found in the *Atlas of Cerebrospinal Fluid cells* of Kölmer[13].

The graphs presented in this chapter indicate the ratio of the different cells found in the slides used for cytology, and do not represent the real cell-count results.

RESULTS

Only in one sample of patients with multiple sclerosis, is a slight increase of acid phosphatase activity demonstrated in monocytes. Plasma cells are present in more than half of the cases (Table 1).

In Guillain–Barré syndrome, only 2 cases show moderate increased enzyme activity of monocytic cells (Table 2) and in subacute sclerosing panencephalitis there is no staining for acid phosphatase (Table 3). A large number of lytic cells, however, are strongly positive. In the patients with cerebral infarcts, acid phosphatase activity can sometimes be demonstrated, mainly when phagocytosis is present. In cases classified as metabolic or toxic encephalopathies, this enzyme activity can rarely be shown.

In the cases of proven bacterial meningitis, strong acid phosphatase staining is present in monocytes, macrophages and to a lesser degree in granulocytes. The reaction is most positive in the first tap, prior to the antibiotic treatment, and becomes negative within a 2-week period.

In patients with viral meningitis or in those in which the infectious agent cannot be demonstrated, the cerebrospinal fluid cells are not stained for the lysosomal enzymes, except at a later stage, in case of severe brain destruction such as in herpes encephalitis.

All cases of leptomeningeal haemorrhage of more than 3 days of age show very intense acid phosphatase activity, mainly in monocytes and macrophages. After one month, the staining for enzyme activity becomes variable in the residual siderophages. In cases of traumatic tap, the acid phosphatase activity is absent.

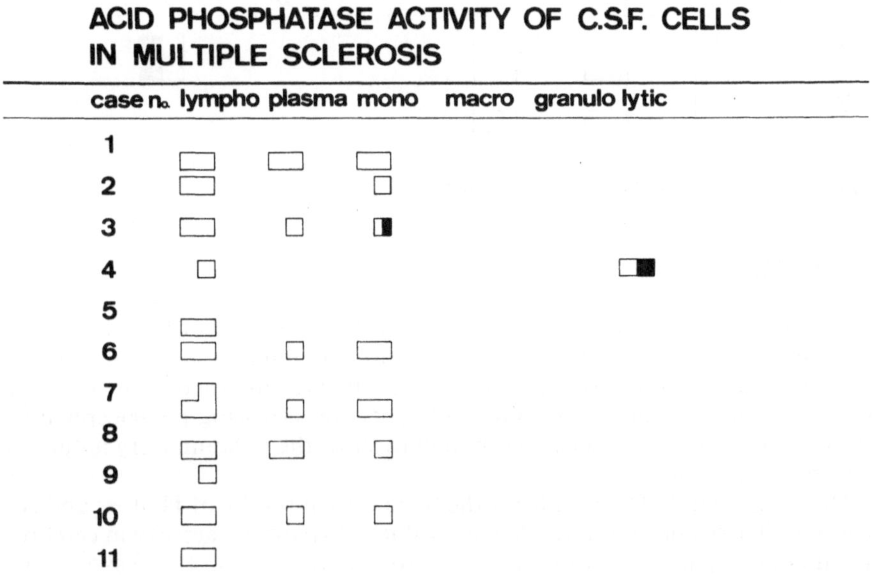

ACID PHOSPHATASE ACTIVITY OF C.S.F. CELLS IN MULTIPLE SCLEROSIS

case n₀	lympho	plasma	mono	macro	granulo	lytic
1						
2						
3						
4						
5						
6						
7						
8						
9						
10						
11						

Figure 1   Only in one sample can acid phosphatase activity be demonstrated in monocytes

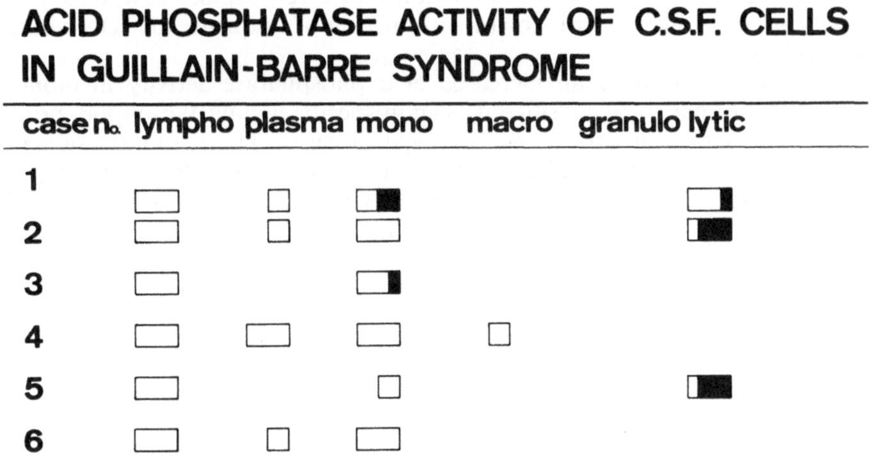

ACID PHOSPHATASE ACTIVITY OF C.S.F. CELLS IN GUILLAIN-BARRE SYNDROME

case n₀	lympho	plasma	mono	macro	granulo	lytic
1						
2						
3						
4						
5						
6						

Figure 2   In the early samples of two patients with Guillain–Barré syndrome, moderate acid phosphatase activity is present in monocytes. Lytic cells have a strong acid phosphatase staining

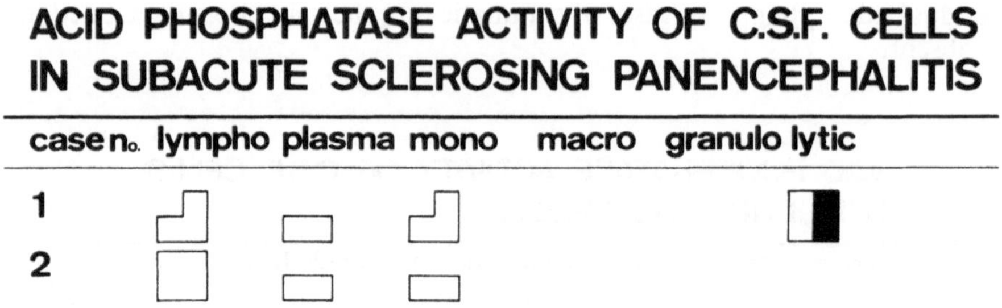

ACID PHOSPHATASE ACTIVITY OF C.S.F. CELLS IN SUBACUTE SCLEROSING PANENCEPHALITIS

case no.	lympho	plasma	mono	macro	granulo lytic
1	⌐	▭	⌐		▮
2	▭	▭	▭		

Figure 3 The acid phosphatase staining is negative

COMMENTS

From this study it appears that the acid phosphatase staining of cerebrospinal fluid cells is not a useful diagnostic method in immunologically induced demyelinating disorders of the central nervous system, such as in multiple sclerosis, Guillain–Barré syndrome, and subacute sclerosing panencephalitis. The method appears not sensitive enough to show the inflammatory nature of this group of diseases.

The present study fully confirms the biochemical results of Hansen and co-workers[2]. These authors show elevated values of lysozyme activity in cerebrospinal fluid of patients with multiple sclerosis and Guillain–Barré syndrome, but also a considerable overlapping between the findings in this group of patients and the normal controls. They also consider the increased cerebrospinal fluid lysozyme values in bacterial meningitis to be mainly due to breakdown of the blood–brain barrier, whereas in the inflammatory demyelinating disorders the increased values of cerebrospinal fluid lysozyme activity are more likely caused by the production of lysozyme, by cells within the meninges.

The demonstration of an increased acid phosphatase activity in mono-histiocytic cells has to be considered as an unspecific hallmark of blood–brain barrier destruction in various neurological diseases. The demonstration of plasma cells can still be considered to be the most specific cytological finding in cerebrospinal fluid of patients with multiple sclerosis[8-12], with Guillain–Barré syndrome[13] and with subacute panencephalitis[14].

References

1. Cuzner, M. L., Davison, A. N. and Thompson, R. H. S. (1981). The demyelinating diseases of the central nervous system. In Davison, A. N. and Thompson, R. H. S. (eds.). *The Molecular Basis of Neuropathology*, pp. 384–411. (London: E. Arnold)
2. Hansen, N. E., Karle, H., Jensen, A. and Block, E. (1977). Lysozyme activity in cerebrospinal fluid. Studies in inflammatory and non-inflammatory CNS disorders. *Acta Neurol. Scand.*, **55**, 418
3. Novikoff, A. (1961). Lysosomes and related particles. In Brachet, J. and Mirsky, A. (eds.). *The Cell. Biochemistry, Physiology, Morphology.* Vol. II, pp. 423–488. (New York: Academic Press)

4. Olisher, R. M. (1971). Der Nachweis der unspezifischen Esterase in Liquorzellen. Eine cytodiagnostische Zusatzuntersuchung. *Z. Neurol.*, **200**, 61
5. Peiffer, J. and Schwarze, E. W. (1971). Beitrag zur Enzymhistochemie der Liquor-und Lepto-meningealzellen. *Nervenartz*, **42**, 267
6. Cardozo, P. L. (1958). Advantages and disadvantages of the May–Grünwald–Giemsa procedure in exfoliative cytology. *Acta Cytol.* (Philad.), **2**, 284
7. Gömori, G. (1950). An improved histochemical technic for acid phosphatase. *Stain Technol.*, **25**, 81
8. Bischoff, A. (1964). Das Vorkommen von Plasmazellen in Liquor cerebrospinalis bei der multiplen Sklerose. *Dtsch. Z. Nervenhk.*, **185**, 606
9. Bammer, H. (1966). Über die Beziehung der Plasmazellen im Liquor zur Activität der multiplen Sklerose. *Verh. Dtsch. Ges. Med.*, **32**, 733
10. Péter, A. (1967). The plasma cells of the cerebrospinal fluid. *J. Neurol. Sci.*, **4**, 227
11. Brucher, J. M., Smidts, W. and Lecuit, J. (1972). L'analyse cytologique du liquide céphalo-rachidien par une méthode de cytocentrifugation. Résultats dans la sclérose en placques. *Acta neurol. Belg.*, **72**, 201
12. Schlote, W. and Roos, W. (1974). Gibt es ein characterisches Liquorzellbild bei der multiplen Sklerose? *Nervenartz*, **45**, 576
13. Kölmer, H. W. (1977). *Atlas of cerebrospinal fluid cells.* 2nd Edn., pp. 1–142. (Berlin: Springer Verlag)
14. Schaltenbrand, G. (1954). Die chronischer Meningitiden. *Dtsch. Z. Nervenhk.*, **171**, 275

21
Influence of human allergic encephalitogenic peptide on platelet aggregation in multiple sclerosis

M. PROSIEGEL and J. NEU

In previous studies we found a significantly increased ADP-and serotonin-induced platelet aggregation (PA) in multiple sclerosis (MS) patients compared with clinically healthy controls[1,2].

Meanwhile we could confirm these results in a greater number of MS patients compared with a control group of patients with other neurological diseases (OND). Again the MS patients showed a highly significantly increased serotonin-induced PA and a less marked increased ADP-induced PA. Neither the results of our own investigations nor of any previous studies provided a conclusive answer to the question whether the platelet alterations are epiphenomena or pathogenetically relevant phenomena of MS.

Consequently we studied the influence of human allergic encephalitogenic peptide (EP) on PA in 20 MS patients and 20 healthy controls. The following is a report on our methods and findings. The MS cases were classified as acute, progressive or in remission. EP was obtained from Interchem, Munich, FRG. Immediately after venipuncture $30 \mu g$ of the peptide were added to 1 ml of citrate blood and incubated for 25 minutes at room temperature. After centrifugation $100 \mu l$ of the supernatant serum were removed and added to $900 \mu l$ of citrated platelet-rich plasma (PRP) of the same patient. Immediately following this procedure PA was measured using the photometric method of Born and O'Brien as modified by Breddin *et al* (see reference 2). The results are shown in Table 1. In six patients the addition of the serum to PRP resulted in an irreversible PA (Figure 1). In 13 patients the addition of the serum to PRP was not able to *induce* a PA, but to *enhance* an ADP-induced PA. In Figure 2 you can see, on the left side, the PA curve induced by ADP alone; the right curve is from the same patient, but was induced by ADP combined with the serum. Compared with curve I PA in curve II is considerably increased (note the deep 2nd aggregation wave as well as the smaller amount of the disaggregation wave).

Table 1 Platelet aggregation (PA)-inducing activity in the serum of MS patients and normal controls after addition of human allergic encephalitogenic peptide to their blood

	Spontaneous PA induced by addition of the serum	ADP-induced PA enhanced by addition of the serum	ADP-induced PA unaltered by addition of the serum
No of MS patients			
(n = 20)	6	13	1
acute (n = 8)	5	3	0
progressive (n = 5)	1	4	0
in remission (n = 7)	0	6	1
No of controls (n = 20)	0	0	20

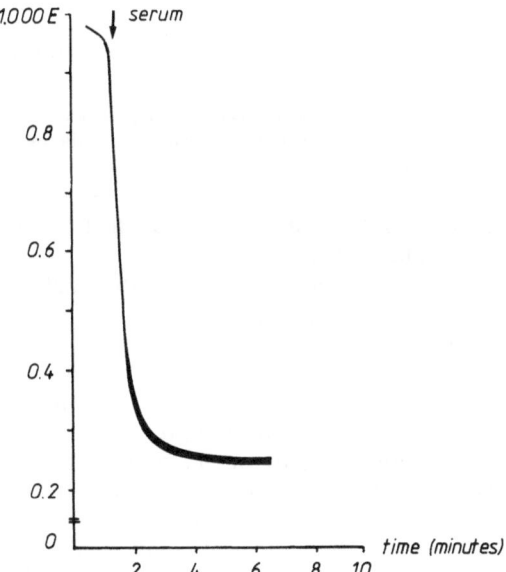

Figure 1 Irreversible platelet aggregation induced by the serum

In one patient and in all controls addition of the serum to PRP did not induce a PA, nor was there any difference between PA induced by ADP alone and PA induced by ADP combined with the serum.

Our results indicate that after the addition of EP to the blood of MS patients a factor X with PA-inducing activity can be demonstrated in the supernatant serum. This factor X is able to induce a PA by itself or to enhance an ADP-induced PA.

In order to exclude the possibility that factor X was released by the platelets themselves after their stimulation with the EP, we added 30 μg of EP to 1 ml of

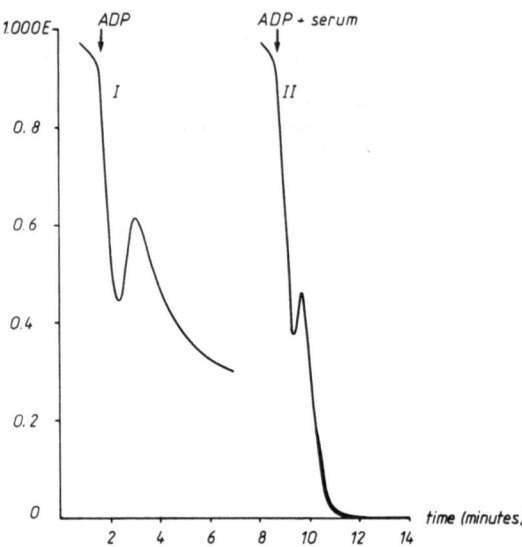

Figure 2 Curve 1: platelet aggregation induced by ADP. Curve II: same patient; platelet aggregation induced by ADP combined with the serum (note the amount of disaggregation being smaller than in curve I).

PRP in all patients and controls; in no case was the EP able to induce a PA or to enhance an ADP-induced PA.

We assume, therefore, that the platelet-activating factor X in the serum was released by the white or red peripheral blood cells of MS patients during their reaction with the EP.

Our results suggest an explanation for the well known fact that thromboses and platelet aggregates occur in the small veins situated at the centre of MS plaques. Our hypothesis is, that platelet aggregates lead to vascular lesions in the cerebral microcirculation, and to an increased vascular permeability in MS patients, thus facilitating the passage of lymphocytes through the vessel walls.

Further studies with a large number of MS patients and a control group of patients with OND and with the basic protein of myelin as antigen are planned to determine the specificity and the possible pathogenetical relevance of the reported findings. In our opinion the interaction between platelets and lymphocytes in MS should be investigated in more depth in future.

References

1. Prosiegel, M., Neu, J., Pfaffenrath, V. and Nahme, M. (1980). Thrombocytenaggregation und Multiple Sklerose. *Narvenarzt,* **53,** 227–230
2. Neu, J., Prosiegel, M. and and Pfaffenrath, V. (1982). Platelet aggregation and multiple sclerosis. *Acta. Nerv. Scand.,* **66,** 497–504.

22
The effect of dietary supplementation of enriched marine oil on serum levels of ω-3 and ω-6 polyunsaturated fatty acids in multiple sclerosis

M. ROSNOWSKA and W. CENDROWSKI

ABSTRACT

The serum fatty acid composition has been investigated in seven patients with slowly progressive multiple sclerosis and in five control individuals. The serum level of tymnodonic (C 20:5 ω-3) and clupadonic acid (C 22:6 ω-3) has been shown to be normal in multiple sclerosis patients. Before diet supplementation with Maxepa there was significant decrease of linolenic (C 18:3) and eicosanoic (C 20:1) acids, as well as an increase of palmitic acid (C 16:0) in sera of MS patients. The variation in the serum fatty acid pattern in MS patients after 1 week diet supplementation with Maxepa has been measured for the first time. There was significant increase in serum clupadonic, tymnodonic and arachidonic acid (C 20:4 ω-6) in MS patients who have been given Maxepa. Linolenic (C 18:3) and eicosanoic (C 20:1) acids remained not supplemented and palmitic acid (C 16:0) was still increased. It has been suggested that the diet supplementation in slowly progressive multiple sclerosis should consist of both ω-3 and ω-6 polyunsaturated fatty acids.

INTRODUCTION

α-Linolenic, clupadonic and tymnodonic acids are polyunsaturated fatty acids that are important components of cerebral grey and white matter as well as retinal lipids. They belong to ω-3 fatty acid series and can not be converted from the ω-6 fatty acid family[1]. In multiple sclerosis (MS) the content of tymnodonic (EPA) in ethanolamine and choline glycerophosphatides from cerebral grey matter was reduced, Gerstl et al[2], Clausen[3] and Andreoli et al[4] found a slight decrease of clupadonic acid (DHA) in plasma lysolecithin of MS patients. More recently Cho, Parker and Utermohlen[5] confirmed that patients with severe MS have lowered proportions of clupadonic and other ω-6 fatty acids in the platelets and serum. Possible deficiency of EPA and DHA in the brain and serum of MS patients may have important biochemical and immunopathological implications[6,7]. Moreover, there were inspiring suggestions that cod-liver oil containing EPA and DHA can improve therapeutic effectiveness of diet supplementation with vegetable oils[8,9]. It was thought reasonable to carry out the trial of diet supplementation in MS patients with enriched marine oil (Maxepa) which is a readily abundant source of C20: 5ω-3 and C22:6 ω-3 fatty acids. The object of the present study was to observe, in MS, the effect on serum ω-3 and ω-6 polyunsaturated fatty acids of enriched marine oil.

CLINICAL MATERIAL and METHOD

Patients and controls

Seven patients with clinically definite, slowly progressive MS were included in the study. The diagnosis was made according to the criteria set forth by Rose *et al*[10]. There were six women and one man aged from 42 to 74 years with the duration of the disease ranging from 7 to 29 years. All patients were severely disabled and the mean grade of disability was seven in Kurtzke's scale[11]. Five controls, aged 40–70 years, who have been without or who show only slight brain damage signs, were also included in the study (two with epilepsy, two with sciatica and one with slight brain ischaemia).

Diet supplementation

10 ml of enriched marine oil (Maxepa, mostly from cod-liver, specially refined and processed by British Cod-Liver Oils, Hull, UK) were given to MS patients three times daily with meals for 1 week. Daily dose of Maxepa contained 2.7 g of EPA and 3.3 g of DHA. The enriched marine oil (Maxepa) was analysed by gas–liquid chromatography for fatty acids composition before use. The results of analysis are shown in Table 1 and Figure 1.

Table 1 Fatty acid composition (% of methyl esters) of the enriched marine oil (Maxepax) fed to multiple sclerosis subjects

Notation	Fatty acids	%	Remarks on levels
C14:0	Myristic acid	6.89	
C16:0	Palmitic acid	15.30	relatively high
C16:1	Palmito-oleic acid	8.02	
C18:0	Stearic acid	4.09	
C18:1	Oleic acid	14.84	relatively high
C18:2	Linoleic acid	1.69	low
C18:3 ω-6	γ-Linolenic acid	0.80	very low
C20:1	Eicosanoic acid	2.85	
C20:4	Arachidonic acid	1.18	low
C20:5 ω-3	Eicosapantaenoic acid (EPA)	19.31	very high
C22:6 ω-3	Docosahaenoic acid (DHA)	11.15	high

Total ω-3 fatty acids over 30%, total ω-6 fatty acids over 3%, ω-3/ω-6 ratio 10:1

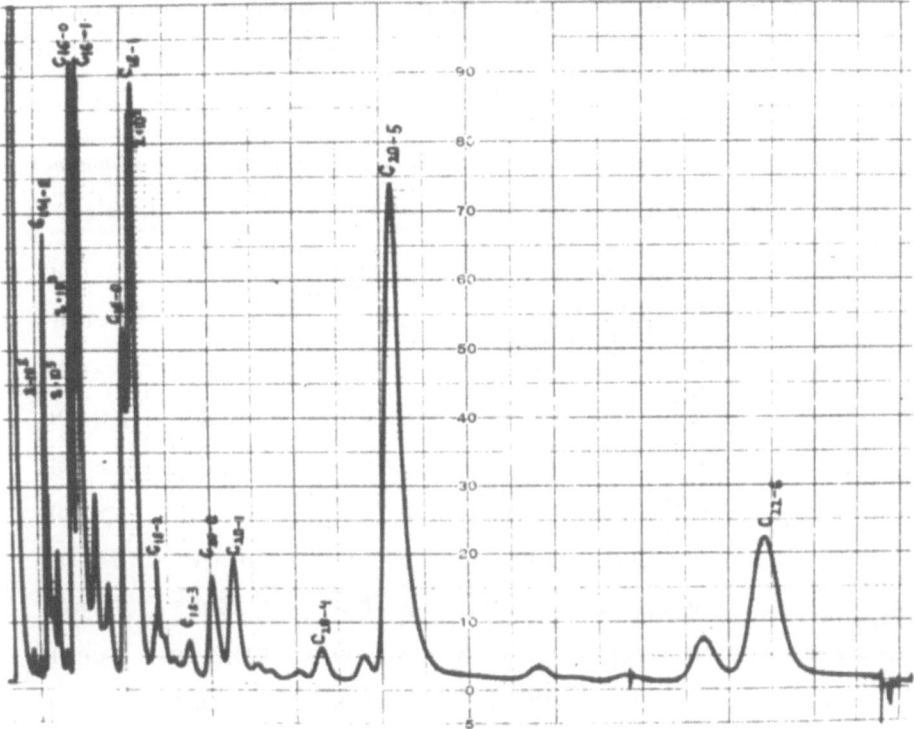

Figure 1 The chromatogram of the enriched marine oil (Maxepa) before use in multiple sclerosis patients. There were relatively high proportions of palmitic acid (C 16:0), oleic acid (C 18:1), tymnodonic acid (C 20:5 ω-3) and clupadonic acid (C 22:6 ω-3).

Fatty acids determination in the sera

Before and after diet supplementation with Maxepa venous blood samples (10 ml) were drawn from seven MS patients who had been fasting from 10 p.m. the previous evening. Venous blood samples were also taken from five fasting controls. Gas–liquid chromatographic analyses of serum fatty acids (FA) were carried out twice, and the mean percentages of FA methyl esters were calculated. The chromatographic procedure was based on the method described previously by Rosnowska et al[12].

RESULTS

Table 2 shows the fatty acid composition of serum in seven MS patients and five control individuals. It is noteworthy that before diet supplementation six out of seven MS patients demonstrated normal levels and the remaining MS patient showed complete absence of EPA and DHA in serum (Figure 2).

This latter abnormality occurred in middle-aged women with advanced,

Table 2 Serum composition of ω-3 and ω-6 fatty acids in seven multiple sclerosis patients before and after 1 week of taking marine oil supplement and in five control individuals

Fatty acids	MS patients before marine oil supplement n = 7	MS patients after marine oil supplement	Statistical significance	Control individuals n = 5	Statistical significance
	A	B	A v. B	C	A v. C
	mean ± SD			mean ± SD	
Myristic C14:0	1.08 ± 0.15	0.95 ± 0.11	$p > 0.01$	0.67 ± 0.19	$p > 0.01$
Palmitic C16:0	24.53 ± 3.01	20.21 ± 1.37	$p > 0.01$	16.60 ± 3.30	$p < 0.01$
Palmito-oleic C16:1	3.57 ± 0.68	3.12 ± 0.49	$p > 0.01$	2.66 ± 0.65	$p > 0.01$
Stearic C18:0	8.27 ± 1.08	8.44 ± 0.97	$p > 0.01$	6.60 ± 0.82	$p > 0.01$
Oleic C18:1	30.5 ± 3.75	23.0 ± 3.66	$p > 0.01$	24.40 ± 3.60	$p > 0.01$
Linoleic C18:2	18.75 ± 3.07	14.12 ± 2.36	$p > 0.01$	14.70 ± 1.60	$p > 0.01$
Linolenic C18:3	0.44 ± 0.12	0.45 ± 0.13	$p > 0.01$	2.0 ± 0.80	$p < 0.01$
Arachidic C20:0	0.27 ± 0.06	0.25 ± 0.08	$p > 0.01$	0.15 ± 0.05	$p > 0.01$
Eicosanoic C20:1	0.54 ± 0.10	0.45 ± 0.06	$p > 0.01$	3.40 ± 1.80	$p < 0.01$
Eicosadienoic C20:2	0.46 ± 0.08	0.27 ± 0.09	$p > 0.01$	0.30 ± 0.07	$p > 0.01$
Eicosatrienoic C20:3	1.35 ± 0.12	0.79 ± 0.17	$p < 0.01$	1.36 ± 0.22	$p > 0.01$
Arachidonic C20:4	4.46 ± 1.02	8.70 ± 0.40	$p < 0.01$	6.35 ± 1.00	$p > 0.01$
Eicosapentaenoic C20:5	0.64 ± 0.11	10.73 ± 1.70	$p < 0.01$	0.58 ± 0.14	$p > 0.01$
Docosahexaenoic C22:6	2.30 ± 1.38	5.05 ± 0.94	$p < 0.01$	1.13 ± 0.27	$p > 0.01$

slowly progressive MS. Before the supplementation with Maxepa there was a significant decrease of linolenic (C 18:3) and eicosanoic (C 20:1) acids, as well as an increase of palmitic acid (C 16:0) in the sera of MS patients ($p < 0.01$). After 1 week of diet enrichment with Maxepa the serum proportion of C 20:5 ω-3, C 22:6 ω-3 acids and arachidonic acid (C 20:4 ω-6) in all MS patients were substantially increased ($p < 0.01$), Figure 3.

However, linolenic (C 18:3) and eicosanoic (C 20:1) acids remained not supplemented, and palmitic acid (C 16:0) was still increased. In all patients Maxepa was well tolerated, but did not change within 1 week any neurological symptoms and signs.

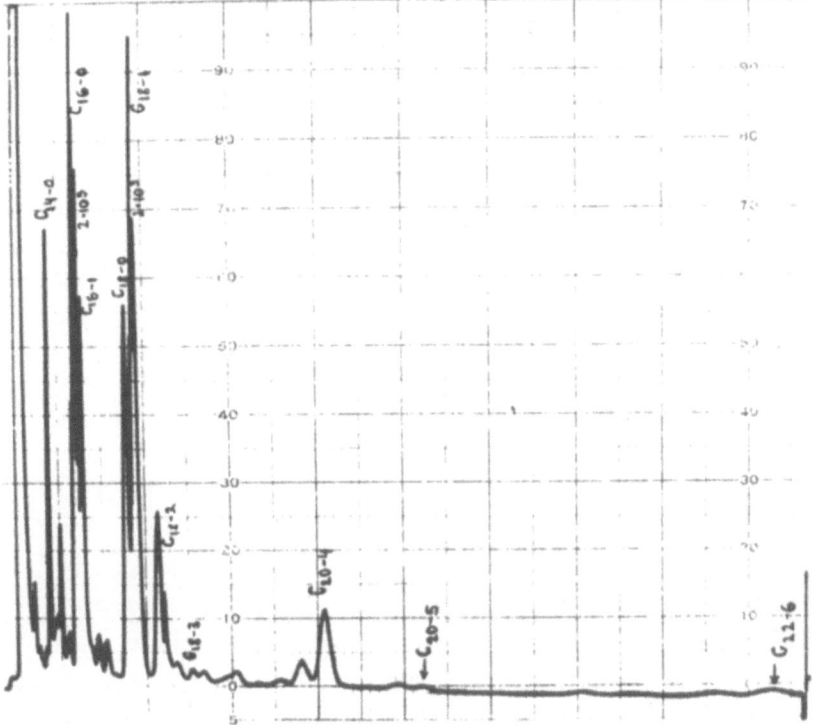

Figure 2 The chromatogram of ω-3 and ω-6 serum fatty acids in MS patients before diet supplementation with marine oil (Maxepa). Note low levels of linolenic acid (C 18:3) and eicosanoic acid (C 20:1) as well as almost complete absence of tymnodonic (C 20:5 ω-3) and clupadonic acid (C 22:6 ω-3) in the serum.

DISCUSSION

The present study demonstrated normally low proportions of ω-3 polyunsaturated fatty acids and significant diminution of some ω-6 polyunsaturated fatty acids in MS patients before the diet supplementation. Low serum level of linoleic acid (C 18:2 ω-6) in severe forms of MS patients was efficiently restored by sunflower seed oil supplement to the diet[12]. Recently Neu, Prosiegel and Autenrieth[13] demonstrated marked deficiency of linoleic and arachidonic acids in the CSF of MS patients. After 1 week of diet supplementation with Maxepa, serum clupadonic and tymnodonic acids were in MS patients surprisingly large, but linolenic and eicosanoic acids remained not supplemented. Similar findings were demonstrated in healthy subjects. Mackerel diet, cod-liver oil or Maxepa provided evident increase in the proportions of free fatty acids (20:5 ω-3 and 22:6 ω-3), in cholesterol esters, phospholipids and triglycerides of plasma[14,15].

The question arises whether ω-3 and ω-6 polyunsaturated fatty acid abnormality has any relevance to multiple sclerosis. The disease is 30 times less

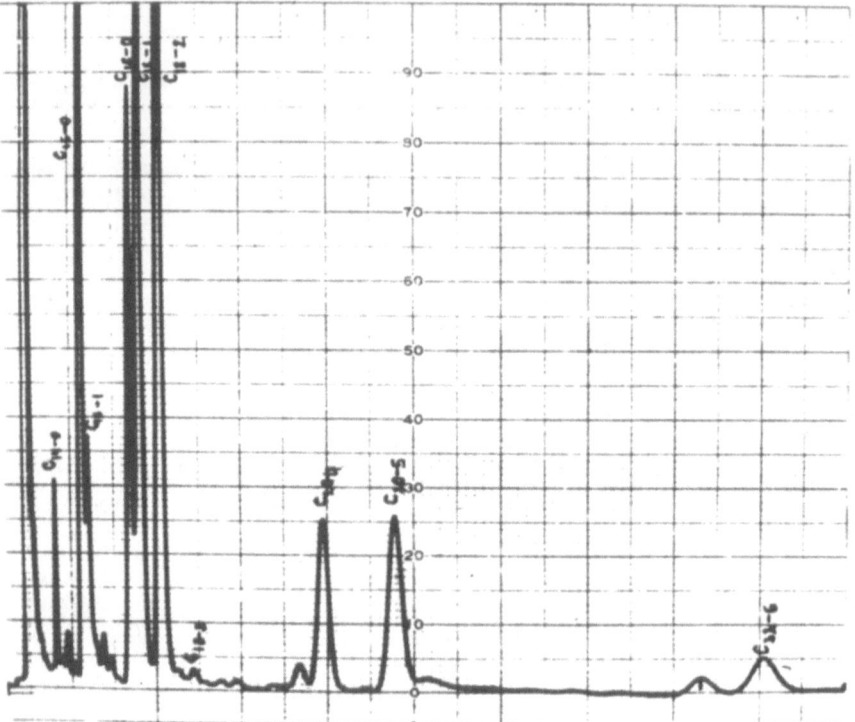

Figure 3 The chromatogram of ω-3 and ω-6 serum fatty acids in MS patients after 1 week diet supplementation with marine oil (Maxepa). There was marked increase in serum arachidonic (C20:4), clupadonic (C22:6 ω-3) and tymnodonic acids (C20:5 ω-3)

prevalent in Greenland Eskimos than in Danes[16]. The natives of Greenland despite the possible lower frequency of DRw2 antigen and perhaps more frequent viral infections before the age of 5 years, show different patterns of serum polyunsaturated fatty acids. They demonstated very high levels of C 20:5 ω-3 in cholesterol esters, phospholipids, triglycerides and as free fatty acid (whereas Danes and possibly Poles showed only traces or very low levels), and reduced levels of C 18:2 ω-6 as well as C 20:4 ω-6 acids[1]. The difference could suggest that a nutritional factor is of importance in multiple sclerosis. However, the exact proportions of EPA and DHA as well as ω-3/ω-6 ratio in the brain white matter and CSF lipids of MS patients taking enriched marine oil is not known. Normal-appearing white matter of MS brains showed substantially less of C 20:1, C 22:4 and C 24:4 fatty acids[17,18]. The significance of the above mentioned findings is not clear. The can either reflect very minute, chemical lesions of myelin sheaths or a local disturbance of the chain-elongation mechanism with acyltransferase specific for C 20 to C 26 fatty acids.

Polyunsaturated fatty acids from ω-3 and ω-6 families exert important immunoregulatory activity, since they suppress experimental allergic encephalomyelitis in guinea-pigs[19]. Yet the therapeutic effectiveness of EPA and DHA in multiple sclerosis is not established[20]. Recently, three independent groups of investigation from Belfast, Newcastle upon Tyne and London are trying to evaluate therapeutic advantages of enriched marine oil in MS patients[20]. However, the supplementation of the diet should be done both with marine and sunflower seed oils, because pure enrichment with large doses of marine oil can produce toxic changes in the myocardium, depletes the body of vitamin E, and does not normalize serum levels of C 18:2, C 18:3 and C 20:1 fatty acids[21]. Budowski[14] suggested that the optimal ratio of ω-6 to ω-3 polyunsaturated fatty acids in the diet is 5:1.

References

1. Dyreberg, J., Bang, H. and Aagaard, O. (1980). Alpha-linolenic acid and eicosapentaenoic acid. *Lancet*, **1**, 199
2. Gerstl, B., Tavaststjerna, M., Eng, L. and Smith, J. (1972). Sphingolipids and their precursors in human brain (normal and MS). *Z. Neurol.*, **202**, 104
3. Clausen, J. (1971). New findings on brain lipids in multiple sclerosis. *Abstracts of III International Meeting of Society Neurochemistry, Budapest* p.15
4. Andreoli, V., Maffei, F., Tonon, G and Zibetti, A. (1973). Significance of plasma lysolecithin in patients with multiple sclerosis: a longitudinal study. *J. Neurol. Neurosurg. Psychiatr.*, **36**, 661
5. Cho, S.-H., Parker, R. and Utermohlen, V. (1982). Platelet arachidonic acid metabolism in multiple sclerosis and healthy control subjects. *Abstracts of MS symposium, Copenhagen* p.11
6. Sinclair, H. (1980). In Field, E. (ed.). *Multiple Sclerosis in Childhood.*, foreword (Springfield: Ch. Thomas)
7. Ericson, K., McNeill, C., Gershwin, E. and Ossmann, J. (1980). Influence of dietary fat concentration and saturation on immune ontogeny in mice, *J. Nutr.*, **110**, 1555
8. Thompson, R. H. (1979). Omega-3 and omega-6 polyunsaturated fatty acids in multiple sclerosis (*personal communication*)
9. Crawford, M. Budowski, P. and Hassam, A. (1979). Dietary management in multiple sclerosis. *Proc. Nutr. Soc.*, **38**, 373
10. Rose, A., Ellison, G., Myers, L. and Tourtellotte, W. (1976). Criteria for the clinical diagnosis of multiple sclerosis. *Neurology*, **26**, 20
11. Kurtzke, J. (1961). On the evaluation of disability in multiple sclerosis. *Neurology*, **11**, 686
12. Rosnowska, M., Cendrowski, W., Piesio, B. and Wieczorkiewicz, M. (1980). Wpływ krótkotrwałego podawania oleju słonecznikowego na poziom kwasów linolowego i arachidnowego oraz lipidów w surowicy krwi chorych ze stwardnieniem rozsianym. *Neurol. Neurochir. Pol.*, **14**, 27
13. Neu, I. Prosiegel, M. and Antenrieth, W. (1983). Essential fatty acids in the serum and CSF of MS patients. *Abstracts of MS Symposium, Brussels*
14. Budowski, P. (1981). Review: Nutritional effects of omega 3-polyunsaturated fatty acids. *Israel J. Med.*, **17**, 223
15. Sanders, T. and Younger, K. (1981). The effect of dietary supplements of omega 3-polyunsaturated fatty acids on the fatty acid composition of platelets and plasma choline phosphoglycerides. *B. J. Nutr.*, **45**, 613
16. Kurtzke, J. (1980). Geographic distribution of multiple sclerosis: an update with special reference to Europe and the Mediterranean region. *Acta Neurol. Scand.*, **62**, 65
17. Göpfert, E., Pytlik, S. and Debuch, H. (1980). 2′-3′-Cyclic nucleotide 3′-phosphohydrolase and lipids of myelin from multiple sclerosis and normal brains. *J. Neurochem.*, **34**, 732
18. Craelius, W., Gurmankin, R., Rosenheck, D. and Schaefer, D. (1981). Free fatty acid patterns in normal and multiple sclerosis white matter. *Acta Neurol. Scand.*, **63**, 197

19. Mertin, J. (1983). Immunological aspects of multiple sclerosis. *Abstracts of MS symposium, Brussels*
20. Cendrowski, W. (1982). Nienasycone kwasy tluszczowe w immunologii i leczeniu stwardnienia rozsianego. *Pol.Tyg.Lek.,* **37,** 225
21. Hornstra, G. (1980). Dietary fats and arterial thrombosis. *Thesis.* Rijksuniversitet. Maastricht.

Section II
Treatment of the Disease

23
Immunological treatments in multiple sclerosis

O. R. HOMMES

It seems to me that, celebrating the 25th anniversary of the Belgian Research Group for Multiple Sclerosis, we are at a critical point in the search for a treatment of multiple sclerosis, and may be also at a critical point in the understanding of the pathogenesis of this disease.

The rationale for an immunological approach to the treatment of MS was discussed yesterday. This approach and its far-reaching consequences seems more convincing than any of the bewildering 120 other therapeutical claims, recently tabulated by the International Federation of MS Societies.

Immunological treatments of MS were started at a time when indications for immunological abnormalities were rather scarce, certainly not as convincing as they are now. At that time, in the mid-1960s, the gap between immunological knowledge of MS and its consequences for clinical treatment was enormous, and most clinicians were not willing to make the jump, especially not after the outcome of the well designed co-operative study in the evaluation of therapy in multiple sclerosis, conducted at that time in the United States. This study stressed the enormous logistic problems in a multicentred trial, and to many people the efforts did not match the outcome. In hindsight however, the methodological spin-off was so great that we should express our highest regards for the careful work that was done there.

At the start of immunological treatments the discussion on what should be the immunological goal of the treatment also commenced: should it suppress the dysregulated immunological activity, or should it enhance it. It can be phrased in another way: is the immunological disturbance a sign of insufficiency or of overactivity of the system. From a comparative point of view the hyperactivity approach was supported by many other human diseases, which were most probably caused by an abnormally active immunological process directed to a tissue or a tissue component, in which a tissue component acted as an antigen. Even at this moment we are not further than that in MS, and some very distinguished workers in this field feel that the immunological activity in MS is not strong enough and should therapeutically be enhanced. However, general immunological knowledge has increased so far that the distinction 'deficient' versus 'overactivity' may be unimportant, as deficiency in one part of the system mostly causes overactivity in another part and *vice versa*.

In this light it may be important to briefly trace what happened in the years since Aimard, Girard and Raveau in 1966 introduced the immunosuppressive treatment of MS with antimitotic drugs[1]. They used cyclophosphamide and later azathioprine in patients with exacerbating remitting type of MS and claimed a good response.

In the following years the Munich group, headed by Frick, studied the effects of various types of immunosuppressive approaches, i.e. anti-lymphocyte globulin, thoracic duct drainage, azathioprine and prednisone, alone or in combinations, in patients with remitting course of the disease. The group from Rennes (Oger, Sabouraud) started a longterm treatment with low doses of azathioprine, as did the group from Würzburg (Mertens and Dommasch). In Melsbroek and Nijmegen, intensive immunosuppressive treatment in the remitting and in the chronic-progressive disease were studied. In 1977, 11 years after the introduction of immunosuppressive treatment, the Melsbroek Symposium tried to summarize the results of these efforts[2]. A great majority of the studies done so far were uncontrolled. And the main problems for all therapeutic research in MS hovered over this symposium, as they did before and continue to do. As it is best to face the enemies I tried to catch them on a slide (Table 1).

Table 1 Main problems for clinical trials of treatment in multiple sclerosis

Cause and pathogenesis
Clinical and laboratory parameters of activity and course of disease
Variability of clinical course; types of clinical course
Non-specific (placebo) response to treatment
Influence of external factors on course of disease

Aimard's group from Lyon reported on their 10 years experience with azathioprine longterm treatment. Gonsette's group and the Nijmegen group reported on 6 years experience with cyclophosphamide. These and other reports indicated a positive response on relapse frequency and speed of deterioration. And a very important issue came up there as Guseo and Jellinger[2a] discussed their pathology findings in immunosuppressed MS patients: a clear reduction of cellular infiltrates in brain tissue and meninges could be demonstrated.

I have listed some data here indicating that of the 45 studies published at that time, details of 560 patients were complete enough to warrant a conclusion: 40% of the patients improved and 25% stabilized for a year or more by these types of treatment (Table 2). The cautious conclusions of the Melsbroek Symposium said that beneficial effects of immunosuppressive treatments were found in uncontrolled studies, and that these studies should continue. A strong need for controlled studies was expressed. The parameters for effectiveness of the treatment and patient selection were discussed. The side effects of the treatment reported at that time did not seem serious and did not block the continuation of the trials (Table 3).

Table 2 Melsbroek symposium on immunosuppressive treatment in multiple sclerosis (1977)

Methods/drugs used so far
Cyclophosphamide
Azathioprine
Myelin basic protein
Cytosine arabinoside
Penicillamine
Anti-lymphocyte globulin
Anti-thymocyte globulin
Chlorambucil

Route of administration
Oral, intravenous, intrathecal

Results
45 Uncontrolled studies: inhibition of progression?
Reduction of frequency and severity of relapses
Details: 520 patients – 40% improved
                   25% stable

Table 3 Melsbroek symposium on immunosuppressive treatment in multiple sclerosis (1977)

Conclusions
Beneficial effects of IS treatments in uncontrolled trials
Uncontrolled trials of IS treatments should continue
Need for controlled trials of IS treatment
Parameters of effectiveness of IS treatment needed
Patient selection: relapsing course
Side-effects not serious

Some very important questions appeared:

(1) When to start a treatment: as early as the diagnosis is suspected, or as the disease is definite and full blown?
(2) How long to continue the low dose treatment, or how frequent to pulse high dose treatment?
(3) Is there anti-mitotic drug dependency?
(4) Is double blind or placebo controlled trial with immunosuppressive drugs possible and justified?
(5) Is immunosuppression really effected and how is it measured?

You see a host of purely clinical problems presented itself to the investigators. And now, 6 years later, these problems are no less, have even increased in size. And the methods of approach have also changed and widened the scope, as plasma exchange, levamisole and interferon trials did, which we can hardly say are immunosuppressive.

In the last few years the results of three controlled trials have been published. Patzold and his colleagues from Hannover studied longterm treatment with azathioprine in all types of MS[3]. Mertin and his colleagues from London studied anti-lymphocyte globulin and azathioprine in the relapsing type of the disease[4]. Hauser and his colleagues from Boston studied the severe progressive type of the disease with high dose intravenous cyclophosphamide

Table 4 Nijmegen workshop on immunosuppressive treatment in multiple sclerosis (1982)

Conclusions
Immunosuppressive treatments probably effective in:
High-dose short; low-dose chronic dosage
Young patients, short duration of disease
Exacerbating–remitting course, chronic–progressive course
Reduction of relapse frequency, inhibition of progression
No serious side-effects reported

Table 5 Nijmegen workshop on immunosuppressive treatment in multiple sclerosis (1982)

Conclusions
Experimental phase not finished
Need for controlled trials
Observation periods 3 years or longer
Re-assessment of patient selection criteria
Side-effects should be carefully studied

combined with ACTH[5]. These studies showed that immunosuppressive treatment was effective on relapse rate and progression rate. Several other controlled studies are in progress or are planned.

In 1982 the Nijmegen Workshop on Immunosuppressive Treatment in Multiple Sclerosis tried to summarize the situation again[6] (Tables 4 and 5). Nearly all the clinicians active in immunosuppressive treatment of MS attended. Immunosuppressive treatment probably is effective as well in its high-dose short course, as in its low-dose chronic dosage. Young patients with a short duration of the disease seemed to improve most. The remitting as well as the chronic progressive course of the disease do respond to this treatment, as demonstrated by reduction of relapse frequency and inhibition of progression. The experimental phase was judged not to be finished. The need for controlled trials was stressed again, although convictions regarding this point sometimes were deeply opposed. General agreement was reached on the point that observation periods should be longer than 3 years, and that patient selection criteria should be reassessed in such a way that by applying strict Schumacher criteria a propitious phase for treatment might be passed over. The problem of side-effects was discussed intensively, but all members of the Workshop agreed that it had not caused serious problems even with the hindsight of more than 10 years experience.

One of the results of this Workshop was the formation of the European Committee on Treatment and Research in Multiple Sclerosis, that will try to co-ordinate European activities in this field. In 1982 in North America the Working Group on Trials of New Drugs in Multiple Sclerosis was formed with the same goals. No doubt the fast developments in the field of immunological treatments in MS have stimulated the organization of these committees, and further work in the immunological treatments will be in the forefront of these committees' interests.

I would like to extend my congratulations to the Belgian Research Group for Multiple Sclerosis with its 25th Anniversary Symposium, the programme for which is an adequate appreciation of the importance of immunological factors in the pathogenesis and treatment of MS. For the president of the group, Dr Richard Gonsette, this Symposium not only will be a great scientific event, but also a great personal satisfaction as he has been one of the pioneers in the field of immunological treatment in MS.

In the coming years some important tasks are waiting for us. I would like to first discuss some more specific aspects that are developing now, then set out to define some wider clinical problems, and finally end with some more general questions regarding MS.

IMMUNOLOGICAL DISORDERS IN MS

One of the most important recent developments is the possibility of typing T-cell populations and their sub-sets with monoclonal antibodies to surface markers of the cells. Studies by Bach and her colleagues[7] from Paris, and Reinherz and colleagues[8] from Boston showed that there is a deficit of suppressor T-cells in active multiple sclerosis. The helper/suppressor ratio for active phases of MS is increased, not only in the relapsing phase, but also in chronic progressive MS as we have shown[9]. This ratio is decreased to normal levels, or even below that, by intensive and chronic immunosuppression[9] by reduction of T-helper and a relative increase of T-suppressor cells, showing that T-helper cells are more susceptible to cyclophosphamide than T-suppressor cells. We were also able to demonstrate in MS brain that cellular cuffs, so characteristic for the early MS lesion, consist predominantly of T-helper cells[10], a fact at the same time demonstrated by Nyland et al[11] who demonstrated an increased helper/suppressor ratio, matching the increased ratio in the blood.

In vitro studies of Oger and Antel[12] on suppressor cell dependent high IgG secretion of B-cells of MS patients, showed a normalization of this secretion under azathioprine treatment. These facts may demonstrate that we could have found markers for the activity of the disease, that are clearly susceptible to immunosuppressive treatment and may indicate the effectivity of this treatment.

A second very interesting development is the relation of prognosis of immunosuppressive treatment to HLA typing. As we demonstrated earlier, DRw2 positive chronic progressive patients tend to have a more favourable response to immunosuppressive treatment than others[13], as they have a more favourable course if untreated[14]. Madigand could also demonstrate this in the remittent type of the disease. We are, therefore, probably faced with the fact that not only age, duration of the disease and type of the disease influences the outcome of the treatment, but also some hereditary factors.

A third important factor, that has shown rapid development but which is still an enigma, is the significance of the intrathecal IgG synthesis. No doubt we have adequate methods now to demonstrate this phenomenon in MS patients. That it has some relation to the immunological process in the brain seems reasonable, but it does not have a clear relation to activity of the disease process.

The problem was placed in a completely different perspective by Nagelkerken from the Central Red Cross Laboratory in Amsterdam, as he demonstrated with anti-idiotype antibodies, that this idiotypic IgG of the spinal fluid is also present in the serum and is produced by circulating lymphocytes and is also produced by some cells in the spleen[15]. It brings attention to the fact that the source of immunological abnormalities in MS may exist outside the brain.

Finally, I would like to draw attention to studies on basic protein in MS. Now that better techniques have become available, more information on basic protein as an antigenic stimulus in MS is needed.

The above mentioned aspects, T-cell typing and helper–suppressor ratio, HLA-typing, IgG and BP studies, together with associated clinical data, may give us more insight into the course and activity of the disease, and in this way may provide useful parameters to monitor the effectivity of the immuno-suppressive treatment. The recent developments of nuclear magnetic resonance (NMR)-scanning in the field of MS, may even make it possible to actually 'see' the effect of the treatment on the lesions. Neurophysiological measurements of latencies of evoked responses may also contribute, in the future, to the measurement of disease activity and progress in the individual patient.

From these specific considerations I would like to go over to more general ones, connected with the execution of clinical trials in MS.

SOME CLINICAL EXPERIMENTAL PROBLEMS

Some possible parameters of disease activity and progression have already been mentioned. They will be of no help to the treatment of the individual patients if they only remain the results of broad statistical considerations. What is really needed, are clinical, immunological, biochemical and neuro-physiological parameters for disease activity and progress in the individual patient. This I think must have priority in all our clinical research on therapy in MS.

Second to this is the careful design of clinical trials. This will be one of the major tasks of the European Committee for Treatment in MS and for the Working Group on Trials of New Drugs. A list of current clinical trials indicates how much work is being done (Table 6). It also shows that large numbers of these trials are now conducted in a well-controlled way. Many of the problems and difficulties in conducting clinical trials are directly related to the establishment of parameters for clinical activity and course of the disease. If these parameters become more reliable, the design of clinical experiments in MS will be much easier.

Another point I would like to bring to your attention is the patient selection criteria. In recent years some evidence has been found that young patients, with a short duration of disease, may react more favourably to immuno-suppressive therapy than others[13]. This brings us to the consideration that maybe the earlier the patient is treated, the better, a point that Frick stressed from the beginning. However, in applying strict Schumacher criteria to the diagnosis of definite MS, we have sometimes to wait for another severe relapse, or for severe chronic progression. Now we could say: we have to wait

Table 6   Current clinical trials on immunological treatment in multiple sclerosis (NMSS-USA)

Drug/Treatment	Number of trials	Control/placebo DB
Immuran	10	8
Cyclophosphamide	7	5
Plasmapheresis	6	3
Lymphocytopheresis	6	0
Interferon	5	3
Total lymphoid irradiation	3	—
Cyclosporin A	2	1
Antilymphocyte serum/globulin	2	—
Thymectomy	2	—
Transfer factor	2	1

Thymosin fraction 15	levamisole
Facteur thymique serique	protease inhibitor
Thymopoietine pentapeptide	corticotrophin
*Poly-unsaturated fatty acid**	4-aminopyridine
*Copolymer I**	
Human immunoglobulin	

*Controlled studies

too long. It would mean that in experimental treatment groups patients should be included with the diagnosis 'possible' MS, or that we should reconsider criteria for 'definite' MS, with the objective of being able to treat, with immunosuppression, the very early stages of the disease. In waiting for several exacerbations to occur, or for several systems to be affected, we may lose precious time to correct the disease in its first stage. Better to reduce Kurtzke 1 to Kurtzke 0, than to reduce Kurtzke 4 to Kurtzke 3. The other end of the Kurtzke Disability Status Scale brings us *ceteris paribus* to comparable considerations. Inclusion of severely disabled patients (DSS 8) in experimental therapeutic groups may completely block all our possibilities of discovering a slight but consistent improvement. Such a slight improvement may be very important if it would continue over many years. Continuing reconsideration of experimental therapeutic design in multiple sclerosis is, therefore, of utmost importance, especially because we cannot afford to waste any medical or clinical resources we have. This brings me to the aspect of public spending and medical involvement in therapeutic trials in MS. It has to be brought to the fore in all possible ways that a treatment for MS may be within our reach; especially at a time in which data reach us that the prevalence of the disease may have increased dramatically in some countries.

SOME GENERAL QUESTIONS ABOUT THE DISEASE

In discussing all these points, we might be on our way to start thinking anew about the disease itself.

(1)   Is it a specific disease entity or some general aspecific reaction of the central nervous system to a variety of causal mechanisms, initially

causing minor inflammatory reactions and minor or imperceptible clinical signs and symptoms, only to start a generalized immunological reaction with demyelination after several silent years?

(2) Is the inflammatory reaction really a focal phenomenon or is it preceded by a general infiltration of the whole CNS with plasma cells, small lymphocytes and monocyte derived microglial macrophages (Tourtelotte: inflamed brain), that shows focal activations over the years, causing clinical disease only then.

(3) Is the course of the manifest disease caused by the same factor over the years or is the initial reaction (inflammatory, immunological demyelination) completely different from a second phase after 4 or 5 years, consisting of axonal degeneration by the lack of oligodendroglial support?

(4) If immunology is deranged shouldn't we study the origin of immunological system: the bone marrow, earlier and more intensely?

(5) As remyelination with oligodendrocytes and Schwann cells is active in the central nervous system after all sorts of demyelination, why is it so scarce in MS, or what blocks sufficient and repeated remyelination in MS? And how could this remyelination be activated and stimulated?

That the Belgian Research Group for Multiple Sclerosis brings us together in this Anniversary Symposium where the immunology of MS is an important subject, demonstrates the active position that Belgian MS Research has in the worldwide fight against this disease. It has complied fully with the original significance of the Greek verb *therapeuoo*, that is: to place yourself at the disposal of the patient; it told the physician to offer his services. Let us, with this *therapeuoo* in mind, continue to offer our services to, and to be at the disposal of, our patients. One of the important aspects of this *therapeuoo* is to look for and study carefully several types of treatment, of which the immunological approach to me seems the most promising to date.

References

1. Aimard, G., Girard, P. F. and Raveau, J. (1966). Sclérose en plaques et processus d'auto-immunisation. Traitement par les anti-mitotiques. *Lyon Médicale*, 345
2. Delmotte, P., Hommes, O. R. and Gonsette, R. E. (1977). *Immunosuppressive treatment in multiple sclerosis*. 224 pp. (Gent: European Press)
2a. Guseo, A. and Jellinger, K. (1975). The significance of perivascular infiltrations in multiple sclerosis. *J. Neurol.*, **211**, 51
3. Patzold, U. and Pocklington, P. (1980). Azathioprine in multiple sclerosis. A 3 years controlled study of its effectiveness. *J. Neurol.*, **223**, 97
4. Mertin, J., Kremer, M., Knight, S. C., Batchelor, J. R., Halliday, A. M., Rudge, P., Healey, M. J. R., Compston, A., Thompson, E. J., Denman, M. and Medawar, P. B. (1982). Double blind controlled trial of immunosuppression in the treatment of multiple sclerosis: final report. *Lancet*, **ii**, 351
5. Hauser, S. L., Dawson, D. M., Lehrich, J. R., Beal, M. F., Kevy, S. V., Propper, R. D., Mills, J. A. and Weiner, H. L. (1983). Intensive immunosuppression in progressive multiple sclerosis. A randomized, three-arm study of high-dose intravenous cyclophosphamide, plasma exchange and ACTH. *N. Engl. J. Med.*, **308**, 173
6. Hommes, O. R., Mertin, J. and Tourtellotte, W. W. (eds.). (1982). Immunosuppression in multiple sclerosis. *Proceedings of the Nijmegen Workshop on Immunosuppressive Treat-*

ment in Multiple Sclerosis, June. Clinical Trials Journal, (supplement) (to be published).

7. Bach, M. A., Phan-Dinh-Tuy., Tournier, E., Chatenoud, L. and Bach, J. F. (1980). Deficit of suppressor T cells in active multiple sclerosis. *Lancet* **ii,** 1221

8. Reinherz, E. L., Weiner, H. L., Hauser, S. L., Cohen, J. A., Distaso, J. and Schlossman, S. F. (1980). Loss of suppressor T-cells in active multiple sclerosis: analysis with monoclonal antibodies. *N. Engl. J. Med.*, **303,** 125

9. Brinkman, C. J. J., Nillesen, W. M. and Hommes, O. R. (1983). T cell subpopulations in blood and cerebrospinal fluid of multiple sclerosis patients: effect of cyclophosphamide. *Clin. Immunol. Immunopath.* (in press)

10. Brinkman, C. J. J., ter Laak, H. J., Hommes, O. R., Poppema, S. and Delmotte, P. (1982). T-lymphocyte subpopulations in multiple sclerosis lesions. *N. Engl. J. Med.*, **307,** 1644

11. Nyland, H., Matre, R., Mørk, S., Bjerke, J. R. and Naess, A. (1982). T-lymphocyte subpopulations in multiple sclerosis lesions. *N. Engl. J. Med.*, **307,** 1643

12. Oger, J. J-F. and Antel, J. P. (1983). Effect of azathioprine on IgG secretion on Con A induced suppressor cells in multiple sclerosis patients. In Hommes, O. R., Mertin, J. and Tourtellotte, W. W. (eds.). *Immunosuppression in multiple sclerosis*. Clinical Trials Journal, symposium (in press)

13. Hommes, O. R., Lamers, K. J. B. and Reekers, P. (1980). Effect of intensive immunosuppression on the course of chronic progressive multiple sclerosis. *J. Neurol.*, **233,** 177

14. Madigand, M., Fauchet, R., Oger, J. and Sabouraud, O. (1981). Sclérose en plaques: corrélation possible entre formes cliniques et groupes HLA. *Nouvelle Presse Médicale*, **10,** 2349

15. Nagelkerken, L. M. and Out, T. A. (1984). *In vitro*-stimulated peripheral blood lymphocytes from MS patients produce idiotypes of oligoclonal CSF IgG (to be published)

24
Multiple sclerosis incidence material data used in the design of clinical trials

O. ANDERSEN

At the present time a number of somewhat divergent clues can be found in the basic sciences on which to base a therapeutic regimen for the treatment of MS[1-3]. Clinical trials have a potential for testing proposed hypotheses, but like other scientific methods, have a number of pitfalls.

One basic quality of a clinical trial to be discussed in this study is its power, that is its capacity to detect a significant difference between control and intervention groups when a real difference exists. If the power is too low – which may happen for instance when patient groups are too small – results tend to be non-significant and there is a risk that efficient regimes will be abandoned.

A clinical trial could rely on clinical or neurophysiological data. In either case it is essential that monitoring of the patients is so complete that febrile and other pseudobouts are differentiated from real exacerbations. Basically, scoring systems have been used to evaluate the course of individual bouts[4] or progress[5]. Relapse rates have been used to measure activity in the remittent phase[6].

The present study concentrates upon relapse rate for the following reasons:

(1) It is a crucial parameter in early stages with the prospect of prolonged latency.
(2) Through well planned combined efforts of patients and investigator it is in many cases possible to monitor the occurrence of a new bout with the time unit of 1 day.
(3) The necessary unbiased longitudinal data on relapses from which many hazard functions can be calculated is available from the Gothenburg incidence material[7], allowing the calculation of power in various planned clinical trials with different patient selection.

Obviously, as high power can be achieved by choosing a highly efficient hypothetical drug, by selecting patients with high event rate, or by working with large patient materials, a salient practical point is the selection of patients with suitable high relapse rates.

Figure 1 shows the relationship between the number of patients, event rate,

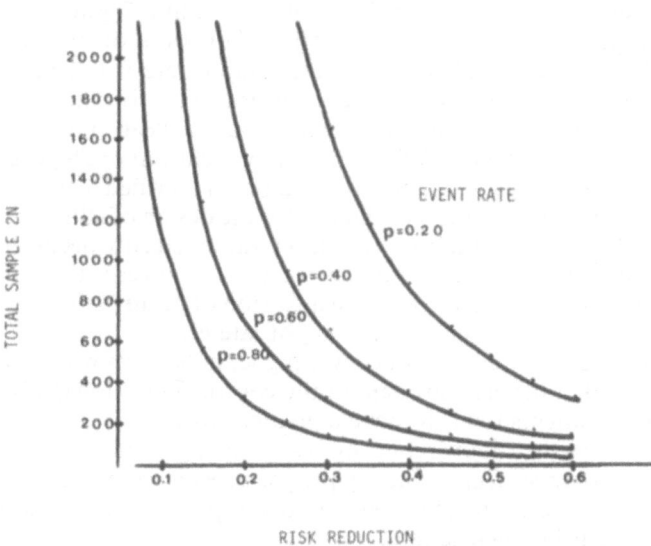

Figure 1 Relationship between event rate (p), total sample size and reduction in event rate in a trial with power 90%. Two-sided 0.05 significance level

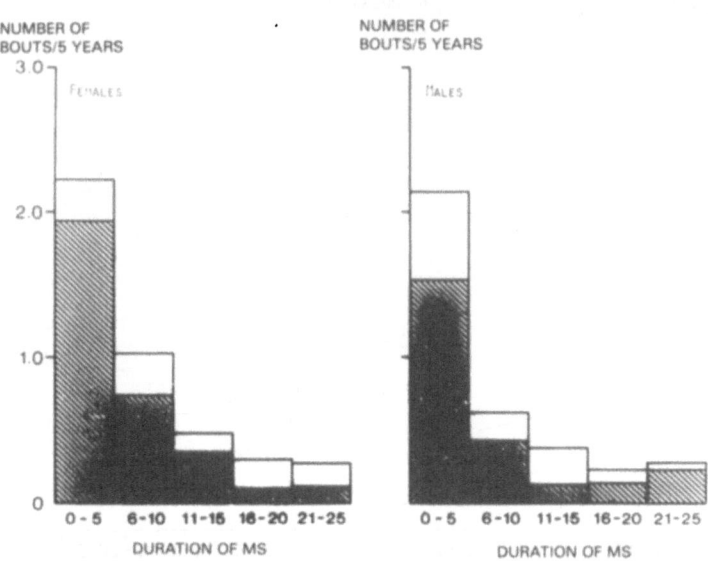

Figure 2 Average number of bouts per 5 year period calculated for all patients with a diagnostic MS probability $\geqslant 3$. Higher values = all kinds of bouts and distinct periods, lower values = distinct bouts only. From Broman, Andersen and Bergmann[7] with permission of the publishers

therapeutic efficiency and power. For instance, if in a 2 year pilot trial only major therapeutic advances, e.g. a 50% reduction of relapse rate, are considered of interest, and the untreated relapse rate is 0.2 per 2 years the number of patients needed to achieve a power of 90% is estimated to be 526.

The Gothenburg MS material[7] includes a 15 year unbiased incidence material with 12–27 years of follow-up. After exclusion of 29 possible cases it consists of 283 probable, clinically definite or verified cases. This paper analyses data from the incidence material for the design of clinical trials in MS.

Figure 2 shows that total bout frequency rather steeply declines. Thus, the planned study tends to be performed with greater power if the monitoring of each patient is not too prolonged. The inclusion of more patients in early bout phase more than compensates censoring of late cases.

Figure 3 reveals that bout frequency is higher in patients with an early onset, a relationship that persists throughout the course. Thus, the study performed in early onset patients tends to have a greater power.

Figure 4 shows that bout frequency is slightly higher if patients are rejected when steady progress occurs. Steady progress seems to inhibit the occurrence of bouts, so censoring in the event of steady progress will tend to increase power in trials using relapse rate.

Figure 5 illustrates the fact that the risk for a new bout decreases with increasing distance from the preceding bout. After about 5 years of freedom from bouts the average relapse rate is reduced to 0.2 per 2 years, which makes

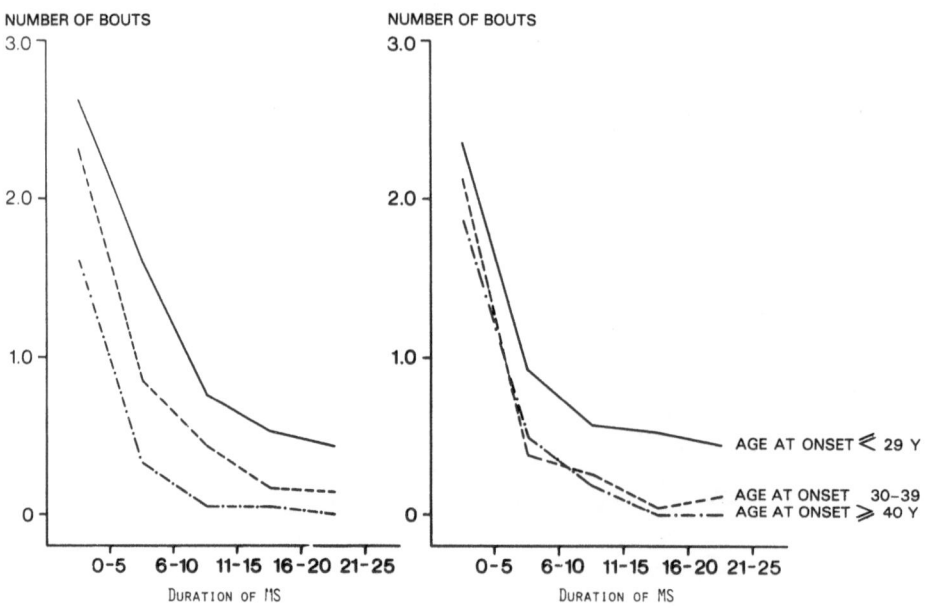

Figure 3 Average number of bouts per 5 year period calculated for each of three age at onset groups. Only the higher values, as used for the patients in Figure 2. From Broman, Andersen and Bergmann[7] with the permission of the publishers

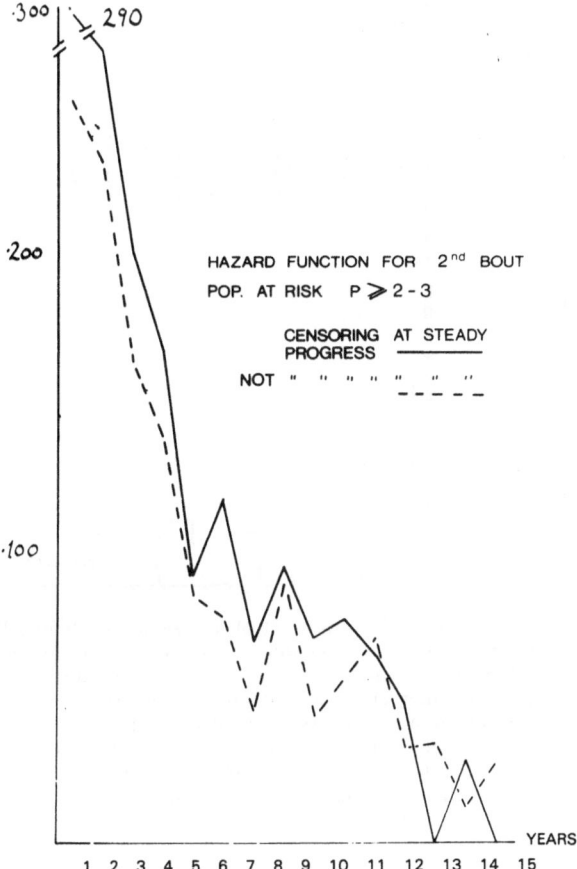

Figure 4 Hazard function for second bout with and without censoring at the occurrence of steady progress, calculated for each of the first 15 years of the disease

large numbers (more than 500 for a moderately efficient agent) necessary if a clinical trial has a preponderance of such patients.

Figures 6–9 show the relationship between the topography of a bout and the risk for a new bout. Risks are slightly higher after optic neuritis than after useless hand and spinal bouts. Given a free choice of patients, the power of a trial might be further increased by the use of topographic criteria.

The purpose of this study was to find optimal criteria of patient selection for clinical trials in multiple sclerosis. Tables 1 and 2 show calculations of relapse rate confined to a 2 year period after a bout.

As bout frequency is declining from onset, the power resulting from the recruitment of patients at the onset bout is of particular interest. Relapse rate for the subsequent 2 years will, according to incidence material data, be approximately 0.4 per 2 years. As may be seen from Figure 1, a considerable

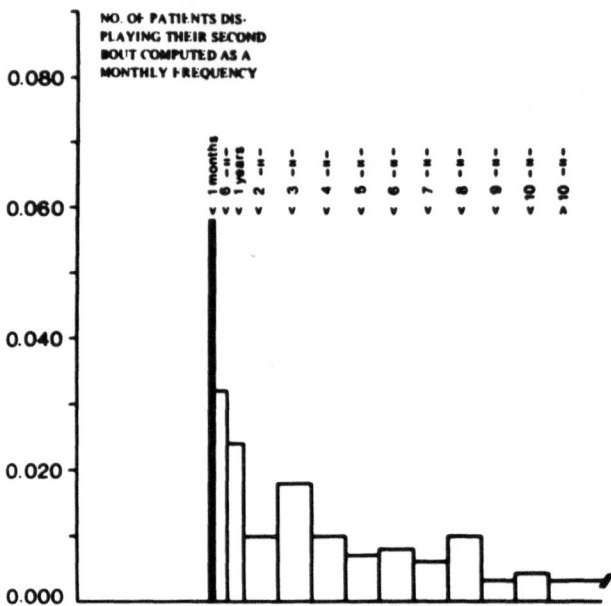

Figure 5 Distribution of time intervals from onset of first significant bout (all topographic categories) to the onset of second significant bout (all topographic categories). First bout occurs at beginning of column designated '<1 month'. The number of patients displaying their second bout is counted in the indicated intervals, i.e.<1 month, 2–5 months, 6–11 months, etc. To compensate for unevenness of intervals, numbers of patients are expressed as monthly frequencies (Figures 4–9) and were computed as hazard functions, see statistical methods[9]. There were 241 patients with a significant first bout and 185 patients with a significant second bout at any time during follow-up. Note the characteristic steeply falling risk after the bout. From Andersen[9], with permission of the publishers

Table 1 Calculations of event rate following three different selection criteria, Polyphasic and migrating bouts are counted as one bout, and bouts type 1, 2, 3, 4 are uses. This classification of bouts was used in a previous publication[9]

	1 year-pairs	2 year-pairs	Onset bout
Number of bout pairs/onset bouts	100	128	193
Relapse within 2 years, number of patients	56	64	79
No relapse within 2 years, number of patients	44	64	114
Number of relapses	100	104	121
2 year event rate (of first relapse)	56%	50%	41%

number of patients is still needed. The power of the study will be further reduced because of loss of patients ultimately not reaching the level of diagnostic probability[7] required in the study. Therefore, more efficient selection criteria were searched for.

If a 'pair' of bouts is defined as two bouts occurring with an interval of less than 1 year, and if only the first 'pair' is counted in each patient, 100 bout 'pairs' are found in the Gothenburg incidence material. With the simple

Table 2 Calculation of power under conditions that in some trials are realistic. Estimations based on four different event rates calculated from incidence data. Fisher's exact test

Event rate	Reduction to	Patient samples	Power
56%	25%	30 + 30	0.60
56%	15%	30 + 30	0.89
50%	20%	30 + 30	0.59
50%	15%	30 + 30	0.77
41%	15%	30 + 30	0.52
41%	10%	30 + 30	0.73
22%	10%	30 + 30	0.13
22%	5%	30 + 30	0.31

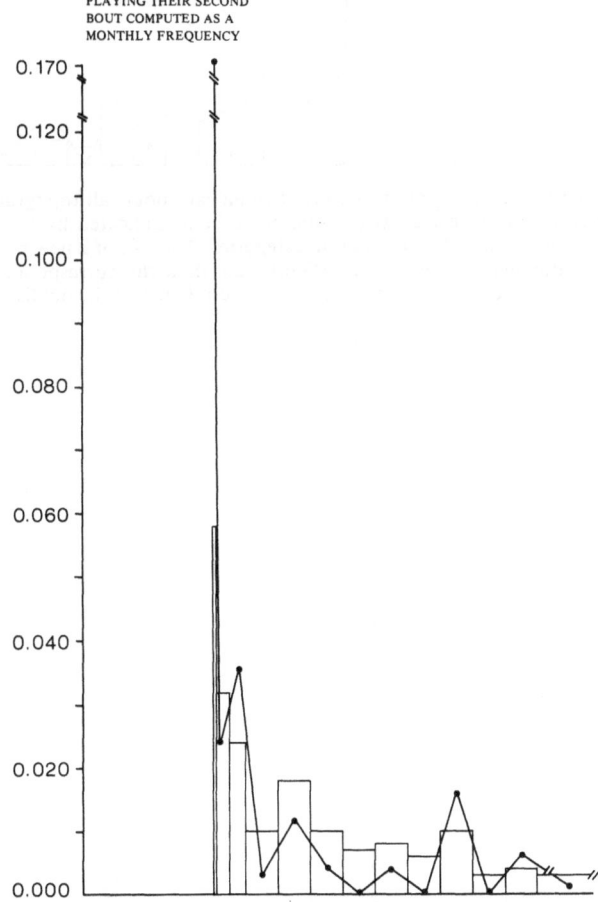

Figure 6 Distribution of time intervals to next significant bout (all topographic categories), $n = 27$, after first significant intracranial optic nerve bout, indicated by •——•. Background: Corresponding distribution for bouts of all categories. The immediate risk of a new bout after an intracranial optic nerve lesion is high. From Andersen[9] with permission of the publishers

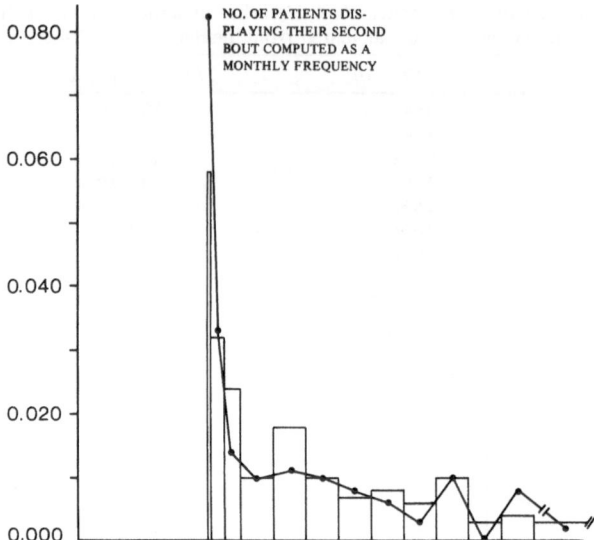

Figure 7 Distribution of time intervals to next significant bout (all topographic categories), $n = 47$, after first significant extracranial optic nerve bout, indicated by •——•. Background: Distribution of intervals after first bout of all categories. The risk of a new bout within a short interval is high, although it seems to be slightly less than the corresponding risk after an unspecified optic nerve bout. From Andersen[9], with permission of the publishers

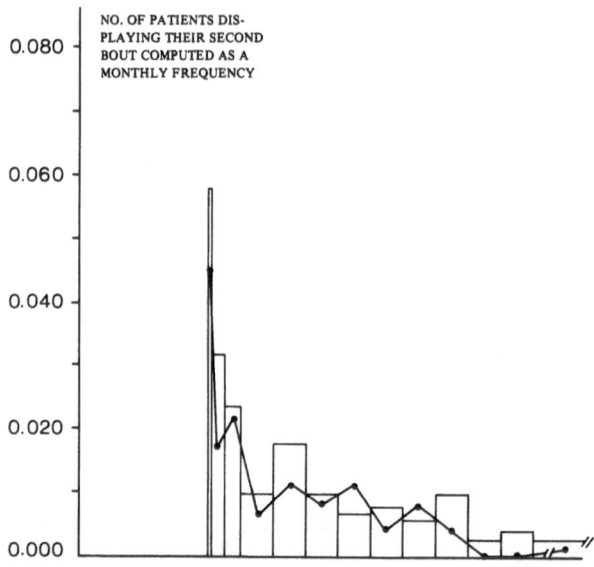

Figure 8 Distribution of time intervals to next significant bout (all topographic categories), $n = 59$, after the first spinal bout (with typical truncal level or sensory dissociation), indicated by •——•. Background, the risk after a bout of any category. From Andersen[9], with permission of the publishers

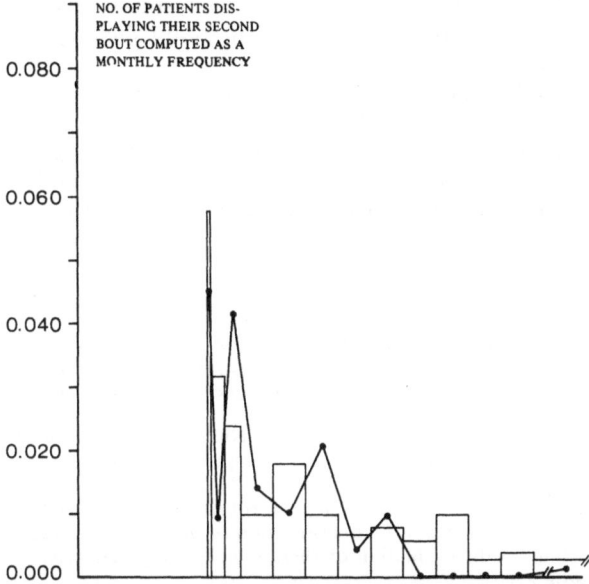

Figure 9 Distribution of time intervals to next significant bout (all topographic categories), $n = 31$, after a useless hand bout, indicated by •——•. Background: The corresponding distribution after a bout of any category. From Andersen[9], with permission of the publishers

entrance criterion a 'pair' the expected relapse rate for the next 2 years is about 56%. If the definition of 'pair' is extended to the occurrence of two bouts within less than 2 years, the expected relapse rate for the subsequent 2 years will be about 50%, somewhat less satisfying for the purpose of clinical trials design.

Table 2 shows with some examples the crucial influence of event rate upon the power of the study. Samples of 30 patients in each of control and intervention groups are considered realistic. At first the event rate of 56% following 1 year-'pairs' is used. Reductions to a relapse rate of 15% following therapy would give a satisfying power of 89% indicating that the design is adequate when moderately or highly efficient therapies are tested. Conversely, if patients with an event rate of 22% are used, a moderate reduction to 10 or 5% will give a catastrophically low power, with the consequence that a therapeutic effect will probably not be detected.

Extreme strictness of criteria tends to cause recruitment problems. The Gothenburg incidence of first 1 year-'pairs' of bouts was 100/380,000/15 years. A combination of basic criteria such as young age onset, censoring when steady progress occurs, and the use of the first year after a bout gives almost as satisfying a power as 'pairs', and patient recruitment for the trial is much faster. Investigators may therefore contemplate the use of two such strata.

It might well be that evoked response or nuclear magnetic resonance data give higher event rates and tend to give higher statistical power than purely clinical event rates. Power calculations on evoked response data are urgently needed. It is not yet known whether evoked response event rate is also a suitable method when increased variability in established MS lesions[8] is taken into consideration.

Although not all clinical trials in multiple sclerosis use relapse rate, the advantage of this parameter is that a number of selection and stratification procedures of patients can be simulated in models using incidence data. Examples show that patients eligible for unicentre trials can be distinguished from patients found unsuitable for such trials by straightforward criteria.

References

1. Raine, C. S., Traugott, U. and Stone, S. H. (1980). Applications of chronic relapsing experimental allergic encephalomyelitis to the study of multiple sclerosis. In Bauer, H. J., Poser, S. and Ritter, G. (eds.) *Progress in Multiple Sclerosis Research* pp. 3–10. (Berlin: Springer)
2. Kristensson, K., Svennerholm, B., Vahlne, A., Nilheden, E., Persson, L. and Lycke, E. (1982). Virus-induced demyelination in herpes simplex virus-infected mice. *J. Neurol. Sci.,* **53,** 205
3. Haase, A. T., Ventura, P., Gibbs, C. J. and Tourtellotte, W. W. (1981). Measles virus nucleotide sequences: Detection by hybridization *in situ. Science,* **212,** 672
4. Cooperative study in the evaluation of therapy in multiple sclerosis. (1970). ACTH vs. placebo. *Neurology,* **20.**
5. Fog, T. (1965). The long-term treatment of multiple sclerosis with corticoids. *Acta Neurol. Scand.* **41,** (Suppl. 13), 473
6. Millar, J. H. D., Zilkha, K. J., Langman, M. J. S., Payling Wright, H., Smith, A. D., Belin, J. and Thompson, R. H. S. (1973). Double-blind trial of linoleate supplementation of the diet in multiple sclerosis. *Br. Med. J.,* **1,** 765
7. Broman, T., Andersen, O. and Bergmann, L. (1981). Clinical studies on multiple sclerosis. I. Presentation of an incidence material from Gothenburg. *Acta Neurol. Scand.,* **63,** 6
8. Cohen, S. N., Syndulko, K., Hansch, E., Tourtellotte W. W. and Potvin, A. R. (1982). Variability on serial testing of visual evoked potentials in patients with multiple sclerosis. *Adv. Neurol.,* **32,** 559
9. Anderson, O. (1980). Restricted dissemination of clinically defined attacks in an MS incidence material. *Acta Neurol. Scand.,* **62,** (Suppl 77)

25
Long term treatment with azathioprine in multiple sclerosis patients

K. LAUER, W. FIRNHABER and D. JOHN

Based upon much clinical and experimental data demonstrating an enhanced immunological response in multiple sclerosis, especially inside the CNS, attempts have been made to influence the disease process by immunosuppressive agents. The substance most frequently used was azathioprine. The results of this treatment were not judged unequivocally. One obvious impression from the literature is that most uncontrolled studies, where only in the treated patients the course under therapy was compared with that before treatment, gave rather impressive results, often in spite of comparatively short periods of treatment. The most frequent finding was a substantial reduction of the relapse rate. In some studies, some effect of azathioprine was also described in chronic progressive cases by demonstrating a comparatively high proportion of cases with a stable course under therapy, but this proportion decreased with the length of follow-up.

On the other hand, many studies using a true control group of untreated patients revealed either no or only a rather slight influence of azathioprine on the disease course. The proportion of positive results in these studies seems to increase with the duration of treatment.

The most important problem is, as discussed previously, to compile a control group matched in sufficient variables to avoid bias caused by different types of the natural disease course in both groups. The epidemiological study which we have performed for 3 years in the southern part of the West German state of Hesse, where all diagnosed cases were also interviewed thoroughly on their disease course including relapses, duration of progressive and stable phases and the development of disablement in daily living, gave us the opportunity to collect a sufficient number of untreated patients.

We investigated the course in 62 MS patients (age $39 \pm 10y$) treated with azathioprine for at least 2 years by a retrospective evaluation of the files of in- and outpatient departments of our own neurological hospital.

The great majority, 54 patients, were classified as 'definite MS' according to the criteria described by Poser and co-workers. Six patients had a probable MS, and two further patients with only 'possible MS' were included. This

119

seemed justified since both had signs for polytopic lesions inside the CNS and an elevated intrathecal IgG synthesis with high-alkaline bands in isoelectric focusing, but they had experienced only one episode after which immuno-suppressive treatment was started.

Forty-six patients had an exclusively intermittent course before therapy, whereas in 16 cases azathioprine treatment was started in a progressive stage. Six of them had a primarily progressive, the remaining 10 patients a second-arily progressive course. The drug was given in a daily oral dosage of 150 mg in the first three months, later on 100 mg per day. Acute relapses were treated with synthetic ACTH or corticosteroids, generally dexamethasone, over 4–6 weeks.

The control group consisted of 59 patients from the epidemiological area. For each treated patient, a control subject of the same sex, age at onset and the same type of clinical course at *that* time after onset at which azathioprine was started in the treated patient, was selected. The group comprised 43 inter-mittent and 16 progressive cases. For 3 treated intermittent cases, no control partner could be found. In both partners respectively, a time-interval corres-ponding to the pretreatment and to the treatment period of the treated partner was followed up. The evaluated parameters were the relapse rate per year, the progression index according to Poser *et al*, defined as the increase of the DSS score (Kurztke) per year, and the proportion of patients developing a second-arily progressive course in the period after onset in which treatment was performed in the treated partner. For the calculation of the relapse rate, the first bout marking clinical onset was omitted, and the degree of progression in the pretreatment period was assessed only to the state before the last bout leading to the initiation of immunosuppression in the intermittent cases.

In the following, the intermittent and the progressive cases are treated separately.

In the patients with an intermittent course, therapy was started on average after almost 6 years duration, whereas the period of treatment lasted 39 months on average, which is a little more than one half of the pretreatment period (Table 1).

If the azathioprine-treated group is regarded as isolated, and the course before, during and (as in 5 cases) after treatment is compared, a very impres-sive and significant reduction of the relapse-rate from 1.0 to 0.48 under treat-ment, and an increase to 1.0 after withdrawal of the agent, is found (Figure 1). The same is true for the progression index which decreased from 0.76 to 0.16 under treatment and increased again to 0.58 after cessation of treatment. These changes are also highly significant.

However, if both parameters in the period of treatment were compared between the azathioprine group and the controls, no significant differences were found (Figure 2). The mean value for the relapse rate was even higher in

Table 1 Intermittent course before therapy ($n = 46$)

Onset age:	12–44 yr	(26 ± 8 yr)
Duration before therapy:	0–456 mon	(69 ± 78 mon)
Duration under therapy:	24–74 mon	(39 ± 15 mon)

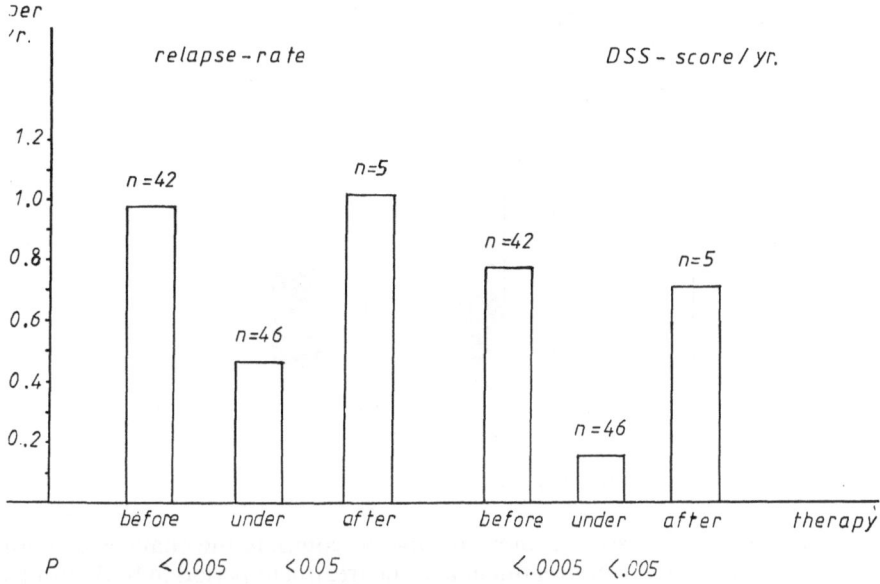

Figure 1   Intermittent course: azathioprine-treated group

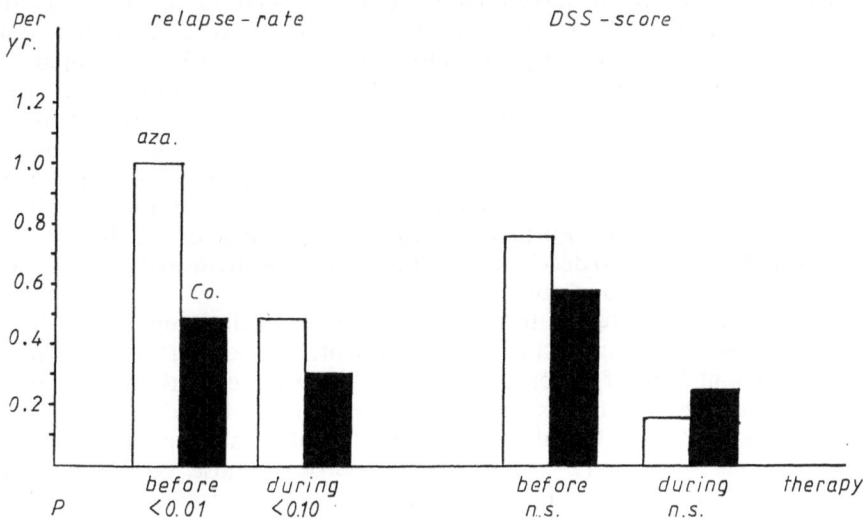

Figure 2   Intermittent course: azathioprine-treated group *vs.* controls

the azathioprine group (0.48 *vs.* 0.32), although not significantly, and the mean progression index was only insignificantly lower in the treated patients (0.16 *vs.* 0.25). However, in the interpretation of these findings, the apparently more active course before therapy in the azathioprine group must be noted, which showed a significantly higher pretreatment relapse rate than the

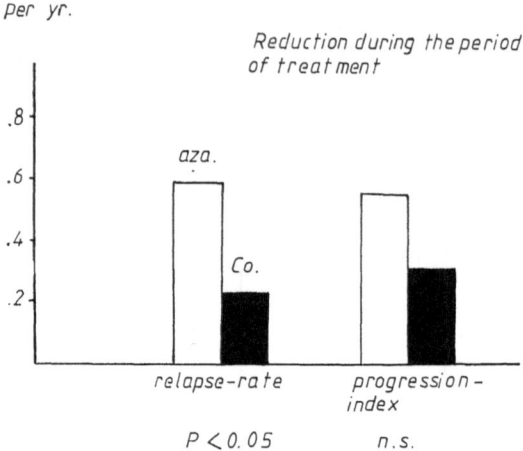

Figure 3 Intermittent course: both groups

controls. Therefore it seemed more reliable to compare the changes of both parameters between the pretreatment and the treatment period in both groups (Figure 3). Then it became apparent that the reduction of the relapse rate under therapy was significantly greater in the azathioprine group than in the control group during a corresponding interval (0.60 *vs.* 0.23; $p<0.05$), whereas the reduction of the progression index was greater but not significantly so in the treated patients (0.57 *vs.* 0.32; $p>0.1$). The apparent discrepancy regarding the therapeutic effect between the uncontrolled and the controlled approach was partially caused by different lengths of the pretreatment and treatment periods. The therapy period is still too short in comparison with the time elapsed before therapy, and the lower proportion of patients with *no* relapse and *no* progression during that shorter period must result in much lower mean values. Furthermore the natural course of the disease has previously been shown to decelerate and the relapse rate to decrease with time. This was confirmed in our study.

Furthermore we evaluated how many patients in both groups respectively experienced *no* relapse in the period of treatment. The percentage was almost identical, about 40%. If the progression index is evaluated in the same way, a higher percentage of patients with no progression was found in the treated group (67% *vs.* 50%). This difference was not statistically significant, but a tendency was obvious ($p<0.1$). The proportion whose course became progressive in the period of treatment was smaller in the azathioprine group, but this difference was, again, not significant, possibly because of the small number of cases (2/46 *vs.* 5/43; $p>0.10$).

Table 2 Progressive course before therapy ($n=16$)

Onset age:	15–48 yr	(34 ± 11 yr)
Duration before therapy:	24–216 mon	(112 ± 51 mon)
Duration under therapy:	24–72 mon	(51 ± 17 mon)

The group of patients with a progressive type at the start of treatment was much smaller and comprised 16 patients only (Table 2). Their age at onset was significantly higher and the treatment as well as the treatment period was much longer than in the intermittent cases. Again the treatment period was about one half of the pretreatment-period (Table 2). To start with, the course before was compared with that during therapy in both groups. Only the progression index was evaluated. As in the intermittent cases, there was a significant reduction of the progression rate in the treated patients, but also in the untreated controls in the same period after onset. The statistical significance was even higher in the controls as the result of a smaller standard deviation (Figure 4).

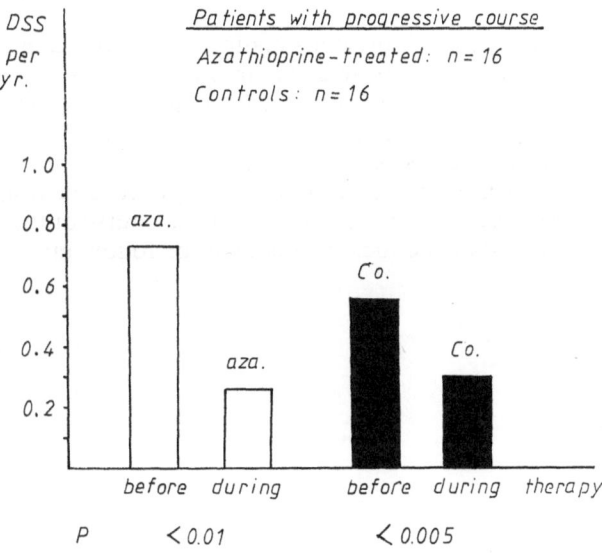

Figure 4 Progressive course: azathioprine–treated group *vs.* controls (progression index)

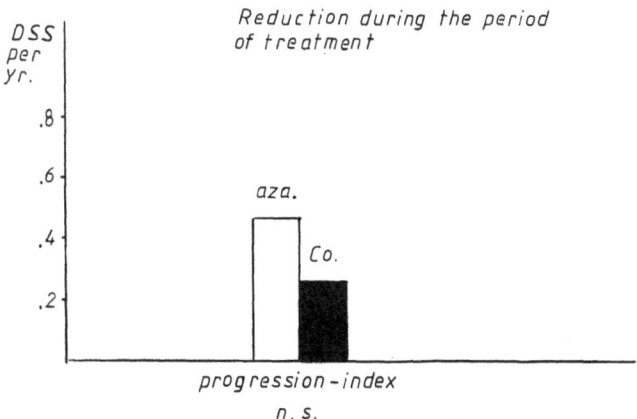

Figure 5 Progressive course: gradient of progression index

123

If, again, the *gradient* of the progression index between pretreatment and treatment periods was compared in both groups, a steeper gradient was found in the azathioprine-treated patients, but no statistical significance was obtained (Figure 5).

The proportion of patients with *no* progression in the treatment period was 3 times as great in the treated group, but the difference was again not significant, probably because of the small figures (6/16 *vs.* 2/16; $p > 0.1$).

Side-effects were comparatively rare and generally slight. No irreversible effects were observed. The most frequent complaints were a stronger tendency towards common colds and nausea. In one case only, a woman with a severe leukopenia, the drug had to be withdrawn.

In summary, our data support previous findings of a significant reduction of the relapse rate in MS patients with an intermittent course, whereas the progression as determined by the Kurtzke scale was not influenced significantly, although a slight tendency towards a milder course was found in both intermittent and progressive cases. Furthermore, it was confirmed rather impressively that only a controlled approach can give reliable results in therapeutic studies in MS as a consequence of the natural course of the disease, and the generally still too short periods of treatment or follow-up.

26
Long-term immunotherapy in MS

E. C. LATERRE, H. HEULLE and C. J. M. SINDIC

Between 1972 and 1982, 42 patients with definite MS, in terms of McAlpine's clinical criteria, and with oligoclonal pattern of IgG in CSF electrophoresis were treated continuously during 36 months either by cyclophosphamide ($n = 22$), azathioprine ($n = 9$), or succession of both drugs ($n = 11$). The doses of cyclophosphamide (mean 75 mg per day) and azathioprine (mean 100 mg per day) were progressively adjusted in each case to obtain a leukocyte count between 3000 and 4000 per mm^3, controlled monthly. Urologic control was performed in cyclophosphamide group. All patients were still ambulant at the beginning of the treatment. The severity of symptoms were graded according to the Kurtzke disability status scale. Twenty patients (mean age: 32.5 ± 2.9) were selected for this trial because of their relapse rate and severity of their residual symptoms uncontrolled by corticosteroid treatment. The 22 other patients (mean age: 48.6 ± 3.1) were in a progressive course at the beginning of treatment. In the first group (remitting progressive form), stabilization or regression of symptoms occurred in 15 patients out of 20. In the second group (progressive form), stabilization occurred in six patients out of 22.

27
Immunosuppression with cyclophosphamide in multiple sclerosis

R. E. GONSETTE, L. DEMONTY, Y. DE SMET and P. DELMOTTE

SUMMARY

Since 1966 cyclophosphamide (Cy) immunosuppression has been used in MS patients.

In the first group of patients, the authors were mainly interested in the possible influence of a single intensive immunosuppression on the annual relapse rate (ARR). When compared to matched non-treated patients, a marked reduction of the ARR was observed in treated cases. However, the beneficial effect was limited in time (2–3 years) and, in the long run, no significant influence on the overall handicap was to be seen.

In the second group of patients, acute Cy immunosuppression was repeated in order to prolong the beneficial effect of the first treatment. Even if the ARR was reduced to some extent, no significant influence on the progressing disability was observed.

In a third group of patients, 'combined' acute and chronic Cy immunosuppression was employed. After a mean follow up period of 4 years, it appears that the reduction of both ARR and progression of the disease is definitely more marked than in patients treated with acute immunosuppression alone.

Combined acute and chronic immunosuppression seems to be the most effective treatment in relapsing–progressive cases with a short evolution, frequent exacerbations, and a likely unfavourable course.

INTRODUCTION

Immunosuppressive therapy in multiple sclerosis (MS) was based at first upon the view that auto-immune mechanisms may be implicated in the pathogenesis of the disease. This notion was supported by a series of indirect arguments including the presence of antibodies (oligoclonal IgG) in the cerebrospinal fluid of the patients, and the experimental demyelinating induced by brain tissue extracts in animals (experimental allergic encephalomyelitis: EAE).

Initially the aim of treatments using cytotoxic drugs in MS was to reduce this hypothetical associated hyperimmunity by suppressing abnormal sensitized lymphocytes which produce adverse immunological events, and particularly the antibody-producing B-cells.

Since then, there is increasing evidence that this effect of cytotoxic drugs on the immune response is due to their influence on lymphocyte function and not simply to cell death, and it has been demonstrated that such responses are subsequently restored when cells are allowed to recover.

When this clinical study was initiated in 1967, the goal was to demonstrate a possible effect of a 'single acute immunosuppression' on the evolution of MS, and particularly on the annual relapse rate (ARR). Therefore, patients frequently relapsing were mostly selected. Immunosuppression was never administered during or immediately (less than 8 weeks) after an exacerbation, and no concomitant corticotherapy was employed.

Cyclophosphamide (Cy) was selected as immunosuppressive agent since, at that time, this cytotoxic drug was used in the treatment of diseases thought to be of auto-immune origin. In the first group of patients, Cy was administered by mouth, as it was assumed to be completely absorbed from the gastro-intestinal tract. It soon became evident, however, that most patients were severely nauseated and that an intravenous (i.v.) intermittent high dose schedule was more tolerable.

MATERIAL AND METHODS

Since 1967, 243 MS cases have been selected from a group of patients hospitalized in the 'Belgian National Centre for Multiple Sclerosis'.

Distribution of the patients according to sex and clinical forms is listed in Table 1.

Table 1 Patient distribution

Number of patients treated:	243
Evaluable cases*:	185
Males:	94
Females:	91
Clinical forms:	
Relapsing–remittent:	46
Relapsing–progressive	139

*Follow-up for 2 years at least

Cy solutions for injection are prepared immediately before use, and dissolved in 500 ml of 5% glucose and water. A first dose of 500 mg Cy is administered i.v. over a 2–3 hour period. In most cases, a transient mild increase in leukocyte count is observed the day after this first infusion. 1–2 g Cy are then infused at 3 or 4 day intervals, in order to produce a lymphopenia under 1000. The lymphopenia (<1000) is maintained for 14 days and when the nadir of the leukopenia is below 2000, the patient is isolated to prevent contact infections.

Individual responses to Cy differ considerably from patient to patient, but a mean dose of 4–6 g is generally effective. Spontaneous recovery of leukocyte depression is usually complete by 21 days after the last infusion of the drug. Cy is relatively platelet sparing and a dramatic depression of the platelet count was seen in only one patient.

Immediate side-effects of Cy were easily controlled. Anti-emetic drugs are given when nausea and vomiting are a significant source of discomfort to patients. Hair loss or complete alopecia occurred quite systematically, but this effect was invariably reversible and rather well accepted by the patients.

Sterile cystitis is prevented by adequate hydration and frequent emptying of the bladder. Haemorrhagic cystitis was observed in two patients, and well controlled by irrigation of the bladder and transfusion to keep up with blood loss. Other severe adverse reactions were never observed.

Because of the wellknown effect of Cy on the gonads, producing azoospermia and amenorrhoea, and the possible teratogenic effect of the drug in pregnant women, patients were asked to practise birth control within the 6 months after the acute immunosuppression therapy.

SELECTION OF PATIENTS

At first, the criteria used for selecting the patients were rather wide, as we did not know at that time which kind of patients would benefit the most. A definite diagnosis of MS, according to the Schumacher's criteria, was requested, and pure relapsing as well as relapsing-progressive forms were included. Pure progressive forms were not treated by acute Cy immunosuppression.

The distribution of treated patients, according to their disability evaluated by the Kurtzke scale, was widely spread allowing an estimation of a possible efficacy according to the severity of the handicap when the treatment was given. In the same way, patients with a widely scattered interval of time between the onset of the disease and treatment (from 1 to 10 years and over) were accepted.

According to the wellknown age distribution of the disease, most of the treated patients were in the third decade of their life. Patients below age 18 or over age 60, patients whose impaired intellectual functioning interfered with a correct evaluation of their evolution, and patients with non-neurological disorders possibly creating a hazard for receiving Cy, were excluded.

MODE OF EVALUATION

As already published[1], our interest in the first part of the study was mainly focused on the possible influence of Cy on the ARR. We know that this is open to criticism and Patzold and Pocklington[2], in a recent publication, feel that the ARR is not suited as a measure for the disease activity, since it decreases as the illness progresses.

This reduction of the ARR is progressive however, and we think that it is possible to partly overcome the difficulty by restricting the evaluation of the ARR to a limited period of time. In our patients, the ARR was therefore calculated over the 2 years before and the 2 years after the acute immunosuppression.

We believe that by calculating the ARR over this restricted period of 4 years, we minimize the risks of interference with the spontaneous ARR reduction, provided that the difference between the two rates before and after treatment is sufficiently marked. However, we agree that relapses and disease progression probably correspond to different pathological mechanisms, and that in the long run, the progression of the handicap is the most important event for the patients. When the progression of the disease is concerned, the evolution of the handicap was evaluated using the Kurtzke scale.

RESULTS

The influence of a single acute i.v. immunosuppression on the ARR was determined in 119 patients (Table 2).

Table 2 Evolution of the annual relapse rate after a single i.v. immunosuppression

Duration of disease before treatment (years)	Number of patients	Annual relapse rate		Decrease ARR %
		Before treatment	After treatment	
1-2	10	2.2	0.3	87
3-5	43	1	0.23	77
6-10	53	0.75	0.26	66
10 and fixed handicap	13	0.46	0.46	0

Table 3 Spontaneous decrease of the ARR in 91 non-treated patients

Duration of disease (years)	Annual relapse rate	Decrease v. 2 precedent years %
1-2	1.44	—
3-4	0.95	35
5-6	0.78	18
7-8	0.68	13
9	0.60	12

It appears that the ARR is markedly reduced in most patients, by 87–66% according to the duration of the disease before treatment. In patients with a long evolution and a fixed handicap, the ARR remained unchanged.

In order to better overcome the problem of using the patient as his own control, this group of treated patients was compared to a group of 91 untreated patients, retrospectively matched according to their sex, age, clinical type and duration of the disease (Table 3).

It appears that the progressive reduction of the ARR in Cy treated patients is definitely more marked when compared to the spontaneous decrease in non-treated patients.

Where the progression of the disease is concerned, it appeared that an improvement of neurological signs and functional disability was observed in 60% of the patients. At that time however, we did not go into the details of the possible influence of a single acute immunosuppression on the evolution of the handicap. As a matter of fact, at the end of this part of the study, we got the impression that a single acute i.v. immunosuppression with Cy was able to reduce the ARR in nearly 70% of the patients, that it was more effective when applied during the first stages of the disease, and ineffective in acute cases, severe or fixed handicaps, or in patients with a long evolution before treatment.

The reduction of the ARR, however, was transient, and in the long run, the effect on the progression of the disease seemed negligible. Moreover, it was striking to observe that after a quiescent period of 2–3 years, the disease seemed reactivated and that, when progressing again, the evolution was definitely faster and more severe in some patients. In those cases, the longterm benefit for the patients was therefore questionable. Thus it appeared necessary to prolong the beneficial effect of the acute immunosuppression with Cy, either by repeating the treatment or by maintaining an oral chronic immunosuppression.

Repeated acute immunosuppression

Pulse intensive immunosuppression was repeated in 22 patients: twice in 19 patients and three times in three patients. This group corresponds to patients rather well stabilized by their first treatment, and asking for a second immuno-suppression either because of new relapses, or in order to prevent a further deterioration. In this group, the interest was mainly focused on the evolution of the handicap determined according to the Kurtzke disability scale. Most of the patients had a rather low disability score at the first treatment. Five years later, 68% are still able to walk, and 10 years later 55% of them are confined to their wheelchair or bedridden.

It is difficult to evaluate the results of this part of the study but, in our opinion, even if the second immunosuppression was still able to decrease the ARR to some extent, in the long run there was no clear-cut influence on the progressing disability. It is possible that the interval of time between two successive acute immunosuppressions was too long and that closer retreatments could be more effective.

Combined pulse and maintained immunosuppression

In the last part of the study, in order to try to influence both ARR and the progressive evolution of the disease, a 'combined' pulse and maintained immunosuppression was begun in 60 patients.

It soon became evident that, because of side-effects, chronic administration of Endoxan in MS patients is not so easy. Isophosphamide, an analogue of cyclophosphamide, has been reported to be better tolerated orally, and this drug was supplied to us for clinical trial by Asta Werke. The metabolism of isophosphamide is similar to that of Cy. Its haematopoietic toxicity appears to be lower, but the renal toxicity is increased and is thus the dose limiting factor.

Immediately after the acute treatment, 24 patients received a daily dose of 50 mg Endoxan (cyclophosphamide) and 36 patients received a daily dose of 150 mg Holoxan (isophosphamide). For both agents, those doses are considered as producing an effective immunosuppression in man. The clinical tolerance of isophosphamide was definitely better in our patients, with the consequence that drop-out in the isophosphamide group was observed in only 30% of the patients, compared to 63% in the Cy group. Reasons for discontinuation in the Cy group were side-effects in 40% of the patients, compared to only 14% in the isophosphamide group. It is possible, however, to partly overcome side-effects due to Cy by slowly increasing the weekly dose, up to 50 mg daily. In both groups, the most frequently observed adverse reactions were: cystitis, gastritis, leukopenia, hepatotoxicity and secondary infections.

Clinical criteria for the selection of patients in this part of the study were more severe. Recruitment was limited to patients experiencing frequent relapses (ARR 1.62) and a short evolution (the mean duration of the disease was 4 years), and presenting a disability no greater than a Kurtzke 6 at entry.

When evaluating the results, our interest was mainly focused on the evolution of the handicap. Patients were regularly tested and evaluation of the functional disability was determined according to the Kurtzke scale (Table 4).

Table 4 Evolution of the handicap in 35 evaluable patients treated with 'acute and maintained' immunosuppression

Duration of treatment (years)	Number of patients	Improved	Stable	Worsened
8	2	—	1	1
6	4	3	1	—
5	5	—	4	1
4	10	1	7	2
3	4	1	3	—
2	10	1	7	2
Total	35	6	23	6

After a mean follow up for 4 years, the handicap was stable or improved in 29 patients, that is 80% of the group. This group was compared to a group of 35 patients treated with a single acute immunosuppression and retrospectively matched as close as possible to the 'combined' treated patients according to sex, the age at onset, the handicap when entering the trial, the interval of time between onset and treatment, and types of course (Table 5).

After the same mean follow up period of 4 years, 12 patients out of 35 remained stable. In other words, in the non-treated group the handicap remained stable in only 35% of the patients, compared to the 80% stable

Table 5 Evolution of the handicap after a single i.v. immunosuppression

Follow up (years)	Number of patients	Improved	Stable	Worsened
8	3	—	1	2
6	3	—	1	2
5	5	—	3	2
4	7	—	1	6
3	12	1	3	8
2	5	—	2	3
Total	35	1	11	23

patients treated by 'combined' acute and chronic Cy immunosuppression. The difference between the two groups is highly significant ($p<0.005$).

DISCUSSION

As mentioned before, when this clinical study was started in 1966, Cy was selected, as it had been demonstrated that B lymphocytes showed marked impairment of their ability to regenerate surface immunoglobulin after treatment with this drug. This effect seems definitely less marked for other immunosuppressive agents and this may be the reason why Cy can induce tolerance more readily. From the initial evidence that Cy possesses an inherent selectivity for B cells, it is now becoming clear that certain T cell populations are even more susceptible, and that Cy causes a marked depression of both cell-mediated and humoral immune responses.

In our preliminary experience, an evaluation of lymphocyte subsets in five patients during intensive i.v. immunosuppression, indicates that T lymphocytes are generally more vulnerable to Cy than B lymphocytes. Moreover, when considering helper and suppressor cells, we observed a higher susceptibility of T-helper to Cy compared to T-suppressor. Which kind of immune response is involved the most in promoting brain tissue injury in MS still remains unknown, and an immunosuppressive agent inhibiting both of them seems therefore particularly advisable.

From a personal experience, for 15 years in nearly 250 MS cases treated with i.v. Cy immunosuppression, we have gained the impression that this treatment is capable of influencing the natural course of the disease, and particularly the ARR in about 70% of the patients. Our impression is based upon a careful and prolonged follow up of the clinical evolution in a very large group of patients. For technical reasons (subjective side-effects for instance), this study could not be blinded. However, when compared to the spontaneous reduction of the ARR in matched non-treated patients, the ARR decrease calculated over the 2 years after an acute immunosuppression is definitely more marked.

There are conflicting opinions in the literature concerning the possible influence of immunosuppressive treatments on the ARR in MS. As a matter of fact, most authors[1,3-8] observed a significant decrease of the ARR after a prolonged immunosuppression (3–4 years and over), whereas no differences were found between treated and non-treated patients[2,9,10] when the follow up period was shorter (2 years or less). The same seems to be true where the progression of the disease is concerned.

Acute i.v. Cy immunosuppression produces a more rapid therapeutic effect than oral long-term daily therapy, but the effect of a single acute treatment is limited in time. This is to be expected since it is assumed that subclinical pathological processes continuously evolve, even in apparently stabilized patients. The association of both acute and long-term immunosuppression theoretically combines the advantages of early and prolonged therapeutic effects. In our experience, when applied in relapsing-progressive cases with a rapid evolution, this scheme of treatment reduces the ARR and the progression of the disease in most of the patients.

However, chronic administration of cyclo- or isophosphamide raises the problem of the long-term toxicity of these substances. Besides minor side-effects and more severe acute adverse reactions, Cy produces severe effects on the gonads. Aspermia and amenorrhoea are observed after prolonged therapy, the ovarian tissue seeming less sensitive to Cy than testicular germinal epithelium. Cy administered during the first trimester of pregnancy could cause fetal death or extremity defects in the fetus but, apparently, Cy has no teratogenic effect when given in the last trimester of pregnancy. When Cy is withdrawn, it is admitted that lesions are reversible and both men and women have become the parents of normal children after documented gonadal atrophy from Cy.

Cy is carcinogenetic in animals, and reports of new tumours in patients treated for cancer with this drug make it almost certain that this complication may occur in man. The problem is that up till now, it seems very difficult to determine to what extent Cy can be considered a serious hazard. A few cases of acute leukaemia following Cy therapy for advanced breast cancer and Sjögren's syndrome have been reported. In those patients however, radiotherapy and polychemotherapy had been used, and therefore the role of Cy in the development of new tumours remains a perplexing problem. Malignant tumours were observed in three out of 243 patients treated with Cy, respectively cancer of lung, gallbladder and urinary bladder. Lung and gallbladder cancers were detected 11 and 13 years after a single acute immunosuppression. Urinary bladder cancer was observed 11 years after an acute immunosuppression followed by oral administration of Cy for 2 years. As a matter of fact, this cancer was observed 9 years after the oral administration had been stopped. We believe that the long interval of time between the drug administration and the development of cancer in our patients makes it unlikely that there is a direct correlation between Cy therapy and cancer occurrence.

Even though maintained oral immunosuppression appears relatively safe and able to stabilize some patients, it is evident that this treatment is not the final solution for MS control. A better understanding of the role of T lymphocytes in the pathogenesis of MS will probably lead to therapeutic applications. In this sense, Brinkman et al[11] have recently demonstrated that EAE could be suppressed in rats by subcutaneous injection of monoclonal antibodies to all peripheral T lymphocytes ($W3/13$) and a clinical study of OKT 12 monoclonal antibody in MS patients seems to be under way in the USA.

At the present time, however, when compared to other therapeutical trials (basic protein, transfer factor and levamisole), immunosuppression appears to be the treatment in favour of which the strongest arguments have been observed, indicating a beneficial effect on the course of the disease. This is the reason why in our department, combined acute and chronic immunosuppression is performed in young patients with a short evolution, frequent exacerbations and rapidly progressing deterioration. In those cases indeed, an unfavourable course is likely to be expected.

References

1. Gonsette, R. E., Demonty, L. and Delmotte, P. (1977). Intensive immunosuppression with Cyclophosphamide in multiple sclerosis. Follow up of 110 patients for 2–6 years. *J. Neurol.*, **214**, 173
2. Patzold, U. and Pocklington, P. (1982). Azathioprine in treatment of multiple sclerosis. Final results of a 4½ year controlled study of its effectiveness covering 115 patients. *J. Neurol. Sci.*, **54**, 377
3. Aimard, G., Confavreux, C., Trouillas, P. and Devic, M. (1978). L'Azathioprine dans le traitement de la sclérose en plaques. Une expérience de 10 ans à propos de 77 malades. *Rev. Neurol.* (Paris), **134**, 215
4. Dommash, D., Lurati, M., Albert, E. and Mertens, H. G. (1980). Long-term Azathioprine therapy in multiple sclerosis. In Bauer H. J., Poser, S. and Ritter, G. (ed.). *Progress in MS Research*, pp. 381–387. (Berlin, Heidelberg, New York: Springer Verlag)
5. Frick, E., Angstwurm, H., Blomer, R. and Strauss, G. (1977). Immunosuppressive Therapie der Multiplen Sklerose. 4. Mitteilung: Behandlungsergebnisse mit Azathioprin und Anti-Lymphocytenglobulin. *Münch. Med. Wochenschr.*, **119**, 1111
6. Hauser, L. H., Dawson, D. M., Lehrich, J. R., Beal, M. L., Kevy, S. V., Propper, R. D., Mills, J. A. and Weiner, L. W. (1983). Intensive immunosuppression in progressive multiple sclerosis. A randomized three-arm study of high dose intravenous Cyclophosphamide, plasma exchanges and ACTH. *N. Engl. J. Med.*, **308**, 173
7. Rosen, J. A. (1979). Prolonged Azathioprine treatment of non-remitting multiple sclerosis. *J. Neurol. Neurosurg. Psych.*, **42**, 338
8. Sabouraud, O., Madigand, M. and Merienne, M. (1982). Continuous immunosuppressive therapy for multiple sclerosis: appraisal of 67 cases treated before 1972. *Workshop on Immunosuppressive Treatments in Multiple Sclerosis*, June 10–12, 1983, Nijmegen, The Netherlands
9. Rudge, P. (1982). Immunosuppressive treatment of multiple sclerosis. *Workshop on Immunosuppressive Treatments in Multiple Sclerosis*, June 10–12, 1983, Nijmegen, The Netherlands
10. Zeeberg, I., Heltberg, A., Krustensen, J. H., Raun, N. E. and Fog, T. (1982). A long-term double blind controlled trial of Azathioprine vs placebo in treatment of progressive multiple sclerosis. *Workshop on Immunosuppressive Treatments in Multiple Sclerosis*, June 10–12, 1983, Nijmegen, The Netherlands.
11. Brinkman, C. J. J., Ter Laak, H. J. and Hommes, O. R. (1983). The effect of monoclonal anti-T cell antibodies on the clinical course of experimental allergic encephalomyelitis in rats. In Gonsette, R. E. and Delmotte, P. (eds.) *Immunological and Clinical Aspects of Multiple Sclerosis*. Chap. 18. (Lancaster: MTP Press)

28
Treatment of progressive multiple sclerosis by the combined application of antilymphocyte serum, azathioprine and prednisone

H. De SAXCE, R. MARTEAU and F. LHERMITTE

INTRODUCTION

This study follows a preceding research, where a group of 50 patients was examined over 4 years. We present here the first results of a 1 year treatment of progressive cases, compared to an untreated group of patients. This study was made in the years 1975–1980.

MATERIAL AND METHODS

Patient selection

The patients suffer from recent, strongly progressive multiple sclerosis; the diagnostic criteria are those internationally used. Only cases having evolved for 5 years or less were considered. The gravity and progressiveness of the disease were decided based upon the frequency of relapses and the prompt deterioration of the functional handicap. All selected patients had first been treated with steroids, with no effect on the progressiveness of the disease.

Group 1 includes 45 patients treated with antilymphocyte serum. 39 patients suffer from incompletely remitting relapses, with permanent deterioration after each relapse. Six patients suffer from directly progressive multiple sclerosis. Group 1 includes 20 men and 25 women averaging 30 years of age.

Group 2 includes 22 patients, 17 with relapsing forms and five directly progressive. The 12 men and 10 women average 31 years of age.

Patients were first selected at random to be in one or the other group. The higher number of patients in group 1 results from the strong demand of patients asking to be admitted to the treatment.

Treatment

The 45 patients of group 1 were treated by the combined application of antilymphocyte serum, azathioprine and prednisone.

The 22 patients of group 2 were treated with azathioprine and prednisone only.

The antilymphocyte serum is prepared by the Institut Mérieux. A 5 ml vial contains 62.5 mg of active proteins. Several lots were used, which are now standardized. The serum is applied through slow intravenous infusion, taking 4-6 hours. The serum is diluted in 250 ml of 0.9% sodium chloride isotonic serum. This dilution is Y-connected to an isotonic serum with higher flow to insure vein permeability.

The treatment includes a 4 week initial treatment and a 1 year continuous treatment. Infusions are made every day for the first 2 weeks then three times a week for the following 2 weeks. The 1 year continuous treatment consists of one infusion per week or four infusions in 1 week per month. The average dose is 2-3 vials (5 ml) per infusion, depending on the clinical and biological tolerance.

To the antilymphocyte serum are systematically combined:

— azathioprine at the rate of $2\,mg\,kg^{-1}\,day^{-1}$, that is on average 100 mg/day,
— prednisone at the rate of 20 mg/day.

After the treatment, azathioprine is administered at the same rate. Prednisone is gradually decreased to 10 mg/day.

Group 2 is treated with the same quantities of azathioprine and prednisone for 1 year, with the same decrease in the rate of prednisone after the first month.

The 2 groups remain on azathioprine during 3 years of follow-up.

Methods

Biological

The leukocyte and platelet ratio was controlled before each infusion. The complete blood composition was determined twice a week. Creatinine clearance was measured before and after the initial treatment, as well as haemostasis (bleeding and clotting). Last, a search for intercurrent infections was systematically called for at any warning sign.

Immunology

The measurement of the serum complement, immune complexes, and rosette formation was performed before and after the initial treatment. The titration of antiglobulin antibodies was calculated every week of the first month. The 10 unit tuberculin, 1/1000 candinine, and 100 unit varidase delayed hypersensitivity tests were also made before and after the initial treatment.

Cerebrospinal fluid (CSF)

Protein and cell studies of the cerebrospinal fluid were performed before the treatment.

Genetic

In some cases a study on HLA tissue groups and on the lymphocytic markers was performed.

Clinical evaluation

Clinical evaluation was performed through the assessment of a functional scale. This scale was always the modified Pedersen scale, which provides a rather complete view of the patient's handicap and of the symptom location. The scores from 0 to 30 were always given by the same clinical team (before treatment, monthly during the first and second year, and then every 2 months). In addition to the score on the Pedersen scale, the number of relapses, whether remitting or not, was also recorded. We believe that in the long-run the change in the functional handicap better describes the progressiveness of the disease than the number of relapses.

RESULTS

Clinical controls

As in our previous study, nearly all patients could be treated according to the protocol.

Treatment had to be discontinued seven times: – five times for 10th day serum diseases, that is for 11% of the patients, – twice for clinical and psychic intolerance.

Treatment was never discontinued for technical reasons. One intercurrent infection necessitated a temporary interruption of the treatment. Various transitory fever and skin reactions were also noted on infusion day or as a result of intravenous injection of prednisolone.

Biological results

The number of red cells and leukocytes was globally not affected by the treatment. The lymphocyte number decreased temporarily. This was already noted in our previous study (decrease of 50% on day 15 for half of the patients).

The platelet number decreased during the treatment due to the anti-platelet effect of the antilymphocyte serum. This temporary decrease was readily adjusted through dosage reductions or momentary interruption of the treatment. No haemorrhagic complications were noted.

Proteinuria was always negative. In addition, creatinine clearance remained unchanged at the end of the initial treatment, as well as in later controls.

Equine antiglobulin antibodies (see Table 1)

Thirty-five files were examined. The antibody titre was measured before, during, at the end of the initial treatment and monthly thereafter. For 21 patients, titres remained negative, regardless of the sampling period. For 12 patients, antibody titres increased sharply between day 10 and day 20. For two patients, titres increased slightly.

Table 1 Equine antiglobulin antibodies (out of 35 patients)

Typical serum accidents:	5 (3 had sharp increase in antibody titre)
Clinical intolerance:	2 patients
Treatment maintained in spite of high antibody titre:	8 patients
Showing aggravation with sharply increased titre:	5 patients
Showing stable condition with average titre:	3 patients

Analysis performed by Laboratoire d'Immunologie Clinique, Pr J. F. Bach, Hôpital Necker, Paris

Three of the patients showing a positive increase in their antibody titre had a patent day 12 serum disease. Two patients had clinical reactions at each infusion, and treatment had to be discontinued. Treatment was maintained for the other patients.

Rosettes – T and B lymphocytes (see Table 2)

31 files were analysed before treatment and 29 at the end of the initial treatment. The rate of E-rosette was regular before treatment for all files. After treatment, this rate decreased in ten cases (seven sharp decreases and three decreases to the lower limit of the normal rate).

The B-lymphocyte rate, which was only analysed in 19 cases, was normal.

Table 2 E-rosettes and B-lymphocytes

E-rosettes, normal before treatment:	31 patients
E-rosettes, decrease after treatment:	10 patients
sharp decrease:	7 patients
lower limit:	3 patients
No analysis for two patients after treatment	
B-lymphocytes unregularly analysed	

Serum complement (see Table 3)

The serum complement (C_3C_4CH50 – CH50 equals total haemolytic complement) was analysed 32 times before treatment and 26 times after 1 month of treatment. The rate of the C_3 and C_4 complement was normal in 31 out of 32 cases before treatment, and in 24 out of 26 cases after 1 month of treatment. The rate of the CH50 was normal in 26 out of 34 cases analysed before treatment. After 1 month of treatment, that rate had increased in 5 out of 19 cases for a first batch, and in 3 out of 15 cases for the second batch.

Table 3 Serum complement

$n = 34$		Result before treatment	Result after 1 month
C_3C_4 analysis		31 normal out of 32	24 normal out of 26
CH50 analysis (total haemolytic complement)	First batch (19)	14 normal	5 increases
	Second batch (15)	12 normal	3 increases
	Total (34)	26 normal	8 increases

Serum immune complex

Out of 29 cases analysed, the amount of precipitate was normal in 25 cases and had increased for four patients.

Therapeutic results

Therapeutic results were always evaluated based upon the functional handicap (modified Pedersen scale). We believe, as many others do, that its results are more significant than the number or frequency of relapses. These last two elements are, however, still taken into account as indicators of the disease activeness.

Group 1 – 45 patients

Five patients had a day 10 serum disease, and treatment had to be stopped. Treatment also had to be stopped for two patients for clinical intolerance. The remaining 38 patients (20 women and 18 men) were treated as planned.

Handicap evolution

After the first month, 17 patients had improved and 21 remained stationary. At the end of the first year, 18 remained improved and 11 stationary. At the end of the second year, 13 were still improved and eight stationary. At the end of the third year, only nine were improved and eight still stationary. The remaining 19 patients (two patients could not be followed-up) were subjected anew to the progressiveness of the disease.

In percentages, the results are as follows:

after 1 year: 47% improved and 29% stable
after 2 years: 34% improved and 21% stable
after 3 years: 50% stable or improved, 50% aggravated

Relapses

There were 11 relapses in the first year and 14 in the following 2 years. Taking into account only those patients suffering originally from incompletely remitting relapses (certain patients had directly progressive multiple sclerosis, that is without steps or relapses but with a continuous progression of the disease), the average frequency of relapses was 0.26 per year over the 3 years. Taking into account all patients, the average frequency of relapses was 0.23 per year. Out of the 36 patients followed-up, 32 were originally of a relapse-type illness.

Group 2 – 22 patients (control group, 12 men and 10 women)

Handicap evolution

After the first year, three patients were improved and 10 stable. At the end of the second year, two remained improved and five stable. After the third year, two were still improved and three stable. The disease progressed for the 17 remaining patients.

In percentages, the results are as follows:

after 1 year: 14% improved and 45% stable
after 2 years: 9% improved and 24% stable
after 3 years: 24% stable or improved, 76% aggravated

Relapses

There were 21 relapses in this group for the first 3 years. The average frequency of relapses (calculated for the 17 patients originally subject to relapses) was 0.41 per year. For the 22 patients, the average frequency was 0.32 per year.

See Tables 4, 5 and 6 for a comparative analysis of the results for the two groups of patients.

Table 4 Comparative analysis

After 1 year	Group 1	Group 2
Improved patients	47%	14%
Aggravated patients	24%	41%

With a χ^2 of 4.25 and 1 degree of freedom (Level of confidence 95%), the difference between improved and aggravated patients appears statistically significant

After 2 years		
Improved patients	34%	9%
Aggravated patients	45%	67%

After 3 years		
Improved patients	24%	9%
Aggravated patients	50%	76%

The differences between group 1 and group 2 were not statistically significant at the end of years 2 or 3

Note: Percentages were calculated on a total of 38 patients for group 1 and on a total of 22 patients for group 2

The statistical analysis was performed by G. Deloche, INSERM U 84, Service du Pr. F. Lhermitte

Table 5 Relapses (comparative analysis)

Number of relapses	Group 1	Group 2
After the first year	11	8
After the second or third year	14	11

The differences between group 1 and group 2 were not statistically significant

Table 6 Comparative analysis

	Group 1	Group 2
After 1 year	$n = 38$	$n = 22$
Improved patients	18	3
Stable condition patients	11	9
Aggravated patients	9	10

$\chi^2 = 3.05$. With 1 degree of freedom, the differences are not significant

	Group 1	Group 2
After 2 years	$n = 38$	$n = 22$
Improved patients	13	2
Stable condition patients	8	5
Aggravated patients	17	15

$\chi^2 = 3.07$. With 1 degree of freedom, the differences are not significant

	Group 1	Group 2
After 3 years	$n = 36$	$n = 22$
Improved patients	9	2
Stable condition patients	8	3
Aggravated patients	19	17

$\chi^2 = 3.48$. With 1 degree of freedom, the differences are not significant

Note: Two patients of group 1 could not be followed-up after year 3. When grouping together stable and improved patients, the differences are still not statistically significant

DISCUSSION

The statistical analysis shows a significant difference between group 1 and group 2 for improved and aggravated patients at the end of the first year, that is at the end of the antilymphocyte serum treatment. The difference is no longer significant in year 2 or 3 when the patients are not subject to the antilymphocyte serum. It should be noted, however, that when the statistical analysis takes into account the patients in stable condition as well as the improved ones, the differences between the two groups are then not considered to be significant for any of the 3 years. As for the number or frequency of relapses, none of the years show any significant difference (see Table 5).

No relapses or aggravations occurred during the intensive treatment. 11 patients of group 1 had no progressive relapse at all during the 3 years (Patients 4, 8, 12, 14, 17, 18, 23, 24, 31, 32 and 37). These patients represent the group of stable and improved conditions. If we consider the progressiveness of the disease for these patients in the 2 years preceding the treatment, it would appear that the antilymphocyte serum or some other part of the treatment would have been beneficial. Five patients, whose condition remained stable after 3 years, had however receding relapses and did not increase their functional handicap (Patients 7, 9, 11, 15 and 21). Ten patients had relapses as soon as the first year, therefore during the treatment (Patients 7, 9, 10, 11, 16, 19, 26, 29, 34 and 38). Four patients had relapses only after the end of the treatment (Patients 6, 15, 20 and 21). Among the 19 aggravated patients after 3 years are the six directly progressive forms of multiple sclerosis. For these six patients, the illness progressed.

11 patients increased their handicap with non or incompletely remitting relapses (Patients 5, 6, 10, 13, 16, 19, 20, 26, 29, 34 and 38). Four patients showed progressive aggravation (Patients 1, 2, 3 and 30).

The directly progressive forms (six patients in group 1) all showed aggravated handicaps after 3 years (Patients 2, 22, 25, 27, 28 and 35). In the control group 2, four cases of this form were clearly aggravated after 3 years while one patient kept a stable handicap. It would appear that the antilymphocyte treatment does not affect the progressiveness of the disease in such cases. This comment was already noted in our previous study. One patient of group 1 died, due to decubitus complications after 3 years.

The beneficial effect of the antilymphocyte serum combined with azathioprine and prednisone appears more clearly in the years of treatment. The psychological impact must be taken into account as patients are followed very carefully, examined every week or every month, and hospitalized for each infusion. This element is non-existent for the control group 2 where patients are not hospitalized and only examined on consultation. The disease progressed anew after 1 year for a number of patients, once the antilymphocyte serum was no longer administered. The patients are then still treated with azathioprine but examined on consultation. This temporary effect of the antilymphocyte serum was already noted in our first study.

Three patients were treated a second time with the antilymphocyte serum after an aggravation of the disease in the second or third year (Patients 6, 31 and 32). No clinical improvement resulted for two of them, and in one case, the equine antiglobulin antibody titre increased sharply. One woman patient was treated every week for 2 years with a stable condition. Her condition aggravated in the third year after interruption of the treatment.

The sharp increase in the equine antiglobulin antibody titre was noted 12 times. Three cases were clinical serum incidents, one was the result of clinical intolerance and treatment had to be stopped. Treatment was continued for the eight other patients. Five of these patients did not respond favourably to the treatment. In one case, treatment was resumed after a progressive relapse, but the second treatment was not at all so effective as the first. For three other patients, the functional handicap was stationary, but the antibody titre, though positive, was not so high (1/256, 1/128). There would, therefore, appear to be a correlation between the increase in the antibody titre and the inefficacy of the treatment, a highly increased antibody titre corresponding to the treatment being ineffective. The reverse proposition is however not verified (see Table 1).

Only ten patients out of 31 showed a decreased E-rosette titre after 1 month of treatment. There is no possible clinical or biological correlation: three patients were in the improved group, two showed a stationary condition, three were aggravated, and one was a serum accident. This E-rosette test appears less adequate than the delayed hypersensitivity skin tests in controlling immunosuppression. This may result from sampling and transportation technical difficulties.

The decrease in the rosette titre is an indicator of cellular immunosuppression and not of therapeutic efficacy. The E-rosette titre was normal in all cases studied before treatment (see Table 2).

The rate of immune complex was regular in 25 cases out of 29, that is in 86% of the cases.

The cerebrospinal fluid analysis, whether for the elements or the rate of proteins and γ-globulins, evidences no significant variation before and after the treatment.

CONCLUSION

Treatment by the combined application of antilymphocyte serum, azathioprine, and prednisone is well accepted by patients under strict technical and surveillance conditions. Seven patients could not be treated according to the protocol, five because of serum accidents and two for clinical intolerances, that is in 17% of the cases. The rosette test was less accurate than the delayed hypersensitivity skin tests used in a previous study.

The complement, immune complex, and rosette titres were normal before treatment with most of the patients studied.

The equine antiglobulin antibody titre increase during the initial treatment was connected either with a serum disease or, when the treatment was continued, with the inefficacy of the treatment.

The comparison with a control group, treated only with azathioprine and prednisone but with the same doses, shows a significant statistical difference in the number of aggravated and improved patients after the first year. The difference is no longer significant in years 2 or 3. Taking into account stable as well as improved conditions, the differences are not significant for any of the 3 years. No differences in the frequency of relapses could be noted, whether for the first year or the following 2 years. The study will be, in any case, pursued for 2 more years, to confirm or refute the above results.

We believe that, in spite of its inconclusive therapeutical results in the long-run, the research on this antilymphocyte serum treatment should be continued for progressive and grievous multiple sclerosis cases. The discussion remains open as to the length of time the treatment could be administered.

References

1. Lhermitte, F., Marteau, R. and de Saxcé, H. (1979). Treatment of multiple sclerosis with antilymphocyte serum. Results of a pilot study on 50 patients followed over a 4-year period. *Rev. Neur.* (Paris), **135**, 389

29
Clinical trials of a synthetic polypeptide (Copolymer I) for the treatment of multiple sclerosis

M. B. BORNSTEIN, A. I. MILLER, S. SLAGLE, V. SPADA, R. ARNON, M. SELA and D. TEITELBAUM

ABSTRACT

A synthetic polypeptide (Copolymer I) composed of alanine, glutamic acid, lysine and tyrosine has been demonstrated to be non-encephalitogenic and non-toxic in laboratory animals. Yet, it is capable of suppressing EAE. This pre-clinical work was performed at the Weizmann Institute for Science, Rehovoth, Israel.

A preliminary open trial examined the ability of COP I to alter the course of multiple sclerosis in 12 chronic-progressive (CP) and 4 exacerbating–remitting (ER) patients. No undesirable side reactions were noted in any patients during more than 2 years of receiving the COP I. Three of the CP and 2 of the ER type of patients are better. These results, which may represent either a placebo effect or a significant response, are now being examined in a randomized, placebo-controlled, double-blind pilot trial.

INTRODUCTION

The understanding of the mechanisms involved in multiple sclerosis (MS), and the search for an effective treatment have been intimately associated with the laboratory model, experimental allergic encephalomyelitis (EAE). The validity of EAE as such a model system has been clearly and convincingly presented by Paterson in a series of scholarly publications[1-5]. Our own work in tissue culture[6-8], also served to relate MS as a naturally occurring disorder to its laboratory counterpart, EAE, further validating the possible extension to MS patients of therapeutic suggestions arising from animal studies.

The synthetic polypeptide, Copolymer I (COP I), was prepared from alanine, glutamic acid, lysine and tyrosine (Table 1) as one of a series of

Table 1 Composition of Copolymer I

Amino acid	N-Carboxyanhydride used for reaction	Amount used in the reaction g	mM	Molar ratio of amino acid in copolymer
Alanine	Alanine	8.6	75	6.0
Glutamic acid	-Benzyl glutamate	6.0	23	1.9
Lysine	,N-Trifluoroacetyl-lysine	14.0	52	4.7
Tyrosine	Tyrosine	3.0	14	1.0
Molecular weight				23 000

compounds which, alone or in combination with various lipids, might simulate the ability of myelin basic protein (MBP) to induce EAE (Sela, personal communication). None of the preparations proved to be encephalitogenic, i.e. capable of inducing EAE, but some, particularly COP I, did suppress EAE in animals challenged with either whole white matter or MBP in complete Freund's adjuvant. The numerous laboratory investigations of the effectiveness of COP I in EAE, involving mice, rats, guinea pigs, rabbits, monkeys, chimpanzees and baboons, are of particular interest to the clinical trials and have recently been reviewed by Arnon and Teitelbaum[9]. In addition, extensive laboratory studies failed to demonstrate any toxicological or other undesirable side reaction in experimental animals exposed to COP I under a variety of testing situations (A. Meshorer, personal communication). Finally, Abramsky et al[10] first examined COP I for its effect on three patients with acute disseminated encephalomyelitis (ADE) and four with terminal MS. The three ADE patients recovered rapidly and completely. The MS patients may have demonstrated slight improvements. What was more important in these first clinical studies was the absence of any significant or undesirable side reactions.

This report presents the data concerning a preliminary trial and its extension into a pilot trial of the effectiveness of COP I in patients with the exacerbating–remitting (ER) and chronic-progressive (CP) types of MS. A preliminary trial is

'conducted for the purpose of establishing dosages, studying toxicity, and obtaining a lead as to the possible efficacy of a new treatment for MS. Such a study is the first organized application of a new treatment which may be a new investigative drug ... Different dosages with different schedules ... are tried on a few patients who are very closely monitored for toxic reactions. For the assessment of therapeutic dosages, the patient with MS will serve as his own control. Therefore, the physician–investigator should be well acquainted with the medical history and past clinical course of MS in each patient ... In most instances, it will not be necessary to involve more than perhaps 10 patients in a given preliminary trial. If the preliminary trial brings forth evidence of therapeutic efficacy and little or no evidence of serious toxicity, it would be reasonable to move onto the next stage of investigation, the pilot trial[11]'.

METHODS AND MATERIALS

The COP I is supplied by the Weizmann Institute. Every preparation of COP I is tested for its ability to suppress experimental allergic encephalomyelitis in guinea pigs and for immunological cross reaction with the basic encephalitogenic protein. On receipt in our laboratory, the sterile, lyophilized material is stored at $-20\,^{\circ}$C until the time of use. At that time, bacteriostatic sodium chloride is injected into the vial to dissolve the polypeptide. The final concentration of COP I in saline has varied from 5 to its present concentration of 20 mg/ml. The solution is distributed into sterile vials, each containing a single, daily dose of the dissolved Copolymer, and frozen. At the time of use, the single dose vials are thawed, and the solution injected subcutaneously.

Sixteen MS patients participated in the preliminary trial. They represented a broad spectrum of neurological involvement ranging from those of the chronic-progressive (CP) type, some of whom were essentially bed or wheelchair bound, to those of the exacerbating–remitting (ER) type who were fully active and employed between attacks. There were four of the ER type and twelve of the CP type. All patients had been well known to the principal investigator (MBB) for years prior to their entry into the study. Some had participated as volunteers in earlier clinical and laboratory studies, while others had been unsuccessfully tried on immunosuppressant therapy.

The preliminary trial was conducted as an open study. All patients were given the COP I and all knew they were receiving it. The evaluating neurologist (AM) was also aware that this was an open study and that all patients were being treated. The initial dosage schedule was suggested by the group at the Weizmann Institute on the basis of their previous studies with laboratory animals[9], such as non-human primates, as well as the brief trial that was performed by Dr Oded Abramsky[10]. Thus, it was planned to prepare the COP I at a concentration of 5 mg/ml of sterile saline solution. This was to be given to each patient intramuscularly five times a week for the first 3 weeks, three times a week for the next 3 weeks, twice a week for the next 3 weeks, and, finally, once a week for the balance of a 6 month period, at which time we originally planned to terminate the trial.

At the time of introduction into the study, the patients were hospitalized at the General Clinical Research Center of The Albert Einstein College of Medicine. They were examined and evaluated by Dr Miller, samples of peripheral blood and cerebrospinal fluid were taken, and the Copolymer injections were started. In the beginning, the patients were hospitalized during the first 3 weeks of treatment, since we had no knowledge as to whether or not there would be any significant local or systemic effects in patients who had multiple sclerosis. We did not, however, note any undesirable side reactions of any significance, and soon found it unnecessary to keep the volunteers in the hospital for any period longer than was prudent following the lumbar puncture, usually 24–48 hours. The patients were seen, however, on an outpatient basis at the Clinical Research Center and their neurological status re-evaluated at various times during the course of the following months.

The specific aims of the preliminary trial were to determine the following:

(1) Did COP I produce any apparent significant or undesirable side reactions?
(2) Did COP I produce any apparent desirable effects?
(3) Could a dosage schedule be established for further (pilot) trials, should they appear to be warranted?

RESULTS

During the institution of the Copolymer treatment, many patients reported and, in fact, demonstrated early improvements in various neurological functions. As time went on, however, and as the dosage of COP I was reduced, these early improvements disappeared and most patients returned to their previous neurological status and continued their chronic-progressive course. Over the period of the next months, the dosage was gradually increased in an effort to determine whether or not the previously observed effect was dose related. By the end of the first 18 month period, those patients who were still on the Copolymer were receiving 20 mg/day in 1 ml of saline, 7 days a week. Twelve patients are still on this schedule – 11 for over 2 years. This is the dosage currently being used in the pilot study.

As for undesirable side reactions, patients rarely reported a transient slight pain, discomfort or itching at the injection site. No local reactions of swelling or redness were noted at that time. No systemic or general reactions of any kind were noted or reported. Examinations of urine were unremarkable. Occasionally, examination of the peripheral blood cellular elements revealed a

Table 2 Results of preliminary trial of Copolymer I therapy in 16 patients with multiple sclerosis

Patient	Type	Age	Sex	Date of entry	Date of termin.	Results
I.Y.	CP	46	F	4/25/78	5/27/81	No effect
R.H.	CP	25	M	5/15/78	5/29/79	No effect
G.T.	CP	35	F	5/30/78	9/20/79	No effect
P.P.	ER	30	F	5/30/78	—	No effect
A.T.	CP	23	M	6/27/78	2/8/79	No effect
P.McL.	CP	39	F	7/18/78	—	Arrested – Marked improvement
J.P.	ER	39	F	7/18/78	10/27/78	Withdrew at time of exacerbation
J.W.	CP	32	M	6/27/78	6/5/79	No effect
K.J.	CP	33	F	7/31/78	12/30/80	No effect
C.N.	ER	32	M	8/7/78	—	Cessation of characteristic attacks
W.R.	CP	49	M	10/3/78	—	Arrest – slight improvement
S.McC.	CP	42	F	10/16/78	—	No effect
H.W.	CP	36	M	10/24/78	11/13/78	No effect
S.R.	CP	38	F	10/24/78	—	No effect
F.H.	ER	27	F	11/7/78	—	Cessation of characteristic attacks
J.M.	CP	34	F	11/20/78	—	Arrest and improvement

CP = Chronic-progressive
ER = Exacerbating–remitting

transient eosinophilia, reaching 16% in one instance. No significant change in blood chemistries appeared. Examinations of blood obtained before and at various times after the institution of COP I administration have revealed no change in lymphocyte transformation in response to COP I, myelin basic protein or phytohaemagglutinin, or in the ability of cells and serum, alone and together, with and without complement to affect CNS myelin in culture. To date, as mentioned above, 11 patients have been exposed to COP I for over 2 years.

Of the 16 patients, two of the ER type withdrew from the study at the time of an acute attack. One later returned. Of the balance all remained in the study for at least 6 months as originally planned. In general, 11 of the 16 patients demonstrated no apparent favourable effects, in that they either had an exacerbation during the course of the study or continued their chronic-progressive course. On the other hand, five of the 16 patients have demonstrated a definite change for the better, please see Table 2.

The longest period of COP I treatment in this group of patients is 36 months. Eleven have received COP I for over 2 years. No patient had any significant or undesirable local or systemic side reaction, but recently there have been side reactions observed by some patients during the pilot trial of COP I in the exacerbating and remitting patients. These occasional reactions consist of local swelling, redness and pain or discomfort at the injection site. Most recently, two patients reported a few instances of a flush, sweating, muscular contractions and a feeling of breathlessness. These occasional reactions lasted from 5 to 10 minutes. Investigations into these reactions are in progress.

Laboratory data

Laboratory examinations have included CBC, routine urinalysis and culture and blood chemistry analyses (SMA 6 and 12) VDRL, CSF protein and glucose and cells. Except for an occasional and transient eosinophilia, reaching 16% in one instance, no significant changes have been noted in any of these clinical tests. There has been no evidence of albuminuria or other evidence of altered kidney function. No pertinent alteration of the patient's serum demyelinating potency on CNS cultured tissues has been observed. Sera have been examined for antibody titres against COP I. In general, they have been elevated. Lymphoblast transformation in response to phytohaemagglutinin, MBP and COP I has not occurred.

The data generated by the preliminary trial appeared to us to warrant the extension of the clinical evaluation of COP I to a pilot trial in the exacerbating–remitting MS patient. This double-blind, placebo-controlled, randomized study was instituted in February, 1980 and is planned to continue until December, 1984 when all 50 patients will have finished their 2 years of participation in the formal trial.

The criteria for enrollment into the pilot trial were as follows:

(1) The patient must have MS of the exacerbating–remitting type with at least one, and preferably two, well-demarcated and well-documented

attacks in each of the 2 years prior to admission to the trial.

(2) Patients must be between the ages of 20 and 35, ambulatory and not previously exposed to immunosuppressant drugs such as azothiaprine or cyclophosphamide. Steroids are allowed.

(3) A psycho–social evaluation must show the patient to be psychologically stable and reliable and capable of participating in the full course of the trial.

On the basis of these criteria, 50 patients were selected from 985 who volunteered, and were considered for participation. Those who were accepted were matched for age, sex, frequency of attacks and degree of disability and randomly distributed into the placebo (0.9% bacteriostatic sodium chloride) or the treated (COP I, 20 mg/ml of 0.9% bacteriostatic sodium chloride) group.

Neurological evaluations are done at the time of entry into the trial, routinely at 3 month intervals, and more frequently at the times of suspected or confirmed exacerbations. The findings are recorded on forms representing the neurological examination, Kurtzke's 8 Functional Systems, and Kurtzke's Disability Status Scale. The data are entered into a computerized data bank and will be evaluated at specified times for the frequency of attacks and the degree of neurological deficit demonstrated by the two groups.

Since the study must remain blinded until its termination, end-point data are not available at this time. However, the available information describing the present status of the trial is shown in Table 3.

Table 3 Baseline characteristics of study population and accumulated time in the study as of April 1, 1983

	Placebo	Cop I	Total
Number entered	25	25	50
Average age	30.96	29.96	30.44
*Sex			
males	10	11	21
females	15	14	29
Race			
white			48
black/Hispanic			2
*Kurtzke DSS:			
0–2	13	13	26
3–4	5	5	10
5–6	7	7	14
mean DSS	3.2	3.2	3.2
*Previous attack rate:			
attacks/year	2.02	1.96	1.99
Time in study:			
total patient months	412	460	872
total patient years	34.33	38.33	72.66
average no. months in the study	18.40	16.48	17.44

*matching variables

On the basis of current end-point data made known to the members of the External Advisory Committee (EAC) and to a few select individuals at the National Institute of Health, a grant request has been approved and funded, as of April 1, 1983, to extend the pilot trial to the chronic-progressive MS patient.

Finally, the EAC has also been unanimous in its decision to permit the organization of a full, multicenter clinical trial of COP I in the exacerbating–remitting MS patient. Hopefully, this will begin within 12–18 months.

ACKNOWLEDGMENTS

This work was supported in part by grant NS 11920 from the NINCDS.

References

1. Paterson, P. Y. (1976). Experimental autoimmune (allergic) encephalomyelitis: induction, pathogenesis and suppression. In Miescher, P. A. and Muller-Eberhard, H. J. (eds.). *Textbook of immunopathology*. 2nd Edn., pp. 179–213. (New York: Grune and Stratton)
2. Paterson, P. Y. (1977). Autoimmune neurologic disease: experimental animal systems and implications for multiple sclerosis. In Talal, N. (ed.). *Autoimmunity. Genetic, immunologic, virologic and clinical aspects*. pp. 643–692, (New York: Academic Press)
3. Paterson, P. Y. (1978). The demyelinating diseases: Clinical and experimental studies in animals and man. In Samter, M., Alexander, N., Rose, B., Sherman, W. B., Talmage, D. W. and Vaughn, J. H. (eds.). *Immunological diseases*, 3rd Edn., pp. 1400–1435 (Boston: Little, Brown)
4. Paterson, P. Y. (1979). Neurological disorders. In Irvine, W. J. (ed.). *Medical immunology*, chapter 14, pp. 361–381. (Edinburgh: Teviot Scientific)
5. Paterson, P. Y. (1980). The immunopathology of experimental allergic encephalomyelitis. In Davison, A. N. and Cuzner, M. C. (eds.). *The suppression of experimental allergic encephalomyelitis and multiple sclerosis*, pp. 11–30. (New York: Academic Press)
6. Bornstein, M. B. (1963). A tissue culture approach to demyelinative disorders. *Nat. Cancer. Inst. Monogr.*, **11**, 197
7. Bornstein, M. B. (1978). Immunobiology of demyelination. In Waxman, S. G. (ed.). *Physiology and pathobiology of axons*, pp. 313–336. (New York: Raven Press)
8. Bornstein, M. B. and Raine, C. S. (1977). Multiple sclerosis and experimental allergic encephalomyelitis: Specific demyelination of CNS in culture. *Neuropathol. Appl. Neurobiol.*, **3**, 359
9. Arnon, R. and Teitelbaum, D. (1980). Desensitization of experimental allergic encephalomyelitis with synthetic peptide analogues. In Davison, A. N. and Cuzner, M. L. (eds.). *The suppression of experimental allergic encephalomyelitis and multiple sclerosis.*, pp. 105–117. (London, NY: Academic Press)
10. Abramsky, O., Teitelbaum, D. and Arnon, R. (1977). Effect of a synthetic polypeptide (COP I) on patients with multiple sclerosis and with acute disseminated encephalomyelitis. Preliminary report. *J. Neurol. Sci.*, **31**, 433
11. Brown, J. R., Beebe, G. W., Kurtzke, J. F., Loewenson, R. B., Silberberg, D. H. and Tourtellotte, W. W. (1979). The design of clinical studies to assess therapeutic efficacy in multiple sclerosis. *Neurology*, **29**, Part 2

30
Lympho-plasmapheresis in multiple sclerosis: effect on clinical and immunological parameters

B. KENNES, C-P. LEROY, J-P. DUMONT, D. BROHÉE, J. JACQUY, G. NOËL and P. NÈVE

INTRODUCTION

Numerous works have brought evidence for the role of immune humoral factors and cytotoxic lymphocytes in the physiopathology of acute and progressive phases of multiple sclerosis (MS)[1,2]. Antibodies against myelin[3], oligodendrocytes[4] or with demyelinating properties[5], immune complexes[6] and changes in blood or cerebrospinal fluid of T cell distribution are observed principally during active MS[7-9]. Also, neuroelectrical blocking IgG antibodies are discovered in MS blood[10]. Furthermore, fragments of neuro-antigens are episodically released[11].

Thus, theoretically, by removing antibodies, immune complexes, antigens and some circulating lymphocytes from blood, chronic lymphoplasmapheresis (L-P) could alter the disease's course of MS. Due to these points and because no preventive measures or definitive treatment may actually be proposed, we analysed the effect of L-P on 34, informed consent and not taking drugs patients with progressive (*PFMS*) or remittent-progressive (*RPMS*: without recent relapse) phase.

MATERIAL AND METHODS

Patients: the details of the population studied are summarized in Table 1. They all experienced a long course and slow worsening disease.

Lympho-plasmapheresis: For each session, 2 litres of plasma were exchanged against physiologic saline mixed with human proteins, and about 10^9 leukocytes (80% of lymphocytes) were removed using Haemonetics 30. L-P was carried out following two types of protocol as shown in Table 2.

151

Table 1 Population of MS (progressive forms)

Age (y ± SD)	Number	Ratio F/M
44 ± 10	34	2

Diagnosis
Slow or step-wise progressive course extending over at least 6 months
Oligoclonal pic CSF
Evocated potentials

Table 2 Design of the study

| | Session of L-P | Number of subjects | | |
		Incorporated	Unrealizable	Renouncement	Treated
Protocol I	1/week for 3 weeks followed by 1/3 weeks for 6 months	26	2	2	22
Protocol II	1/week for 3 months	8	0	1	7
		The programme was stopped because two cases worsened (Weariness ?)			

Symptoms and neurologic (with functional scores) examinations were collected prior to L-P initiation and before each session. At days 0, 30 and after 6 months, immune investigations were realized.

Twelve subjects completed a daily questionnaire of self-assessment.

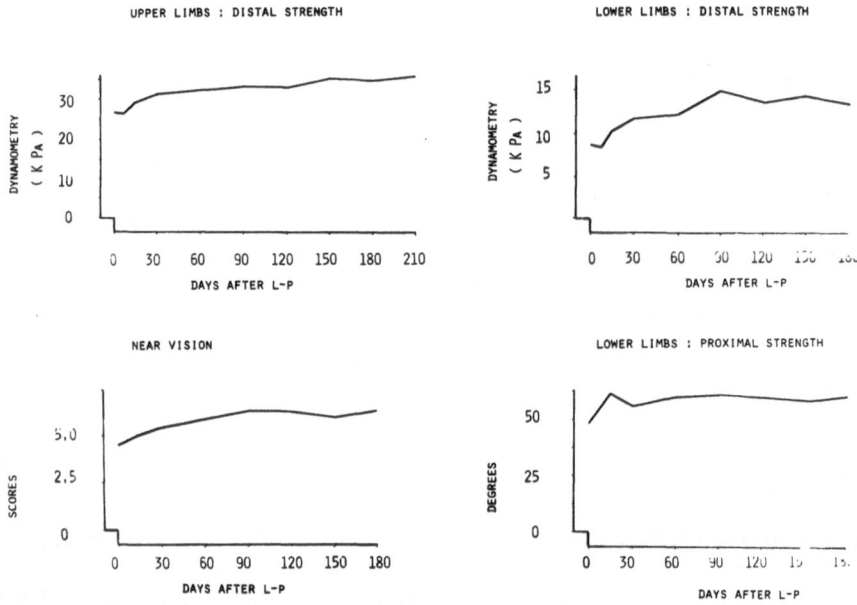

Figure 1 Clinical effects of L-P

RESULTS

The treatment was unrealizable in two cases for vein access reasons and two subjects renounced L-P after 3–6 sessions.

In protocol II, two cases out of the eight treated worsened after 2 months and the programme was stopped.

Effect of L-P on neurologic tests

As illustrated in Figure 1, a significant but modest improvement was observed for upper or lower muscular strengths and visual testings.

The visual acuity measured with the near vision method of Jaeger, showed increased scores in 62% of patients. The improvement became to be significant after 2 months ($p \leqslant 0.02$) and remained so during the next 5 months.

The distal muscular strengths of upper and lower limbs were evaluated by dynamometry. An enhancement of the scores was obtained in 78% of patients for both upper (UL) and lower limbs (LL) while the values remained unchanged in 17% (UL) and 22% (LL), worsened in 4% (UL) and 0% (LL). The statistical significance of the effect was obtained after 15 days for both UL and LL ($p \leqslant 0.01$).

The proximal muscular strength of the legs was tested by estimating the capacity to lift up the overstrained legs from the bed. Only 41% of patients enhanced their score but 59% remained stable. The statistical significance of the changes was only reached after 2 months.

Effect of L-P on self assessment scores

The self assessment scores obtained in 12 MS patients scarcely increased, but with statistical significance ($p < 0.05$–$p < 0.005$) (Table 3). Indeed, 9 of the 12 patients improved their values. Each score corresponded to the sum of the monthly mean's score collated daily from 5 to 6 self-evaluating tests, based on walking, continence, manual and working skills.

Table 3 Self-evaluation scores during L-P

| | \multicolumn{6}{c}{Months} | | | | | |
	1	*2*	*3*	*4*	*5*	*6*
Scores:						
M	12.0	12.8	13.9	14.3	14.2	14.0
SD	4.2	4.1	3.9	3.9	4.7	4.2
N	12	12	12	12	9	8
P		0.05	0.02	0.001	0.005	0.01

The subjective and miction trouble evaluations after 6 months L-P are shown on Table 4. No worsening of subjective impressions could be observed. Interestingly, 10 MS became asymptomatic for miction trouble after several weeks of treatment.

Table 4 Subjective and miction troubles evaluation after 6 months lymphoplasmapheresis

	Worsened	Unchanged	Improved	Asymptomatic
Subjective impressions ($n = 22$)	0	6	16	0
Miction troubles ($n = 14$)	0	1	3	10

n = number of subjects

Effect of L-P on humoral and cellular immunity

The levels of immunoglobulins and complement fractions fell to 50% of basic values, immediately after L-P (Table 5). Normal values were restored for IgG, which remained scarcely lowered at 6 months (17 days after the last session).

Table 5 Effect of L-P on blood imunoglobulin and complement levels

	Levels			
			Times	
	0	0 + L-P	1 month	6 months
IgA'	195 ± 47	82 ± 17^{xxx}	152 ± 36^{x}	196 ± 36
IgG'	930 ± 110	404 ± 41^{xxx}	658 ± 87^{xxx}	708 ± 86^{xxx}
IgM'	166 ± 51	76 ± 36^{xxx}	162 ± 47	178 ± 35
C_3'	66 ± 13	37 ± 3^{xxx}	64 ± 35	64 ± 13
C_4'	93 ± 11	48 ± 3^{xxx}	92 ± 8	92 ± 9
Ct"	31 ± 9	18 ± 3	32 ± 13	33 ± 12

' = mg%ml   " = CH100/ml

Table 6 Role of the immune status on clinical response to L-P

	Low responders	High responders
Clinical response	88 ± 35 (8)	100 ± 70 (6)

Clinical response was evaluated by calculating the increase of total scores after 6 months L-P and expressed in % of total scores before starting the treatment ($\pm$ SM).
In parenthesis: number of subjects evaluated.
Detailed studies for each test did not show any significant difference between the two groups (one way variance analysis test).

Changes in cell mediated immunity are described in another paper in this book. It should be pointed out here that the clinical scores and clinical responses to L-P were not correlated with the status of low or normal proliferative response to T mitogens (Table 6).

DISCUSSION

The results presented in this work suggest that longterm L-P may improve some clinical and immunological parameters in progressive or remittent–progressive (without recent acute relapse) phase.

The functional changes were modest, observed as early as 15 days, and persisted during the 6 month period of treatment. The selection of non-acute forms makes the spontaneous remissions improbable. In addition, since the treatment was realized on ambulant subjects and did not require hospitalization for more than 3–4 hours at each L-P session, there were no changes in life habits. Nevertheless, the authors cannot exclude a placebo effect in response to therapeutic effort. Within the aim to minimize such a factor, a longitudinal study is actually performed, comparing the disease's evolution during or after L-P regimens.

Symptom improvements have already been reported with plasmapheresis[12-15] associated or not with immunosuppressive drugs. The treatment could act by removing neuroelectrical blocking agents[16] and has been demonstrated to reduce IgG levels in cerebrospinal fluid[13].

Some works reviewed by McFarland and Rose[17] suggest that lymphocytapheresis could also stabilize patients with a slow progressive course. These observations are in contrast with those from Giordano et al[18] who found a better response in relapsing–remitting diseases.

Since L-P combined plasmapheresis and lymphocytapheresis, the question whether the first or the second form of the therapy is active in our study remained to be determined. Indeed, on the one hand, analysis of the cell mediated immune parameters, published elsewhere in this book[19] indicates that L-P correct reduced proliferative response to mitogens in some deficient subjects. However, we have been unable to establish a relation between immune parameters and clinical status. On the other hand, our patients were exposed to decreased levels of immunoglobulins from half of the blood levels to normal values. It is difficult to attribute to such a minor change of humoral immunity, the principal action of L-P.

Thus the mode of L-P activity on PFMS or PRMS remains to be elucidated.

SUMMARY

Thirty four MS patients who gave informed consent, were submitted to a long course of lympho-plasmapheresis (L-P) (Protocol I: 1 L-P/week for the first 3 weeks, followed by 1 LP/3 weeks for 6 months = P1; Protocol II: 1 L-P/week during 3 months: P2). Only remitting–progressive or progressive forms of L-P were selected. Symptoms and neurologic (with functional scores) examinations were collected prior to each L-P session. Twelve subjects completed a daily checklist of self-assessment on their functional activity. The treatment was not realized in four cases for vein access difficulties or renouncement.

In P1 (22 MS) no exacerbation could be observed and symptoms, neurologic testings and miction troubles improved in about 70%. A significant effect of L-P appeared as soon as after 2 weeks, persisting during the 6 months.

In P2 (8 MS), 2 cases worsened after 2 months and the programme was stopped.

Finally, the clinical benefit induced by L-P on PFMS or PRMS was not correlated with immune changes observed during the course of therapy.

References

1. McFarlin, D. E. and McFarland, H. F. (1982). Multiple sclerosis I. *N. Engl. J. Med.*, **307**, 1183
2. McFarlin, D. E. and McFarland, H. F. (1982). Multiple sclerosis II. *N. Engl. J. Med.*, **307**, 1246
3. Lisak, R., Zweiman, B. and Norman, M. (1975). Antimyelin antibodies in neurologic diseases. *Arch. Neurol.*, **32**, 163
4. Abramsky, O., Lisak, R., Silverberg, D., Pleasure, D. and George, J. (1977). Antibodies to oligodendroglia in patients with multiple sclerosis. *N. Engl. J. Med.*, **297**, 1207
5. Wolfgram, F. and Duquette, I. (1976). Demyelinating antibodies in multiple sclerosis. *Neurology*, **26**, 68
6. Tachovsky, T., Lisak, R., Koprowski, H. Theofilopoulos, A. and Dixon, F. (1976). Circulating immune complexes in multiple sclerosis and other neurological diseases. *Lancet*, **ii**, 997
7. Arnason, B. and Waksman, B. (1980). Immunoregulation in multiple sclerosis. *Ann. Neurol*, **8**, 237
8. Reinherz, E., Weiner, H., Hauser, S., Cohen, J., Distaso, B. and Schlossman, S. (1980). Loss of suppressor T cells in active multiple sclerosis. *N. Engl. J. Med.*, **303**, 125
9. Cashman, N., Martin, C., Eizenbaum, J. F. and Degos, J. D. (1982). Monoclonal antibody-defined immunoregulatory cells in multiple sclerosis cerebrospinal fluid. *J. Clin. Invest*, **70**, 387
10. Schauf, C., Schauf, V. and Davis, F. A. (1978). Complement dependent serum neuroelectric blocking activity in multiple sclerosis. *Neurology*, **28**, 426
11. Cohen, S., Herndon, R. and McKahnn, G. (1976). Radioimmuno-assay of myelin basic protein in spinal fluid: an index of active demyelination. *N. Engl. J. Med.*, **295**, 1455
12. Schauf, C., Stefoski, D., Davis, F. and McLeod, B. (1979). Concerning the application of plasmapheresis to multiple sclerosis. *Plasma Therapy*, **1**, 33
13. Weiner, H. and Dawson, D. (1980). Plasmapheresis in multiple sclerosis: preliminary study. *Neurology*, **30**, 1029
14. Dau, P., Petajan, J., Johnson K., Panitch, H. and Bornstein, M. (1980). Plasmapheresis in multiple sclerosis: preliminary findings. *Neurology*, **30**, 1023
15. Tindall, R., Walker, J. Ehle, A., Near, L., Rollins, J. and Becker, D. (1982). Plasmapheresis in multiple sclerosis: prospective trial of pheresis and immunosuppression versus immunosuppression alone. *Neurology*, **32**, 739
16. Stefoski, D., Schauf, I., McLeod, B., Haywood, C. and Davis, F. (1982). Plasmapheresis decreases neuroelectric blocking activity in multiple sclerosis. *Neurology*, **32**, 904
17. McFarland, H. and Rose, J. (1982). Lymphocytapheresis in the treatment of multiple sclerosis. *Plasma Therapy*, **3**, 411
18. Giordano, G., Masland, W., Ketchel, S., Holland, K., Tilmann, K., Wallace, B. and Jones, R. (1982). An investigation of lymphocytapheresis in multiple sclerosis. *Plasma Therapy*, **3**, 417
19. Kennes, B., Leroy, C. P., Dumont, J. P., Faverly, D., Brohée, D., Jacquy, J., Noël, G. and Nève, P. (1983). Cell mediated immunity in progressive forms of multiple sclerosis treated by lympho-plasmapheresis. In Gonsette, R. E. and Delmotte, P. (eds.). *Immunological Aspects of Multiple Sclerosis*. chap. P11. (Lancaster: MTP Press)

31
Plasmapheresis in multiple sclerosis: cerebrospinal fluid changes after treatment

R. CAPPARELLI, D. INZITARI, D. SITÀ, B. M. GUARNIERI, L. FRATIGLIONI, L. AMADUCCI, G. AVANZI, C. FRANCO and R. LOMBARDO

INTRODUCTION

Although the pathogenesis of multiple sclerosis (MS) is unknown, much evidence suggests that MS is an immunologically mediated disorder in which demyelinating factors have been detected in serum and in cerebrospinal fluid (CSF)[1-4]. In MS sera 'blocking factors', possibly auto-antibodies, have been shown to affect nerve conduction in vitro[5]. Unconcentrated CSF from MS patients in acute relapse can produce demyelination of tadpole optic nerves[6]. Moreover, circulating immune complexes have been described in MS[7,8]. Preliminary reports indicated a possible benefit from plasma exchanges (PE) in MS patients[9,10]. In order to study the effect of PE in CSF and serum IgG, we studied 18 MS patients, treated with a cycle of PE.

MATERIALS AND METHODS

18 patients (Table 1) with definite MS, 11 in the active phase and 7 in the inactive phase, sex ratio M/F 6/12, were submitted to PE.

Table 1 Plasmapheresis in MS

Patients	(n)	18
Sex ratio	(M/F)	6/12
Average age	(years)	39 ± 9
Duration of disease	(years)	11 ± 7
Stage:		
active	(n)	11
inactive	(n)	7

The CSF and serum analysis was carried out before and after six PE associated with azathioprine at biweekly intervals. Azathioprine, 2.5 mg/kg, was given at the onset of PE, and continued during the treatment. Approximately 3 litres of plasma were changed each time. CSF and serum albumin, CSF and serum IgG, CSF/blood albumin ratio[11] and IgG index[12] were analyzed using radial immune diffusion[13]. CSF oligoclonal IgG bands were detected by agar gel electrophoresis[14]. CSF cell count was performed using a Nageotte camera.

RESULTS

No significant differences in serum and CSF albumin, CSF/blood albumin and cell count were found (Tables 2, 3 and 4). CSF oligoclonal bands remained the same after PE in all patients. Significant differences in serum IgG were detected (Table 3). The mean value of serum IgG showed a marked decrease after PE: from 1030 ± 190 mg/dl vs. 470 ± 140 mg/dl ($p < 0.001$). Also the mean CSF IgG value decreased significantly after PE: 7.2 ± 6 mg/dl before vs. 5.9 ± 6.5 mg after ($p < 0.005$). The mean Link IgG index value increased (almost doubled) after PE: 1.08 ± 0.6 before vs. 2.06 ± 2 after ($p < 0.02$).

Table 2 Plasmapheresis in MS. CSF parameters before and after treatment

| | | | Treatment | |
		Before	After	p
Albumin	(n.v. < 33.1 mg/dl)	22.7 ± 8.9	22.6 ± 10.5	n.s.
IgG	(n.v. < 5.2 mg/dl)	7.2 ± 6	5.9 ± 6.5	<0.005
IgG/albumin	(n.v. < 0.20	0.3 ± 0.18	0.26 ± 0.2	n.s.
Cell count/mm^3	(n.v. < 3 mm^3)	3.3 ± 2	2.7 ± 1.9	n.s.

n.s. = not significant   n.v. = normal values

Table 3 Plasmapheresis in MS. Serum parameters before and after treatment

| | | Treatment | | |
		Before	After	p
Albumin	(n.v. 2950–4800 mg/dl)	3540 ± 390	3620 ± 440	n.s.
IgG	(n.v. 700–1800 mg/dl)	1030 ± 190	470 ± 140	<0.001

n.s. = not significant   n.v. = normal values

Table 4 Plasmapheresis in MS. CSF/blood ratios before and after treatment

| | Treatment | | |
	Before	After	p
CSF/blood albumin ratio (n.v. < 0.0087)	0.0064 ± 0.0027	0.0074 ± 0.0068	n.s.
IgG index (Link) (n.v. < 0.61)	1.08 ± 0.64	2.06 ± 2.18	<0.02

n.s. = not significant   n.v. = normal values

DISCUSSION

We studied the changes of some CSF and serum parameters in a group of MS patients treated with PE.

The therapeutical efficacy of PE in MS has not yet been completely proved[9,10,15-17].

According to the findings of Dau[9] and Weiner[10] our data show that PE lowers the CSF IgG level significantly and in a short time: such a finding could be a consequence of the drastic reduction of serum IgG level determined by PE[9].

In the same connection, the increase of IgG index value is possibly due to the fact that serum IgG levels decrease more than CSF IgG.

The finding that PE lowers the CSF IgG level appears important because several studies have shown some possible correlations between high CSF IgG levels and MS clinical activity[18,19]. However, the immunologic significance and the role in relation to MS of removed IgG, need to be further investigated.

References

1. Lisak, R. P., Zweiman, B. and Norman, M. (1975). Antimyelin antibodies in neurological diseases. *Arch. Neurol.*, **32**, 163
2. Bornstein, M. B. and Raine, C. S. (1977). Multiple sclerosis and experimental allergic encephalomyelitis: specific demyelination of CNS in culture. *Neuropathol. Appl. Neurobiol.*, **3**, 359
3. Ryberg, B. (1978). Multiple specificities of antibrain antibodies in multiple sclerosis and chronic myelopathy. *J. Neurol. Sci.*, **38**, 357
4. Panitch, H. S., Hooper, C. J. and Johnson, K. P. (1980). Cerebrospinal fluid antibody to myelin basic protein: measurement in patients with multiple sclerosis and subacute sclerosing panencephalitis. *Arch. Neurol.*, **37**, 206
5. Schauf, C. L., Schauf, V., Davis, F. A. et al. (1978). Complement-dependent serum: neuroelectric blocking activity in multiple sclerosis. *Neurology*, **28**, 426
6. Tabira, T., Webster, H. de F. and Wray, S. H. (1976). Multiple sclerosis cerebrospinal fluid produces myelin lesions in tadpole optic nerves. *N. Engl. J. Med.*, **295**, 644
7. Tachovsky, T. G., Lisak, R. P., Koprowski, H. et al. (1976). Circulating immune complexes in multiple sclerosis and other neurological diseases. *Lancet*, **2**, 997
8. Goust, J. M., Chenais, F., Carnes, J. E. et al. (1978). Abnormal T-cell population and circulating immune complexes in the Guillain–Barré syndrome and multiple sclerosis. *Neurology*, **28**, 421
9. Dau, P., Patajan, J. H., Johnson, K. P., Panitch, H. S. and Bornstein, M. B. (1980). Plasmapheresis in multiple sclerosis: preliminary findings. *Neurology*, **30**, 1023
10. Weiner, H. L. and Dawson, D. M. (1980). Plasmapheresis in multiple sclerosis: preliminary study. *Neurology*, **30**, 1029
11. Tourtellotte, W. W. and Booe, I. M. (1978). Multiple sclerosis: the blood–brain barrier and the measurement of *de novo* central nervous system IgG synthesis. *Neurology*, **28**, 76
12. Tibbling, G. H., Link, H. and Ohman, S. (1977). Principles of albumin and IgG analyses in neurological disorders. 1. Establishment of reference values. *Scand. J. Clin. Lab. Invest.*, **37**, 385
13. Mancini, G., Carbonara, A. D. and Heremans, J. F. (1956). Immunochemical quantitation of antigens by single radial immunodiffusion. *Immunochemistry*, **2**, 235
14. Lowenthal, W., Van Sande, M. and Karcher, D. (1960). The differential diagnosis of neurological diseases by fractionating electrophoretically the proteins. *J. Neurochem.*, **6**, 51
15. Warren, K. G., Gordon, P. A. and McPherson, T. A. (1982). Plasma exchanges of malignant multiple sclerosis. *J. Can. Sci. Neurol.*, **9**, 27

16. Hauser, S. L., Dawson, D. M., Lehrich, J. R., Beal, M. F. *et al.* (1983). Intensive immuno-suppression in progressive multiple sclerosis. *N. Engl. J. Med.,* **27,** 173
17. Tindal, R. S. A. (1981). Plasmapheresis in multiple sclerosis: prospective randomized trial of pheresis and immunosuppression. *Neurology,* **31,** 137
18. Bradshaw, P. (1964). The relation between clinical activity and the level of gamma globulin in the cerebrospinal fluid in patients with multiple sclerosis. *J. Neurol. Sci.,* **1,** 374
19. Olsson, J. E., Link, H. and Muller, R. (1976). Immunoglobulin abnormalities in multiple sclerosis. Relation to clinical parameters: Disability, duration and age of onset. *J. Neurol. Sci.,* **27,** 233

32
Transfer factor treatment in MS: A 3 year prospective double-blind study (1982–1985)

H. VAN HAVER, F. LISSOIR, P. THEYS, Chr. DROISSART, J. VAN HEES, P. KETELAER, H. CARTON, K. GAUTAMA, I. VANDEPUTTE and C. VERMYLEN

Several clinical trials with transfer factor (TF)[1-3] carried out in the 1970s, showed no beneficial effect on multiple sclerosis (MS) patients.

However in 1980, Basten et al[4] published a clinical study performed in 60 MS-patients, showing a reduction of the progression of MS in patients treated with TF. The reason why Basten could show positive results could have been first because he followed his patients for a much longer period (24 months), the difference becoming significant only after 18 months. A second reason might have been that he used TF from relatives and not from random donors.

In 1981 another promising trial with TF was published by Lamoureux et al[5]. We decided to set up a new prospective study, (1) over a longer follow-up period (3 years) and (2) to look for a possible differential effect of TF from MS relatives and TF from random donors. In addition we chose other immunological parameters.

PATIENTS

Patients had to fulfil the criteria of Schumacher[6], to enter the study. Relapsing–remitting as well as chronic progressive cases were admitted, but patients with no disease progression for more than 3 years were excluded. Only patients able to walk (with or without canes, crutches or braces) were admitted (maximum disability score on Kurtzke scale of 6). All patients were in a stable phase for at least 3 months before the start of the therapy. We started with 105 patients (49 men and 56 women) divided into three groups: a placebo group, a group receiving TF from random donors and a group receiving TF from relatives. Patients were randomized, taking into account the age of the patients, the sex and the disability.

The mean age of disease onset in our patients is 31.6 years: the mean age at entering the trial is 39.84 years. 80.6% of the patients have or had a relapsing–remitting type of disease course: 19.4% a chronic progressive disease from onset. All patients are typed for HLA-A-, B-, C- and D-haplotypes.

Therapy

The total duration of treatment is planned to be 3 years. The frequency of administration is the same as in Basten's study[4]: every 2 weeks for 1 month, then every 4 weeks during 6 months, finally every 8 weeks (= 25 injections in total, each containing 5×10^8 cell equivalent). TF is prepared by the blood transfusion center in Leuven (Red Cross of Belgium).

Besides TF or placebo each patient receives the normal treatment, e.g. muscular relaxants, physical therapy and, if required, steroids. Other immunosuppressive treatment is excluded.

Evaluation

The evaluation is double-blind.

(1) Every time the patient receives an injection he is asked about the side-effects of the treatment, and relapses during the previous interval. Duration and severity of the relapses are scored.
(2) Before entering the trial, and every 9th month, an extensive evaluation is performed.

Clinical evaluation:

Neurological examination
Functional and overall disability scoring (Kurtzke scale) performed by the same neurologist.
Melsbroek disability scale performed by a physical therapist, and which in addition codes for activities of daily living.

Electrophysiological evaluation:

Visual, brainstem and somatosensory evoked potentials, scored according to scale given in Table 1.

Immunological evaluation:

Measurement of the interferon production
in vivo: measurement of the 2.5 oligo-adenylate synthetase concentration
in vitro: measurement of the endogenous interferon production after stimulation with Sendai virus and Concanavalin A.
Evaluation of the natural killer cell activity.

Table 1 Scores of evoked potentials in MS

VEP: each eye is evaluated separately
      0 : normal
      1 : normal latency of P1$\overline{0}$0, but abnormal configuration of the response (form and amplitude)
2.0–2.9 : increased latency of P1$\overline{0}$0 at 200 ms (with or without abnormal configuration)
      3 : increased latency of P1$\overline{0}$0 more than 200 ms or no answer detectable

Maximum score for one eye = 3

BAEP: each ear is evaluated separately
      0 : normal
      1 : prolonged I–III ⎫ additive
      1 : prolonged III–V ⎭
      1 : prolonged I–V (without prolonged I–III or III–V)
      1 : abnormal low amplitude of IV–V complex (less than half wave I)
      3 : absence of wave V or of wave IV and V or of wave III, IV and V

Maximum score for ear = 4

SSEP: scoring each limb

N. medianus:
– normal   0
– normal latency for N$\overline{2}$0 but abnormal configuration   1
  (too low amplitude, absence of one or more waves)
– absence of N$\overline{2}$0   2
– abnormal latency but less than 40 ms   2.0–2.9
  (with or without abnormal configurations)
– latency greater than 40 ms or no response detectable   3

N. peroneus or N. saphenus:
– normal   0
– normal latency but abnormal configuration   1
– prolonged latency but less than 100 ms   2.0–2.9
– latency greater than 100 ms or no response detectable   3

TOTAL SCORE: 0–26

RESULTS

After 1 year of therapy without breaking the code of the double-blind study we can give only some impressions.

(1) *Drop-outs*: two patients dropped out: one committed suicide, another became pregnant.
Basten[4] also noted a small number of drop-outs. This compares very favourably with the results of immunosuppressive studies. For example Patzold[7] noted up to 25% of drop-outs after 1 year of treatment. Although he doesn't give an explanation for this high number of drop-outs, we believe that side-effects and toxicity of azathiaprine play an important role.

(2) *Side-effects*: we didn't note any major side-effect with transfer factor after 1 year of therapy. But about one fifth of the patients complained of fatigue, headache, injection pains, erythema.

(3) *Disability scores* (*Kurtzke scale*)
 mean disability score at onset: *3.48*
 (min.: 1, max.: 7, SD: 1.80)
 mean disability score after 9 months: *3.51*
 (min.: 0, max.: 7.5, SD: 1.95)
 changes in disability score:
  65% of the patients remain stable
  17.5% improve
  17.5% get worse.

 Melsbroek disability scale
 mean disability score at onset: *171.55*
 (min.: 7, max.: 895, SD: 161.10)
 mean disability score after 9 months: *181.563*
 (min.: 0, max.: 1027, SD: 189.278)
 changes in disability score: see (3)
  45.6% remain stable
  27.2% improve
  27.2% get worse.

(4) *Relapses*:

0 relapses	:	71.84%	– 74 patients
1 relapse	:	23.30%	– 24 patients
2 relapses	:	3.88%	– 4 patients
3 relapses	:	0.97%	– 1 patient
mean = 0.33			

One can expect this number of relapses in a normal MS population without specific treatment.

The clinical data were correlated with sex, pattern of evolution (relapsing–remitting or chronic progressive) and HLA-DR2 haplotype. However, no significant correlation has been found.

Electrophysiological evaluation

Visual evoked potentials:
 20.58% get worse
 17.66% improve
 61.76% remain stable

Somatosensory evoked potentials:
 34.3% get worse
 15.7% improve
 52.0% remain stable

Brainstem auditory evoked potentials:
 13.7% get worse
 9.8% improve
 76.5% remain stable

Concerning the electrophysiological results we note no evolution. There was no correlation between the changes in disability and the changes in evoked potentials.

CONCLUSIONS

After 9 months of therapy there is no significant progression in the group taken as a whole. Furthermore, the number of improvements equals the number of deteriorations. Since we didn't break the code it is impossible to interpret these results. They could be the result of a placebo effect on all patients, or the effect of TF on a portion of the patients.

References

1. Behan, P. O., Meluille, I. D., Durward, W. F., McGeorge, A. P. and Behan, W. M. H. (1976). Transfer factor therapy in multiple sclerosis. *Lancet*, 988
2. Fog, T. *et al.* (1978). Long-term transfer factor treatment for multiple sclerosis. *Lancet*, 851.
3. Collins, R. C., Espinoza, L. R., Plank, C. R., Ebers, G. C., Rosenberg, R. A. and Rabriskie, J. B. (1978). A double-blind trial of transfer factor vs. placebo in multiple sclerosis patients. *Clin. Exp. Immunol.*, **33**, 1
4. Basten, A., McLeod, J. G., Pollard, J. D., Walsh, J. C., Stewart, Q. J., Ganick, R., Frith, J. A. and Van Der Brink, C. M. (1980). Transfer factor in treatment of multiple sclerosis. *Lancet*, 931.
5. Lamoureux, G., Cosgrove, J., Duguette, P., Lapierre, Y., Jolicoeur, R. and Vanderland, F. (1981). A clinical and immunological study of the effects of transfer factor on multiple sclerosis patients. *Clin. Exp. Immunol.*, **43**, 557
6. Schumacher, G. A. *et al.* (1965). Problems of experimental trials of therapy in multiple sclerosis. *Ann. NY. Acad. Sci.*, **122**, 552
7. Patzold, V., Hecker, H. and Micklington, P. (1982). Azathioprine in treatment of multiple sclerosis. *J. Neurol. Sci.*, **54**, 377

33
Experiences with immunoglobulin-G infusions in the treatment of acute multiple sclerosis

W. GUENTHER, I. S. NEU, N. KOENIG and U. ROTHFELDER

SUMMARY

In the course of the 12 month trial, 20 patients (14 male, 6 female) aged between 18 and 42 years, and suffering from multiple sclerosis showing an intermittent course of exacerbations and remissions, were treated at 2 month intervals with a preparation of immunoglobulin G, administered by intravenous infusion.

There was a highly significant fall in the FOG-scale scores, from 28.8 to 21.3. Particular improvement was seen in cranial nerve functions and in symptoms due to brainstem lesions. The mean exacerbation rate was 1.13 before treatment and fell to 1.02 after 6 months and to 0.99 after 12 months treatment with IgG. In addition to the clinical parameters (which also included self-ratings of the patients), other parameters were assessed, such as immunological data, latencies of acoustically induced brainstem potentials and the cytotoxicity of lymphocytes.

The results are compared to those of immunosuppressant therapy, and possible modes of action are discussed.

INTRODUCTION

This line in the treatment of patients with multiple sclerosis (MS) is based on reports that the cytotoxicity of lymphocytes against basic myelin sheath protein can be demonstrated in 80% of cases during an acute exacerbation and in 50% of cases between exacerbations[1-3]. Additionally, it is based on clinical observations, that acute exacerbations of MS can be influenced by the administration of human immunoglobulin G (IgG).

Treatment with IgG could possibly be explained on the basis that the IgG molecules might change the cytotoxicity of lymphocytes in MS. To clarify the question, whether an intravenously administered compound of the IgG class is able to penetrate the cerebrospinal fluid (CSF) barrier, despite its high molecular weight, pre-investigation studies have been made[4].

Twelve anti-HBs negative patients received 20 ml each of a β-propiolacton treated IgG compound with a high anti-HBs-titre (1 : 115 000) as a marker. Four patients having an inconspicuous CSF condition were included as controls. Five patients were suffering from slight disturbances and three others from severe disorders of the blood–CSF–barrier function resulting from inflammatory diseases of their central nervous system. CSF was collected by lumbar puncture or drainage for the determination of anti-HBs. Simultaneously, the concentration of antibodies in the serum was determined.

Table 1 shows the results in healthy controls.

With regard to the calculation of the γ-globulin concentration in CSF presented in Tables 1–3, we feel the following explanation is needed.

In a healthy adult we find γ-globulin levels of 9.8%, with a standard deviation of 2.88%, in the lumbar fluid in relation to the total protein content. This corresponds to an (absolute) concentration of 1.3–5.3 mg γ-globulin per 100 ml CSF. On the other hand, the serum contains an average of 1160 mg γ-globulin per 100 ml. Thus, 0.10–0.45% of the γ-globulin concentrations present in the serum are evident in the CSF.

Presuming that the shares of major immunoglobulin classes found in the CSF correspond to the serum values, the concentration of the IgG class in the CSF of individuals not suffering from barrier disorders may be assumed to amount to 1.1–4.7 mg per 100 ml.

Regarding the percentage of IgG anti-HBs immunoglobulin of the simultaneous serum concentration present in the CSF of individuals, who had been administered the hyperimmunoglobulin, it seems to be evident that the values are within the limit of the theoretical estimates (Table 1). However, the marker protein could only be proven evident in the CSF of two of the four patients examined, the level of the marker in the others being too low to be traced by our laboratory methods.

Table 2 summarizes the analogous values in patients suffering from slight barrier disturbances. It is obvious that the percentage of anti-HBs titre in the CSF is higher in these patients, compared to the healthy controls (Tables 1 and 2, last column).

The negative findings after 9 and 13 days, respectively, in patients 8 and 9 can be explained by the considerable drop of the titres in the CSF below the traceable level, supported by the wellknown halflife of IgG molecules[5]. Table 3 lists the titres found in patients suffering from severe barrier disorders. Distinctly increased anti-HBs titres were found in all these patients with severe barrier disorders due to serious inflammatory CSF syndromes.

Thus, based on the results of this pre-investigation study, it could be presumed that intravenously administered γ-globulins penetrate the CSF barrier, and may have a therapeutic influence in the case of inflammation and infection of the central nervous system.

Table 1 Control patients without blood-brain-barrier disturbance

No.	Name	Diagnosis	Cell count	CSF protein mg/100 ml	Sample with-drawal time	Reciprocal in serum	Anti-HBs titre in CSF	% anti-HBs in CSF
1	G.W.	Unspecific headache	12/3	38	4 d	1200	neg.	neg.
2	T.S.	Anterior spinal artery occlusion syndrome	8/3	26	2 d	120	neg.	neg.
3	B.H.	Cerebral contusion	12/3	45	3 h	512	neg.	neg.
					6 h	512	2	0.39
					9 h	1000	2	0.20
					12 h	512	2	0.20
					24 h	512	2	0.20
					48 h*	512	1	0.20
					3 d	512	± pos.	pos.
					5 d	256	neg.	neg.
4	W.G.	Condition after bacterial meningitis (liquor sterile)	8/3	26	3 h	512	2	0.39
					6 h	512	1	0.2
					9 h	512	2	0.39
					12 h	512	1	0.2
					24 h	512	2	0.39
					36 h	512	2	0.39
					48 h*	256	2	0.39
					3 d	256	2	0.78
					5 d	256	2	0.78

*CSF drainage

168

Table 2 Patients with mild blood-brain-barrier disturbance. CSF cell count up to 500/3 cells, total CSF protein up to 100 mg/100 ml

No.	Name	Diagnosis	Cell count	CSF protein mg/100 ml	Sample with-drawal time	Reciprocal in serum	Anti-HBs titre in CSF	% anti-HBs in CSF
5	V.R.	Multiple sclerosis	41/3	58	24 h	980	7	0.71
6	L.V.	Zoster meningoencephalitis	58/3	52	3 d	580	8	0.74
7	P.G.	Meningoencephalitis	100/3	80	24 h	1400	12	0.86
8	Sch.H.	Encephalitis	18/3	54	24 h	390	1 or 2	0.26 or 0.51
					72 h*	145	2	1.38
					9 d	62	neg.	neg.
9	U.R.	Meningoencephalitis	500/3	71	24 h	512	1	0.78
					54 h	512	4	0.78
					76 h*	512	4	0.78
					6 d	128	1	0.78
					13 d	32	neg.	neg.

*CSF drainage

Table 3 Patients with severe blood-brain-barrier disturbance. CSF cell count over 500/3 cells, total CSF protein over 100 mg/100 ml

No.	Name	Diagnosis	Cell count	CSF protein mg/100 ml	Sample withdrawal time	Reciprocal in serum	Anti-HBs titre in CSF	% anti-HBs in CSF
10	N.C.	Meningoradiculitis	1123/3	184	9 d	600	23	3.83
11	L.R.	Meningoencephalitis	1410/3	161	4 d	512	8	1.56
					14 d	128	4	3.13
					21 d	64	2	3.13
12	E.A.	Meningogoccal meningitis	2000/3	192	3 h	512	4	0.78
					6 h	512	4	0.78
					9 h	512	4	0.78
					12 h	512	4	0.78
					24 h	512	8	1.56
					36 h	512	8	1.56
					48 h*	512	8	1.56
					3 d	256	8	3.13
					5 d	128	4	3.13

*CSF drainage

EXPERIMENTAL PROCEDURE AND METHODS

Our pilot study to assess therapeutic effects of IgG-infusions in the treatment of acute MS included 20 patients, 14 females and 6 males, aged between 18 and 42 years. The criterion for admission to the clinical trial was the presence of a disease pattern characterized by exacerbations, with at least three exacerbations prior to the admission. Criteria for exclusion were a disease course which was primarily chronic and progressive, longterm treatment with azathioprine and/or steroids or severe associated disease.

Each patient received an infusion of human immunoglobulin in a preparation suitable for intravenous use (Intraglobin R, 100 ml $\hat{=}$ 5 g–Biotest, Frankfurt, FRG), at 2 month intervals. The clinical treatment extended over a period of 12 months.

The following investigations were carried out at the beginning of the study and after the end of the course of infusions after 1 year:

(1) The usual serum and laboratory investigations, such as enzymes, substances excreted in the urine, serum lipids, electrolytes, differential blood count, coagulation parameters, serum electrophoresis and immunoglobulins G, A, M, and E

(2) The determination of HLA-A at the beginning

(3) Latency time of acoustically induced brainstem potentials

(4) Clinical neurological examination, using the FOG-scale[6]

(5) Calculation of the mean yearly exacerbation rate (obtained numerically by the number of exacerbations to date – less the first one – divided by the number of years since onset of the MS up to the end of the trial) and comparison of this figure with the exacerbation rate up to the end of the trial

(6) Cytotoxicity test[7,8]

(7) Assessment of the course of the disease on the basis of the patient's notes.

The statistical method applied was the variance analysis of dependent variables.

RESULTS

(1) There were no abnormal findings in the laboratory serum investigations carried out at 6 month intervals. The quantitative measurements of immunoglobulins showed the presence of an antibody deficiency syndrome in four of the cases, and in all of them this returned to normal after therapy with IgG.

A striking finding was a mean significant increase in IgE, which could be interpreted as evidence of an allergic reaction.

(2) Determination of the histocompatibility antigens showed A3 in six patients (30%) and B7 in eight patients (40%). HLA and A1 and 2 were each found in eight patients (40%).

171

(3) Measurements of acoustically-induced brainstem potentials permit functional and topical diagnosis in the region of the brainstem, if there is damage to the afferent auditory tracts as a result of direct or indirect affecting processes. Measurement before treatment showed normal findings in nine patients and pathological changes in another nine.

In one female patient it was possible to demonstrate waves 1–3, and in the remaining eight there was an objectively demonstrable prolongation of the latency between waves 1 and 5. After treatment with immunoglobulins there was a return to normal in the latency in three patients, whereas no change was found in the others.

(4) Clinical neurological examination, using the FOG-scale, showed highly significant reduction in the total and partial scores (Figure 1).

The total score of the FOG-scale (Figure 1) showed a highly significant reduction from 28.8 to 21.3 after 6 months treatment. The same trend

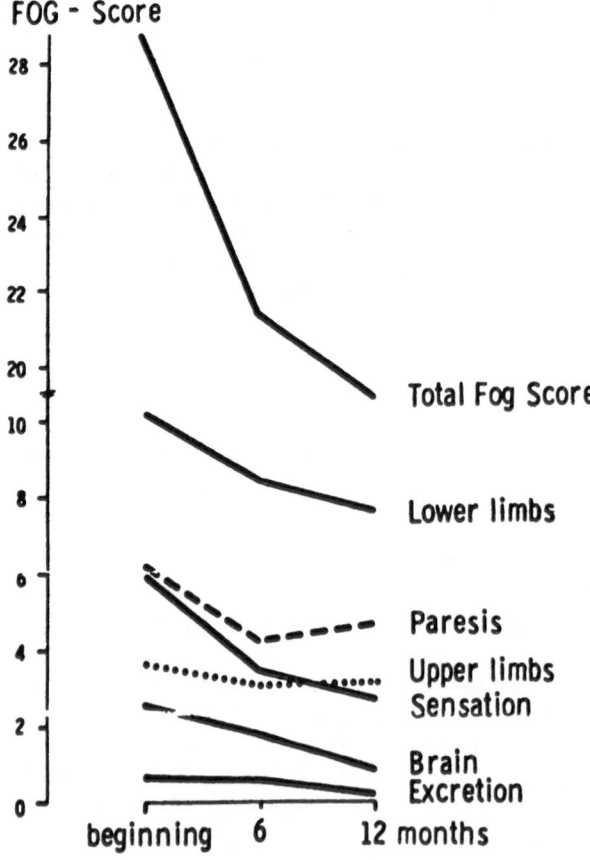

Figure 1 FOG-scores of the clinical neurological examinations during therapy with immunoglobulins

was seen, though to a less pronounced degree, after the second 6 months treatment, with a further reduction to 19 ($p < 10\%$).

Analysis of the data obtained showed the presence of two subgroups, each of which happened to contain just 50% of the patients. One subgroup contained patients who had shown a marked improvement in their FOG-scale scores. Subgroup 2 consisted of patients who had shown only very slight improvements. Interestingly enough, the 'responder'-subgroup contained mostly patients whose symptoms were due to brainstem lesion, although this finding cannot be interpreted yet.

(5) The mean exacerbation rate before treatment was 1.13, and it fell to 1.02 after 6 months and 0.99 after 12 months treatment.

Our assessment of the exacerbation rate, however, must be viewed with caution, since exacerbations are commoner in spring and autumn and these seasons were asymmetrically included in our trial. It must be remembered that an observation period of 1 year is very short in MS-studies.

(6) Before treatment the cytotoxic activity was positive in five patients (25%), while it was negative in all cases at the end of treatment. Further, the cytotoxic activity was increased in one patient after the beginning of the treatment, but was normalized later. Myelin antibodies were found in six patients (30%). After treatment with immunoglobulins they were no longer evident in two patients, whereas they were present in one patient, in whom they had been negative at the beginning.

(7) Self-ratings of the patients in their notes showed slight improvements in both 6 month periods, in the respect, that the majority of them felt psychologically more stable, had greater confidence in their own ability, and some of them had returned to work. One patient recorded deterioration during the treatment. Better psychiatric–psychological investigations in this important field seem to be especially necessary.

DISCUSSION

Among the aetiologic factors involved in the development of MS, it has been suggested that possibly a clinically latent infection with a regionally bound pathogen might have occurred in childhood, which, like a slow virus infection could cause clinical symptoms years later.

The results of immunologic investigations of experimental allergic encephalomyelitis (EAE) in comparison to MS, have given support to the hypothesis that MS too might have an immunological basis, which could possibly be initiated – 'triggered' – by, e.g. viruses or other as yet unknown factors.

Thus, it is possible to isolate serum antibodies against brain lipids and against a basic myelin sheath protein, which indicate the existence of an auto-immune process. In addition, the serum, the CSF and particularly the foci of demyelinization contain glial or myelin toxic antibodies of the γ-globulin types 19S and 7S, which are believed to attack, selectively, the myelin sheath. Above all, however, immunocompetent lymphocytes can be found, which in transfer trial or in tissue culture are able to destroy myelin sheath and glial cells[1-3,9,10].

Based on the theory – supported by animal experiments – that immuno-pathologic reactions play an important role in MS, anti-allergic and immuno-suppressant therapeutic methods have been gaining importance[11-15]. These methods of treatment have not been able to produce too impressive results in the treatment of acute MS so far; furthermore, the treatment is somewhat problematic and hazardous in the respect that it is associated in some cases with severe side-effects.

For the therapeutical action of the immunoglobulin G it could be assumed that receptors on the cell surface of CNS tissue could be competitively inhibited by the antibodies and the immunoglobulins. Furthermore, it should be kept in mind that antibodies which have a cytotoxic effect on target cells in the *in vitro* experiment have this effect suppressed by high levels of IgG. This could have been the possible underlying therapeutic mechanisms in this pilot study designed to gain first clinical experiences in the treatment of acute MS by infusions of immunoglobulin G.

The presented results of our study should be interpreted with particular caution, especially in view of the short observation period of only 12 months. However, the results suggest to a varying degree, that the treatment of acute MS with infusions of IgG is effective, particularly in regard to a significant decrease in the FOG-scale scores of the patients.

The results of the investigations of the cytotoxic activity can, at the moment, neither exclude nor confirm the possibility that the therapeutic effect of IgG in acute MS might be due to a reduction of this activity.

Further investigations are necessary, to establish a possible therapeutic effect of infusions of IgG in the management of acute MS, in particular a blind-randomized–controlled clinical study, which we are beginning at the moment at our Munich clinic.

References

1. Frick, E., Stickl, H. and Zinn, K. H. (1974). Lymphozytentransformation bei multipler Sklerose. Nachweis einer Sensibilisierung gegen basisches Markscheidenprotein. *Klin. Wschr.,* **52,** 238
2. Frick, E. and Stickl, H. (1977). Zur Pathogenese der Multiplen Sklerose. Antikörperabhängige Zytotoxizität von Lymphozyten gegen basisches Protein der Markscheide bei Multipler Sklerose. *Fortschr. Med.,* **95,** 2235
3. Frick, E. and Stickl, H. (1982). Specificity of antibody-dependent lymphocyte cytotoxicity against cerebral tissue constituents in multiple sclerosis. Studies with basic protein of myelin, encephalitogenic peptide. Cerebrosides and gangliosides. *Acta Neurol. Scand.,* **65,** 30
4. Guenther, W. and Neu, J. S. (1983). Investigations of the blood-brain barrier for IgG immunoglobulins in inflammatory CNS-syndromes. *Eur. Neurol.* (in press)
5. Glöckner, W. M., Siebert, H. G., Eggers, H. and Kurz, H. (1980). *Hepatitisprophylaxe durch intravenöses Hyperimmunglobulin. Mitt. der Arbeitsgemeinschaft fur Klinische Nephrologie.* (Göttingen: Vandenhock & Ruprecht)
6. Fog, T. (1965). A scoring system for neurological impairment in multiple sclerosis. *Acta Neurol. Scand.,* **41,** 551

7. Mar, P., Gradl, T. and Dörner, C. (1979). A longitudinal study of immunological parameters in multiple sclerosis. Cytotoxic antibodies. *J. Neurol. Sci.,* **41,** 369
8. Simon, J., Mar, P., Neu, I., Kamm, S. and Schrader, A. (1980). Längsschnittstudie immunologischer Parameter bei Multiple-Sklerose Kranken. *Nervenarzt,* **51,** 176
9. Waksman, B.H. (1980). Experimental allergic encephalomyelitis and the 'autoallergic' disease. *Int. Arch. Allergy.* (Suppl.) **14**
10. Lumsden, E.C. (1972). *Multiple sclerosis.* (London: Churchill Livingstone)
11. Frick, E., Angstwurm, H. and Späth, G. (1971). Immunsuppressive Therapie der Multiplen Sklerose. 1. Vorläufige Mitteilung der Behandlungsergebnisse mit Azathioprin und Antilymphozytenglobulin. *Münchn. Med. Wschr.,* **122,** 221
12. Ring, J., Seifert, J., Lob, G., Coulik, K.., Angstwurm, H., Frick, E., Brass, P., Mertin, J., Backmund, H. and Brendel, W. (1974). Intensive immunosuppression in the treatment of multiple sclerosis. *Lancet,* **2,** 1093
13. Brendel, W., Seifert, J. and Ring, J. (1975). Die klinische Anwendung von Antilymphożytenglobulinen (ALG). *Münchn. Med. Wschr.,* **117,** 1361
14. Lance, E.M., Kremer, M., Abbosh, J., Jones, V., Knight, S. and Medawar, P.B. (1975). Intensive immunosuppression in patients with disseminated sclerosis. I. Clinical response. *Clin. Exp. Immunol.,* **21,** 1
15. Mertin, J. (1977). The evidence justifying immunosuppression therapy in multiple sclerosis. *Proc. R. Soc. Med.,* **70,** 871

34
Dietary supplementation with polyunsaturated fatty acids in acute remitting multiple sclerosis

R. H. DWORKIN, D. BATES, J. H. D. MILLAR, D. W. PATY
and D. A. SHAW

SUMMARY

Fifty eight patients with acute remitting multiple sclerosis were included in a double-blind controlled trial of dietary supplementation with polyunsaturated fatty acids. Patients in the 'treatment' group received a spread containing linoleic acid and those in the 'control' group received oleic acid in a similar spread. There were no significant differences between the composition of the 'treatment' and 'control' groups, nor was there any significant difference in rate of clinical deterioration or frequency of acute exacerbations. There was evidence that exacerbations were of shorter duration and lesser severity in patients whose diet was supplemented with linoleic acid than in 'control' patients.

This cohort of patients was then included in a total series of 172 patients with clinically definite acute remitting multiple sclerosis from centres in Belfast, Newcastle upon Tyne and London, Ontario involved in similar trials. The suspicion that some of the differences noted in the individual trials might vary with respect to severity of the disease has been confirmed by the combined analysis from the three centres. These and other results from the combined figures are discussed and possible reasons for the effects of this therapy identified.

INTRODUCTION

The original suggestion of an association between multiple sclerosis (MS) and the consumption of edible fats was based on epidemiological data relating the prevalence of the disease to variation in diet of different populations[1-4]. Biochemical studies later showed that unsaturated fatty acids were deficient in the brain, serum and red blood cells of patients with multiple sclerosis[5-7]. A specific deficiency of linoleic acid (C18:2ω6) in serum was identified by Thompson[8] though this has not been a constant finding in all groups of patients studied[9,10].

The accumulated evidence, both epidemiological and biochemical, led to a controlled trial of linoleic acid as a dietary supplement in groups of patients with multiple sclerosis in Belfast and London[11]. Seventy five patients completed this trial, 36 in the treatment group who received two doses of sunflower seed oil emulsion providing a total of 17.2 g of linoleic acid per day, and 39 in the control group in which the linoleic acid was replaced by oleic acid to a total of 7.6 g per day. All patients in this trial could walk with or without mechanical aid (Kurtzke Disability Status Score 0–6)[12]. The trial ran for 2 years and the results suggested that relapses were less frequent, less severe and of shorter duration in the linoleic acid supplemented group than in those receiving oleic acid. There was no evidence that the overall rate of clinical deterioration differed in the two groups.

The results of the Belfast/London study[11], although not conclusive, were sufficiently encouraging to prompt the setting up of further trials. In 1974 a trial was begun in Newcastle upon Tyne in which one group of patients was given linoleic acid supplementation as a spread in comparable dosage to the original trial, and a second group which received oleic acid in similar doses[13]. A further trial was begun in London, Ontario in which the vehicles were identical to those used in the original trial[14].

PATIENTS AND METHODS

Fifty eight patients attending the Royal Victoria Infirmary, Newcastle-on-Tyne, with clinically definite acute remitting multiple sclerosis were included, of whom 16 were male (mean age 34 ± 7 years) and 42 female (mean age 33 ± 8 years) (Table 1). Patients were randomly allocated to one of two groups as follows:

Treatment

Patients received linoleic acid in a dose of 23 g/day provided in the form of a spread. Control patients had a similar spread which they took in the same dose as the treatment group, and which provided them with 16 g of oleic acid per day.

On admission to the trial and at approximately 6-weekly intervals patients underwent detailed neurological and functional assessment. The period of follow-up lasted for 2 years and neither patients nor observers knew whether they belonged to a 'treatment' or 'control' group. Overall disability was scored on the Kurtzke Disability Status Scale[12]. All relapses were recorded with particular reference to their duration, site and severity. Relapse severity was scored by the method described by Millar et al[15].

Table 1 Composition of trial groups

| | Acute remitting | |
	Treatment	Control
Patients	29	29
Male	5	11
Female	24	18
Age (M ± SE years)	34 ± 8	33 ± 5
Duration of history (M ± SE years)	7 ± 5	6 ± 3

At entry to the trial, and at between 12 and 24 months thereafter, fasting blood samples were withdrawn from selected patients for fatty acid estimations. Total lipids were extracted with methanol and chloroform and the methyl esters, prepared by acid catalysed transesterification, were examined by gas–liquid chromatography on SP 2340 and EGSS-Y columns. Peaks were identified by comparison with standard and reference retention data and also by comparison with the previous analyses of serum samples. These studies were performed by Professor Gunstone in the Department of Chemistry, St Andrew's University, Scotland.

RESULTS

Table 1 shows the composition of the trial. The age and length of history of patients in the two groups are similar, the sex distribution is uneven within the groups but since there was no evidence of difference in behaviour of the disease between the sexes this is unlikely to have influenced the outcome.

During the 2 years of the trial no patients died and only one was lost to follow-up (Table 2). Analysis of the changes in Kurtzke Disability Status Scale[12] is shown in Table 3 from which it can be seen that there was no significant difference in overall outcome between the groups. Table 4 shows a comparison of the total number of attacks occurring in patients in each of the groups and the slight reduction in the treatment group is not significant. How-

Table 2 Acute remitting outcome

| | Acute remitting | |
	Treatment	Control
Patients completing trial	29	28
Died	0	0
Withdrawn	0	1

Table 3 Acute remitting Kurtzke

| | Acute remitting | |
	Treatment	Control
Kurtzke DSS improved	8	7
Kurtzke DSS unchanged	13	12
Kurtzke DSS deteriorated	8	10

Table 4 Acute remitting relapses

	Acute remitting	
	Treatment	Control
Patients having no attacks	3	4
Patients with 1–2 attacks	12	8
Patients with 3 attacks	14	17
Attacks per patient year	1.0	1.2
Score per relapse	8.2	18.9

Table 5 Serum fatty acids (expressed as percentages) before and during supplementation

	Treatment		Control	
Fatty acid	Before	During	Before	During
Palmitic 16:0	21.5	17.8	20.4	21.0
Oleic 18:1	26.7	18.2	27.9	28.5
Linoleic 18:2ω6	28.2	39.0	28.1	28.0
Arachidonic 20:4ω6	5.6	7.8	7.2	5.0

ever, when the 'attack score'[15], expressed in terms of mean score per attack per patient is compared between the groups, a Mann Whitney U test shows a significant difference in favour of the treatment group. Further analysis has shown that the difference is due predominantly to a reduction in the duration of relapses and only partly to a reduction in their severity.

Table 5 shows the results of total fatty acid estimations in patients before treatment and after an interval of 24 months. The effect of therapy can be seen, in that the percentage of linoleic acid (C18:2ω6) and arachidonic acid (C20:4ω6) increased significantly in those patients taking the linoleic acid spread.

Combined results

The suggestion in 1981[16] that some of the findings from the three trials in Belfast, Newcastle and London, Ontario might be explained in view of differences in the severity and duration of the disease in patients in the trial has been tested by a re-analysis of the original data from 172 patients from those three trials. All patients from Belfast and Newcastle upon Tyne had acute remitting multiple sclerosis as did most of those from London, Ontario. Unfortunately, some of the patients from London, Ontario may have had a more chronic form of the disease but it was not possible to identify these at this late date. Since patients in the three trials were randomly allocated to treatment or control groups, and since the treatment and control medications were essentially similar, assessments have been made by combining the data from the linoleic acid treated groups in the three trials and those from the control groups. Assessments have been made at entry to the trial and at 28 months after onset. In order to examine the relationship between patient characteristics and the effectiveness of linoleic acid patients were divided into groups based on disability at entry to the trial and duration of illness at entry to

Table 6   Combined patient characteristics

	Treatment	Control
Number of patients	87	85
Males	31	37
Females	56	48
Age at onset (years)	30.23	28.51
Age at entry (years)	40.83	40.00
Duration of disease (years)	10.60	11.49
Kurtzke DSS at entry	3.33	3.15
Kurtzke DSS at end	3.79	3,93
Percentage of patients with one or more relapse	63	59
Mean relapse score	15.29	26.47
Mean number of relapses per year	0.66	0.61
Mean duration of trial in months	28.09	28.15

Table 7   Combined figures – Effect of disability at entry

Disability score at entry	Mean change in disability scores		Mean relapse score		Mean number of relapses per year	
	Treatment	Control	Treatment	Control	Treatment	Control
0–2	0.12	0.81	12.16	22.78	0.77	0.94
3–6	0.71	0.76	18.77	32.48	0.58	0.34

Table 8   Combined figures – Effect of duration of illness at entry

Duration at entry to trial	Mean change in disability scores		Mean relapse score		Mean number of relapses per year	
	Treatment	Control	Treatment	Control	Treatment	Control
0–5	0.14	0.57	12.64	25.40	0.97	0.91
6–10	0.52	1.00	18.35	29.63	0.75	0.57
11 and over	0.57	0.74	14.94	24.86	0.45	0.48

the trial. On initial disability, patients with Kurtzke Disability Status Scores of 0, 1 or 2 (minimal disability) were separated from those with Kurtzke Scale Scores of 3, 4, 5 and 6 (moderate to severe disability). Three groups of patients were created on the basis of duration of illness: those with durations of 0–5 years, 6–10 years and 11 or more years of illness at entry to the trial.

For each of these two levels of disability and three levels of duration of illness the statistical significance of the differences between the treated and control groups was tested for each of three variables (viz change in Kurtzke Disability Status Scale scores from the beginning to the end of the trial, average relapse score per relapsing patient and average number of relapses per year). Mann Whitney U tests were used to assess significance because of the ordinal level of measurement and the distribution of these three variables.

The total cohort examined is shown in Table 6 and includes 87 patients in the treatment group and 85 in the control group. There were no significant differences between the groups at entry to the trial.

Table 7 shows the change in disability scores, mean relapse score and mean number of relapses as a function of disability at entry to trial. It can be seen that the differences are most evident with respect to the change in disability score and mean relapse score in patients who had minor disability at entry to the trial. There were scarcely significant differences in the more severely disabled group.

In Table 8 the effect of linoleic acid treatment as a function of the duration of illness at entry to the trial is considered, and again it can be seen that those patients with the shorter durations of illness appear to benefit more in terms of reduced disability and lower relapse scores.

DISCUSSION

The evidence in support of an abnormality of fatty acid metabolism in multiple sclerosis is substantial and has recently been reviewed by Mertin and Meade[17]. The possibility of an impaired absorption of polyunsaturated fatty acids from the gut has been refuted[18]. There is epidemiological support for the suggestion that the deficiency in serum polyunsaturated fatty acids relates to a reduced dietary supply[19], and there is some suggestion of a possible inborn error of fatty acid metabolism[8,20]. Whatever the cause of the abnormality the empirical attempt to improve dietary supply of linoleic acid by supplementation with sunflower oil produced results which were encouraging but not conclusive[11].

In the Newcastle trial there was a benefit from dietary supplementation in patients with acute remitting multiple sclerosis who had attacks of shorter duration and less severity than the controls[13]. This finding was not confirmed by others in London, Ontario[14].

The re-analysis of data from three double-blind trials of linoleic acid in the treatment of multiple sclerosis suggests that patients with minimal or no disability at entry to the trials treated with linoleic acid had a significantly smaller increase in disability over the course of the trial than did control patients. This effect of linoleic acid on overall disability was not reported by any of the original trials. In addition, we confirmed the earlier finding that treatment with linoleic acid significantly reduced the severity and duration of relapses regardless of disability and duration of illness at entry to the trial.

The clinical significance of this beneficial effect of linoleic acid on the progression of multiple sclerosis and on the severity and duration of relapses must remain in some doubt until the mechanism of its action is known. Although various hypotheses have been proposed the role of linoleic acid in the aetiology and course of multiple sclerosis remains uncertain[17].

That the dietary supplementation has an intended effect in increasing the percentage of polyunsaturated fatty acids in the serum is confirmed by the analysis of free fatty acids in serum. In some respects the way in which the polyunsaturated fatty acids affect multiple sclerosis is akin to that documented with ACTH[21]. This finding would be in keeping with the suggested immuno-suppressive function of polyunsaturated fatty acids[17] and, since serum lipids can be fairly rapidly altered by dietary supplementation, there might be some point in using a high polyunsaturated fatty acid diet as an acute treatment during exacerbations of multiple sclerosis.

Recent evidence suggests that polyunsaturated fatty acids protect guinea pigs from experimental allergic encephalomyelitis (Mertin, personal communication). This effect may be achieved by their incorporation into lymphocyte membranes, or alternatively because they are prostaglandin precursors which, especially those of the E series, can act as immuno-suppressants both *in vivo* and *in vitro*[22]. In recent experiments performed by Mertin (personal communication) the amount of polyunsaturated fatty acid used as a dietary supplement has been relatively greater than in the present trial. He originally gave diets containing 2000 mg/kg of linoleic acid per day but more recently has reduced the level to 500 mg/kg per day and still finds a protective effect. If species differences are ignored, the lower dose can be compared to the 250 mg/kg per day used in the Belfast and London, Ontario trials and the 350 mg/kg per day in our treatment group.

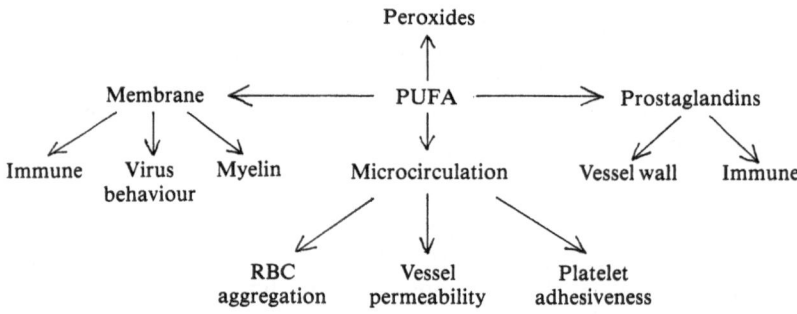

Figure 1 The role of polyunsaturated fatty acids

It cannot, however, be assumed that the role of polyunsaturated fatty acids is necessarily immunological, and the ways in which they could exert their effect upon multiple sclerosis are shown in Figure 1 including the formation of peroxide, a direct effect upon membranes or as precursors of prostaglandin or by an effect upon the microcirculation.

Figure 1 here

References

1. Swank, R. L. (1950). *Annu. J. Med. Sci.,* **220**, 421
2. Swank, R. L., Lerstad, O., Strom, A. *et al.* (1952). *N. Engl. J. Med.,* **246**, 721
3. Swank, R. L. (1953). *Arch. Neurol Psychol.,* **69**, 91
4. Sinclair, H. M. (1956). *Lancet,* **1**, 381

5. Gerstl, B., Kahnke, M. J., Smith, J. K. *et al.* (1961). *Brain,* **84,** 310
6. Baker, R. W. R., Thompson, R. H. S. and Zilkha, K. J. (1970). *J. Neurol. Neurosurg. Psychiatry,* **33,** 506
7. Gul, S., Smith, A. D., Thompson, R. H. S. *et al.* (1970). *J. Neurol. Neurosurg. Psychiatry,* **33,** 506
8. Thompson, R. H. S. (1966). *Proc. R. Soc. Med.,* **59,** 269
9. Love, W. C., Cashell, A., Reynolds, M. *et al.* (1974). *Br. Med. J.,* **3,** 18
10. Wolfgram, F., Myers, L., Ellison, G. *et al.* (1975). *Neurology,* **25,** 786
11. Millar, J. H. D., Zilkha, K. J., Langham, M. J. S. *et al.* (1973). *Br. Med. J.,* **1,** 765
12. Kurtzke, J. F. (1961). *Neurology,* **11,** 686
13. Bates, D., Fawcett, P. R. W., Shaw, D. A. *et al.* (1978). *Br. Med. J.,* **2,** 1390
14. Paty, D. W., Cousin, J. K., Read, S. *et al.* (1978). *Acta Neurol. Scand.,* **58,** 53
15. Millar, J. H. D., Vas, C. J., Noronha, M. J. *et al.* (1967). *Lancet,* **2,** 429
16. Dworkin, R. H. (1981). *Lancet,* **1,** 1153
17. Mertin, J. and Meade, C. J. (1977). *Br. Med. Bull.,* **33,** 67
18. Belin, J., Pettet, N., Smith, A. D. *et al.* (1971). *J. Neurol. Neurosurg. Psychiatry,* **34,** 25
19. Alter, M., Yamoor, M. and Harshe, M. (1970). *Arch. Neurol.,* **31,** 267
20. Thompson, R. H. S. (1977). *Biochemical Society Symposium,* **35,** 103
21. Miller, H. G., Newell, D. J., Ridley, A. R. *et al.* (1962). *Br. Med. J.,* **1,** 1726
22. Pelus, L. M. and Strausser, H. R. (1977). *Life Science,* **20,** 903

35
Essential fatty acids in the serum and cerebrospinal fluid of multiple sclerosis patients

I. S. NEU

SUMMARY

Statistical evaluation of essential fatty acids (determined by gas chromato-graphy) in the serum and cerebrospinal fluid of patients with definite MS and acute CCT showed marked differences to those of healthy subjects. It was also evident that the decrease of essential fatty acids in MS patients differed from that of CCT patients. Whereas the fatty acid levels in the serum of MS patients revealed only minor differences as compared to the controls and CCT patients, MS patients did show a clear decrease, especially of linoleic and arachidonic acids, in the CSF. This difference was most pronounced in cholesterol esters in the CSF. One absorption study with safflower oil demonstrated normal enteral absorption of essential fatty acids and the ability to cross the blood–CSF barrier.

INTRODUCTION

Since the announcement in 1963 by Baker and co-workers of lipid changes in the white matter of multiple sclerosis (MS) brains[1] and the report in 1964 of deficiency levels[2], especially of linoleic acid, in the serum as well as in the red and white blood corpuscles of MS patients, various authors have reported on follow-up results that are in part divergent. A depression of the linoleic acid level in the plasma of patients with craniocerebral trauma (CCT) was also reported.

Detailed analyses were performed of essential fatty acids in both serum and CSF, and the results were compared with those from healthy controls and patients with CCT[5].

The present communication is devoted to a study on the level of linoleic acid (C18:2) and arachidonic acid (C20:4) in serum and the cerebrospinal fluid.

Therefore, the objectives of the present analysis should be:

(1) Do the proportions of saturated and unsaturated fatty acids in MS patients reveal typical deviations as compared to the control groups?

(2) Are there significant deviations, as far as they are significant, similar to those found in craniocerebral trauma (CCT) or significant differences?

(3) Do the analyses yield divergent findings for phosphatides and cholesterol esters depending on whether serum or CSF was examined?

(4) Are there sex-specific differences that could be significant?

(5) Is age a contributory factor?

(6) Are there typical relations among the various proportions of fatty acids, and do these differ between MS patients and healthy control subjects?

(7) Is enteral absorption and the ability of essential fatty acids to cross the blood-brain barrier impaired in MS patients?

PATIENTS

The age distribution of the MS patients with acute exacerbations and remissions was between 20 and 40 years with an average of 33 years; that of the control groups was also between 20 and 40 years with an average of 32 years. The clinical diagnoses were based upon the criteria on Fog[3].

For the statistical analysis the results of the fatty acid distribution (methyl esters) in the serum of 56 definite MS patients and of 10 persons serving as healthy controls were evaluated. The fatty acid pattern was evaluated, furthermore, in phosphatides and cholesterol esters of serum and CSF. A patient group of 11 MS patients was compared with 11 healthy controls.

A further possibility of comparison was provided by the data of 10 patients with acute CCT. Thus the following data material were available:

Total fatty acids (methyl esters) in serum
MS patients   ($n = 56$; n female $= 44$)
Control group   ($n = 10$; n female $= 5$)

Phosphatides in serum and CSF
MS patients   ($n = 11$)
Control group   ($n = 11$)

Cholesterol esters in serum and CSF
MS patients   ($n = 11$)
Control group   ($n = 11$)

The blood sampling process was standardized in all subjects. The time interval between the last meal and blood sampling, together with lumbar puncture was at least 14 hours. (Blood and CSF sampling under vacuum and on ice, then frozen $-80\,°C$.)

METHOD OF STATISTICAL ANALYSIS

On the basis of the data material the mean values of the various fatty acid proportions were analyzed for significant differences in the respective groups. The technique applied was Student's t-test. With the aid of the resulting graphs questions 1–3 could be answered, and suitable hypotheses formulated. Questions 4–6 were approached with the help of 'factor analyses'.

METHODS

Technique for gas chromatographic analysis of the fatty acid methyl esters

The technique applied for the extraction of serum lipids was a modification of the method described by Folch[4].

Technique for gas chromatographic analysis of the phosphatides and cholesterol esters in the serum and CSF

The lipids were extracted from 4 ml of serum or 10–15 ml of CSF in accordance with Sperry's modification[4a] of the Folch method[4].

RESULTS

Fatty acid methyl esters in serum (Figure 1)
(results of mean-value comparison)

MS group vs. control group are compared in Figure 1 which shows the patterns of the four saturated and six unsaturated fatty acids for the 56 MS patients as compared to the 10 control subjects. Due to their low percentage values the mean values of the fatty acids C14:0, C16:1, C20:3 and C22:6 were multiplied by a factor of 10 in the graph and C12:0 by a factor of 100. The unsaturated fatty acids C18:2, C18:1 and the saturated fatty acid C16:0 accounted for the greatest absolute portion. Despite the relatively small sample size of the control group, the differences are significant for most of the fatty acids examined. Significantly higher in the MS group were the proportions of myristic acid (14:0) ($p = 0.001$), lauric acid (C12:0) ($p = 0.01$), C16:1 ($p = 0.01$) and oleic acid (C18:1) ($p = 0.001$).

Significantly lower in the MS group, on the other hand, were the proportions of linoleic acid (C18:2) ($p = 0.001$) and arachidonic acid ($p = 0.05$).

Phosphatides and cholesterol esters in serum

No significant differences could be traced for phosphatides in the MS group vs controls vs CCT group (Figure 2). However, the MS patients showed a significant elevated proportion of saturated fatty acids and a depressed

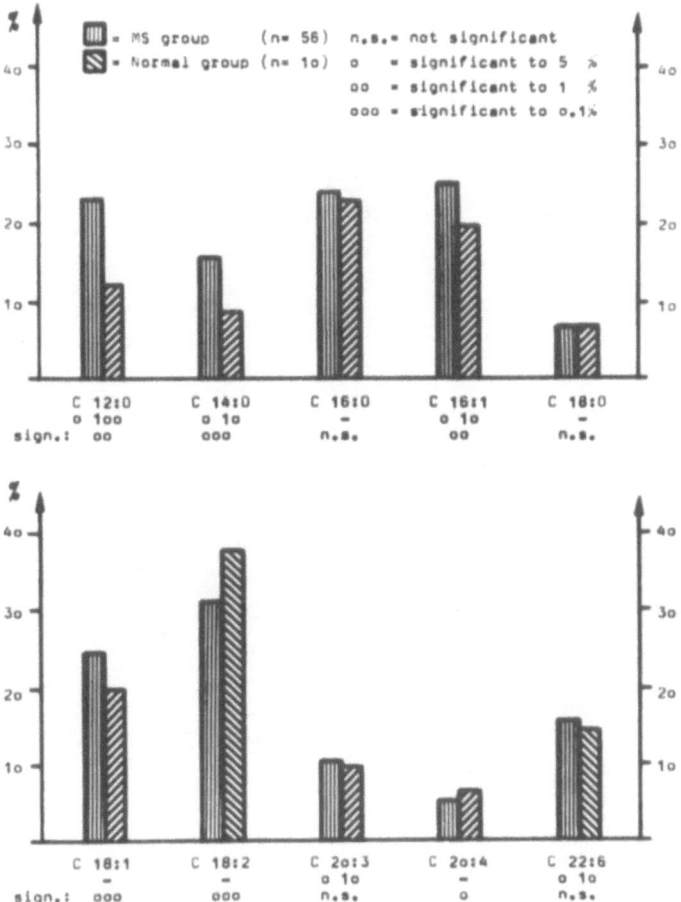

Figure 1   Analysis of fatty acid methyl esters in serum

proportion of polyunsaturated fatty acids. Differences to the CCT group, however, were significant, but these relate only to the unsaturated fatty acids. The proportions of oleic acid ($p = 0.1$) and C20 : 3 ($p = 0.05$) were lower, but not that of arachidonic acid.

Phosphatides: acute vs remissive cases of MS

By comparison of acute cases of MS to that of the control group to remissive cases it was possible to detect differences in unsaturated fatty acid levels despite the small sample size. The proportion of C20 : 3 was higher ($p = 0.1$), than that of C22 : 6 lower ($p = 0.1$).

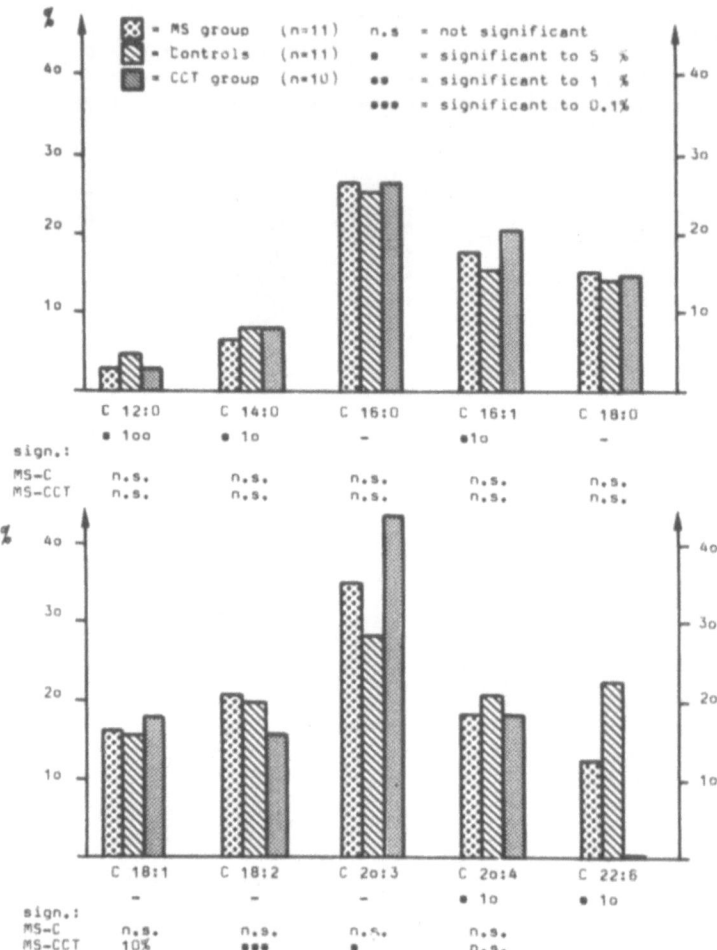

Figure 2 Comparison of serum phosphatides ($n = 32$)

Cholesterol esters in serum

MS groups vs controls vs CCT group (Figure 3).
Significant changes were only traced for unsaturated fatty acids. No
differences were seen in the saturated fatty acids. Among the MS group the
proportion of linoleic acid was greater ($p = 0.01$), but that of oleic acid
($p = 0.1$) and arachidonic acid ($p = 0.05$) were smaller. More significant
changes could, however, be traced in comparison to the CCT group,
suggesting that the disturbances in MS are unrelated to those of CCT. Here the
proportions of linoleic acid ($p = 0.001$) and stearic acid ($p = 0.05$) were
greater. The proportions of oleic acid ($p = 0.01$) and of C16:1 and C20:3
($p = 0.05$) were smaller than in the CCT group.

ESSENTIAL FATTY ACIDS

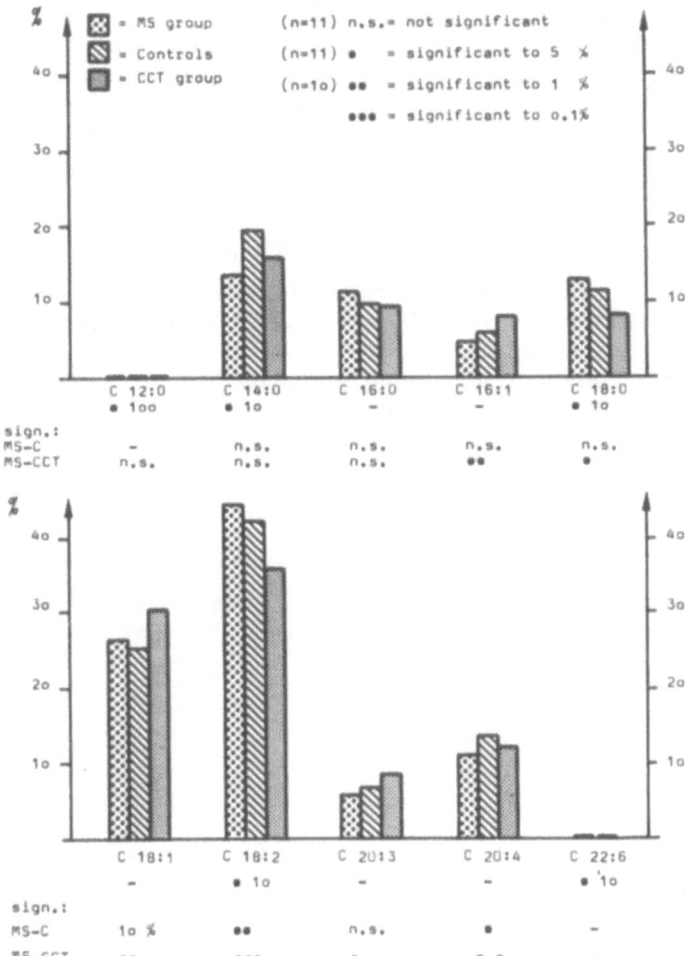

Figure 3 Analysis of serum cholesterol esters ($n = 32$)

Cholesterol esters, acute vs remissive cases of MS

The pattern underwent no appreciable change when the observations were limited to comparison of acute and remissive cases of MS. Owing to the small number of samples any differences were not significant. Nevertheless, there is a tendency.

Phosphatides and cholesterol esters in CSF

Phosphatides

MS groups vs controls vs CCT group.
The MS group revealed significant levels of the saturated and mono-un-

189

saturated fatty acids palmitic acid ($p = 0.05$), stearic acid (C18:0) ($p = 0.01$) and oleic acid (C18:1) ($p = 0.05$). The unsaturated fatty acids C18:2–C20:4 were depressed, although significance could not be demonstrated.

In contrast to the serum analysis, the difference to the CCT group was less pronounced. No significant differences were found with respect to the saturated fatty acids. Only in the analysis of linoleic acid were slight deviations among the CCT group noted ($p = 0.1$).

Phosphatides: acute vs remissive cases of MS (Figure 4)

Comparison of acute to remissive cases of MS showed that among the saturated fatty acids higher concentrations were found in the acute MS group, the difference being significant for stearic acid. Among the unsaturated fatty acids lower concentrations were found among the MS group, the difference being weakly significant for arachidonic acid.

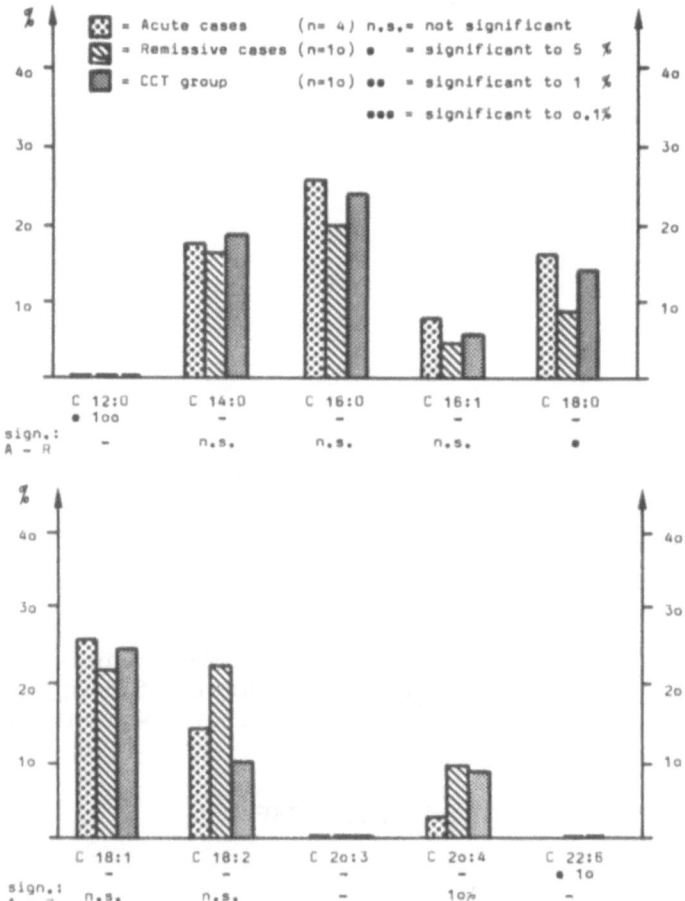

Figure 4 Analysis of CSF phosphatides ($n = 24$)

Cholesterol esters: MS group vs controls vs CCT

Whereas the saturated fatty acid concentrations were significantly greater in the MS group than in the control group, the opposite was the case for the unsaturated fatty acids. Higher proportions of palmitic acid (C16:0) ($p=0.001$), C16:1 ($p=0.001$) and stearic acid (C18:0) ($p=0.05$) were found in the MS group.

In the MS group lower concentrations of linoleic acid (C18:2) ($p=0.001$) and arachidonic acid (C20:4) ($p=0.01$) were observed.

The corresponding results of fatty acid analysis in the CSF resembled those of the CCT group more closely than those of the control group, although significant differences exist here as well.

The proportion of C16:0 ($p=0.01$) and that of C16:1 ($p=0.05$) were

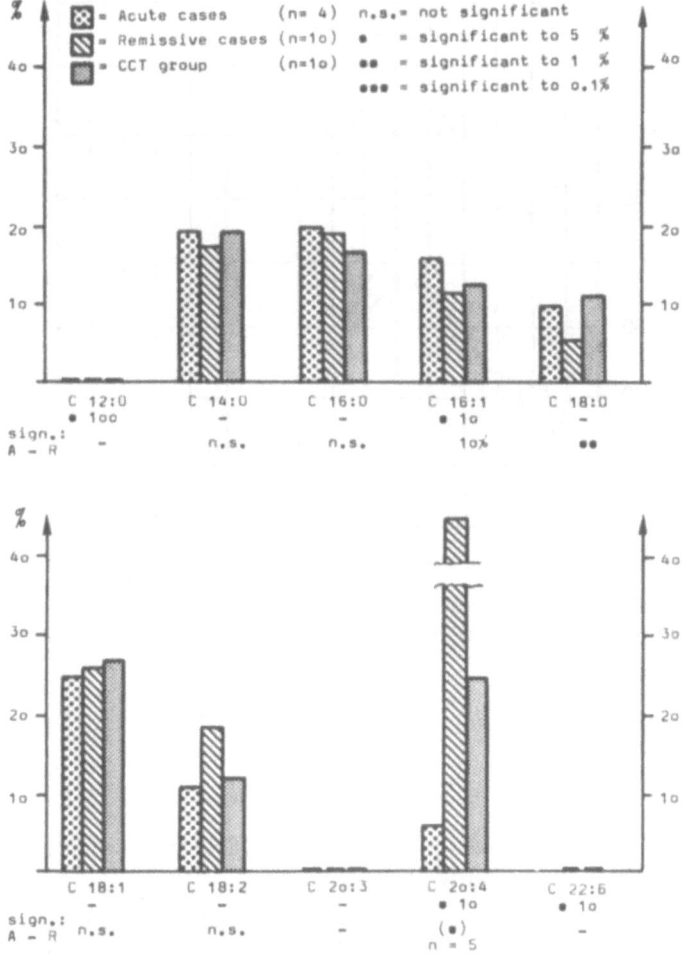

Figure 5 Analysis of CSF cholesterol esters ($n=24$)

greater in the MS than in the CCT group. The proportion of unsaturated fatty acids was lower in the MS group than in the CCT group; however, significance could not be shown.

Cholesterol esters, acute vs remissive cases of MS (Figure 5)

The results among the subgroups 'acute vs remissive' were similar. The differences, however, were significant only for stearic acid, which was significantly higher in the acute MS group than in the remissive controls, and for arachidonic acid, which was significantly lower in the acute MS group than in the remissive controls.

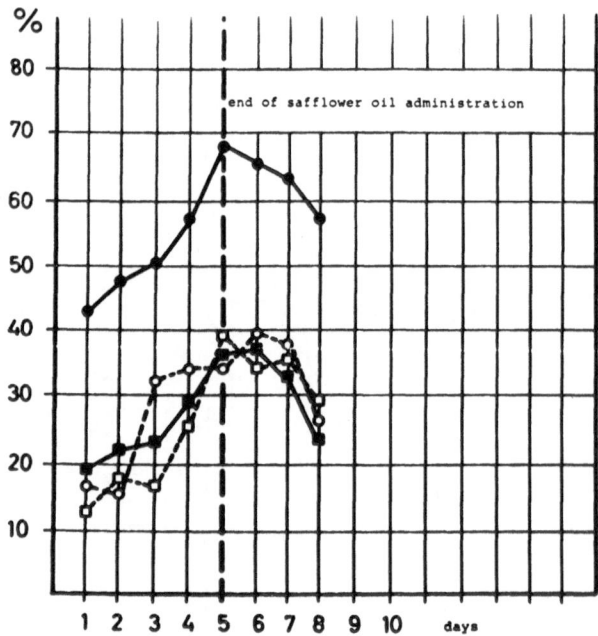

Figure 6 Behaviour of cholesterol esters and phosphatides in serum and CSF following administration of 80 g of safflower oil/24 h to a patient with an acute course of multiple sclerosis.
O Cholesterol esters, CSF
● Cholesterol esters, serum
□ Phosphatides, CSF
■ Phosphatides, serum

Determination of linoleic acid in serum and CSF after oral administration of essential fatty acids in MS (Figure 6)

An MS patient having a significant depression of linoleic acid in serum and CSF was given 80 g of safflower oil/24 h on 5 consecutive days by means of a nose probe. Controls for changes in cholesterol and phosphatide fatty acid pattern of serum and CSF were carried out daily. The increase of individual fatty acids in serum and CSF was on the average significant the 3rd day after administration of the safflower oil. After safflower oil was discontinued on the 6th day, owing to increasing emesis and diarrhoea, a pronounced decrease in serum and CSF fatty acid levels occurred.

DISCUSSION

The results of our determinations of essential fatty acids showed differences, some significant, in MS patients as compared to control subjects and CCT patients. Among the MS patients this was particularly true for the low levels of linoleic acid and arachidonic acid levels and was most pronounced in the fatty acids of cholesterol esters in the CSF. Since a depression of unsaturated fatty acids in the serum of patients suffering from CCT had already been described[5], we compared this additional control group with the MS group in order to establish whether a comparable pattern of fatty acid depression occurs in MS patients. On the basis of statistical analysis, however, it can be assumed that alterations of the fatty acid pattern in the serum and CSF of CCT patients are dissimilar. In MS patients there is apparently a tendency towards a dis-equilibrium in the relationship between saturated and monosaturated fatty acids on the one hand and unsaturated fatty acids on the other. This tendency is even more pronounced during acute MS exacerbation.

The results of our study on the absorption of safflower oil in one MS patient conclusively demonstrate that neither impaired enteral absorption nor disturbances in the blood–brain barrier account for the depressed fatty acid levels found in the CSF and serum of the MS patients.

Several authors have reported on the lipid composition in demyelination foci and in the macroscopically and microscopically normal white matter of MS brains[6,7]. In the demyelination foci depressed values for total phospholipids, cholesterol and cerebrosides were found[8]. The histologically and macroscopically normal white matter of MS brains also revealed a loss of phospholipids[6,7] as well as a decrease in unsaturated fatty acids having three double bonds[7]. These findings suggested that MS patients suffer from impaired brain-lipid metabolism as well as disturbances in the fatty-acid-elongation system[9].

Few neurologic conditions involving a depression of essential fatty acids in the serum are described in the literature, and no satisfactory explanation of the underlying pathomechanism has been presented. Such conditions include CCT[5], hydrocephalus aresorptivus (Neu and Wolfram, unpublished) and Friedreich's ataxia[10]. Nor have the causes of impaired fatty acid metabolism in MS been elucidated. An increase in lipolysis through cyclic AMP is conceiv-able. Recently, it has also been assumed that the lipotrophin–endorphin mechanism leads to activation of lipases and to a rapid release of essential fatty acids. Finally, the hypothesis that activation of macrophages via a decrease in prostaglandin synthesis leads to lipolytic enzyme activation with consecutive linoleic acid breakdown has yet to be experimentally corroborated.

The depression in levels of long-chain unsaturated fatty acids found in MS patients could lead to impairment of vital pleomorphic functions in biologic membranes[11] with the membrane-sealing function of fatty acids on the myelin sheath being of notable importance.

Apart from the possibility of a pre-existing chemopathy, this approach in MS research has been supplemented by immunologic findings, beginning with the findings of Clausen et al[12], in 1976, who showed that a deficiency of poly-unsaturated fatty acids can favour the course of experimentally induced allergic encephalomyelitis (EAE). Then Turnell et al[13] demonstrated in 1973 that free fatty acids act as mediators to influence lymphocytolytic corticosteroid activity. These findings support the hypothesis that fatty acids have a regulatory function in the immune system. Elevated serum levels of essential fatty acids could accordingly exert a suppressive influence on the mechanisms of cellular immune response; depressed serum concentrations, on the other hand, could intensify them[14,15].

References

1. Baker, R. W. R., Thompson, R. H. S. and Zilkha, S. K. J. (1963). Fatty acid composition of brain lecithins in multiple sclerosis. *Lancet*, 1, 26
2. Baker, R. W. R., Thompson, R. H. S. and Zilkha, S. K. J. (1964). Serum fatty acid in multiple sclerosis. *Br. Neurosurg. Psychiatry*, 27, 408
3. Fog, T. (1965). A scoring system for neurological impairment in multiple sclerosis. *Acta Neurol. Scand.*, 41, 551
4. Folch, J., Lees, M. and Sloane Stanley, G. H. (1957). A simple method for the isolation and purification of total lipids from animal tissue. *J. Biol. Chem.*, 226, 496
4a. Sperry, W. H. (1963). *J. Lipid Res.*, 4, 221
5. Troll, U. and Rittmeyer, P. (1973/74). Veränderungen im Fettsäuremuster der Serum-gesamtlipide bei Katabolie. *Infusionstherapie*, 3, 20
6. Cumings, J. N. (1955). Lipid chemistry of the brain in demyelinating diseases. *Brain*, 78, 554
7. Gerstl, B., Kahnke, M. J., Smith, J. K., Tavastjerna, M. G. and Hayman, R. B. (1961). Brain lipids in multiple sclerosis and other diseases. *Brain*, 84, 310
8. Cumings, J. N. (1969). The lipid composition of pure myelin in some demyelinating disorders. *Neuropat. Pol.*, 3, 255–260
9. Neu, I., Woelk, H. (1982). Investigations of the lipid metabolism of the white matter in multiple sclerosis. *Neurochem. Res.*, 7, 727
10. Davignon, J., Huang, Y. S., Wolf, J. P. and Barbeau, A. (1979). Fatty acids profile of pa-tients with Friedreich's ataxia. *J. Can. Soc. Neurol.*, 6, 275
11. Stoffel, W., Dörr, W. and Assmann, G. (1978). Pleomorphe Funktionen von hochungesättigten Phospholipiden in biologischen Membranen und Serumlipoproteinen. *Med. Welt.*, 29, 124
12. Clausen, J. and Möller, J. (1976). Allergic encephalomyelitis induced by brain antigen after deficiency in polysaturated fatty acids during myelination. *Acta Neurol. Scand.*, 43, 375
13. Turnell, R. W., Clarke, L. H. and Burton, A. F. (1973). Studies in mechanism of cortico-steroid-induced lymphocytolysis. *Cancer Res.*, 33, 203
14. Mertin, J., Hughes, D., Shenton, B. K. and Dickinson, J. P. (1974). *In vitro* inhibition by unsaturated fatty acids of the PPD and PHA-induced lymphocyte response. *Klin. Wochenschr.*, 52, 248
15. Mertin, J. and Meade, C. J. (1977). Relevance of fatty acids in multiple sclerosis. *Br. Med. Bull.*, 33, 67

36
The effect of large dose prednisone therapy on intrathecal IgG production in multiple sclerosis

M. WENDER, A. WAJGT, G. MICHALOWSKA and E. TOKARZ

SUMMARY

Several findings support the hypothesis that intrathecal synthesis of IgG is related to the production of multiple sclerosis lesions. Accordingly, one of the goals of an effective therapy in MS should be the eradication of this IgG synthesis. 50 MS patients in an active phase of the disease were treated with 3960 mg of prednisone, over a period of 54 days. The initial dose was as high as 200 mg per day. As a result of this treatment we have found a marked drop of both the absolute and relative plasma IgG levels in as much as 82% and 96% respectively of treated patients. A similar effect, i.e. a significant decrease of the absolute and relative IgG concentrations was found in the CSF. The latter effect is largely due to the decrease of plasma IgG concentration, but inhibition of intrathecal IgG synthesis has contributed as well. In 48% of patients which showed an abnormal starting IgG index, and in 59% of cases with an abnormal starting KL/LL ratio in CSF – a full normalization of indices of the local immunoglobulin production was achieved. Negligible changes, i.e. a slight decrease of the CSF IgG level were found in MS patients which demonstrated a normal CSF IgG spectrum before the treatment. The obtained results thus seem to indicate that the CSF IgG spectrum could be a valuable test for the qualification of MS patients for high dose prednisone therapy, that should be preferentially applied in cases showing a distinct intrathecal synthesis of immunoglobulins.

INTRODUCTION

Recent findings support the hypothesis that CNS synthesis of IgG is related to the production of multiple sclerosis (MS) lesions[1-6]. Accordingly, one of the goals of an effective therapy in MS may be the eradication of CNS IgG synthesis and suppression of intrathecal antimyelin antibody activity[1,3,5,7]. The present clinical trial was designed to test the above hypothesis, and to determine whether prednisone, the drug commonly applied in MS, could suppress IgG synthesis in the central nervous system of MS patients.

MATERIAL AND METHODS

35 clinically definite and 15 clinically probable MS patients, with no other medical problems, were selected according to the criteria of Rose et al[8]. Duration of MS ranged from 3 weeks to 5 years. All patients were in the active stage of the disease, either in the relapsing–remitting phase (33 cases) or in the chronic progressive course of the disease (17 cases). 3960 mg of prednisone was given to all patients during the period of 54 days. The initial dose was as high as 200 mg per day. CSF and blood samples were collected concomitantly, immediately before and after the high dose prednisone medication. In 50 cases the CSF and serum IgG and albumin level, and the CSF KL/LL chain ratio has been estimated by means of the technique presented by Mancini[6,9,10]. The IgG quotient and IgG index were also calculated.

The results were statistically evaluated using the Student's t test for paired values, as well as by an analysis of yes–no data (enumeration data).

Table 1 The influence of prednisone medication on serum IgG and albumin level in MS. Every patient received 3960 mg of prednisone during 54 days

	IgG level mg/dl ($\bar{x} \pm SE$)	Albumin level mg/dl ($\bar{x} \pm SE$)	$\dfrac{IgG}{alb} \times 100\%$ ($\bar{x} \pm SE$)
MS cases before therapy ($n = 50$)	1443 ± 91.5	4507 ± 200.2	32.4 ± 1.5
MS cases after therapy ($n = 50$)	985 ± 62.8	4400 ± 285.3	23.0 ± 0.8
Statistical significance (Student's 't' test for paired values)	$p < 0.001$	n.s.	$p < 0.001$
Statistical significance (analysis of yes–no data enumeration data)	$r = 9$ $p < 0.01$	$r = 21$ n.s.	$r = 2$ $p < 0.01$

n.s. = not significant

RESULTS

Table 1 shows the influence of prednisone medication on serum IgG and albumin level in MS patients. As a result of applied medication we have noticed significant lowering of the serum IgG level and serum IgG quotient, without any changes in the serum albumin concentration. The decrease of the serum absolute and relative IgG levels was found in a significant number of patients (in 41 and 48 cases, respectively, out of 50 patients subjected to prednisone medication).

Table 2 shows the influence of prednisone medication on CSF IgG and albumin level, as well as on intrathecal IgG synthesis estimated from the IgG quotient and IgG index value. The lowering of CSF IgG mean level was statis-

Table 2 The influence of prednisone medication on intrathecal IgG synthesis in MS. Every patient received 3960 mg of prednisone during 54 days

	IgG level mg/dl ($\bar{x} \pm SE$)	Albumin level mg/dl ($\bar{x} \pm SE$)	$\frac{IgG}{alb} \times 100\%$ ($\bar{x} \pm SE$)	Index IgG ($\bar{x} \pm SE$)
MS cases before therapy (n = 50)	5.01 ± 0.91	17.9 ± 1.40	27.9 ± 4.0	1.0 ± 0.1
MS cases after therapy (n = 50)	2.84 ± 0.4	18.0 ± 1.8	15.8 ± 1.9	0.80 ± 0.09
Statistical significance (Student's 't' test for paired values)	$p < 0.01$	n.s.	$p < 0.001$	$p < 0.02$
Statistical significance (analysis of yes–no data enumeration data)	$r = 4$ $p < 0.01$	$r = 31$ n.s.	$r = 7$ $p < 0.01$	$r = 16$ $p < 0.05$

n.s. = not significant

Table 3 The influence of prednisone medication on CSF IgG spectrum in MS cases characterized by intrathecal IgG production before treatment (IgG > 3.15 mg/dl, or $\frac{IgG}{alb} \times 100\% > 24\%$, or Index IgG > 0.70)*

	IgG mg/dl ($\bar{x} \pm SE$ n = 27)	$\frac{IgG}{alb} \times 100\%$ ($\bar{x} \pm SE$ n = 24)	Index IgG ($\bar{x} \pm SE$ n = 23)
CSF IgG spectrum before treatment	7.88 ± 1.5	50.5 ± 6.9	1.69 ± 0.2
CSF IgG spectrum after treatment	4.15 ± 0.7	27.1 ± 3.2	1.13 ± 0.1
Statistical significance (Student's 't' test for paired values)	$p < 0.01$	$p < 0.001$	$p < 0.001$
Statistical significance (analysis of yes–no data enumeration data)	$r = 0$ $p < 0.01$	$r = 0$ $p < 0.01$	$r = 2$ $p < 0.01$
Complete normalization in	17 of 27 cases	12 of 24 cases	11 of 23 cases

*values 3.15 mg/dl, 24%, 0.70 are equal to $\bar{x} \pm 2SD$ in control neurotics

197

Table 4 The influence of prednisone medication on CSF IgG spectrum in MS cases characterized by normal CSF IgG level and normal CSF IgG Index value before treatment (IgG<3.15 mg/dl, or $\frac{IgG}{alb} \times 100\% < 24\%$, or Index IgG<0.70)*

	IgG mg/dl ($\bar{x} \pm SE$ $n=23$)	$\frac{IgG}{alb} \times 100\%$ ($\bar{x} \pm SE$ $n=26$)	Index IgG ($\bar{x} \pm SE$ $n=27$)
CSF IgG spectrum before treatment	1.63 ± 0.14	12.2 ± 1.11	0.41 ± 0.04
CSF IgG spectrum after treatment	1.31 ± 0.15	9.3 ± 0.88	0.51 ± 0.06
Statistical significance	n.s.	n.s.	n.s.
(Student's 't' test for paired values)	$p<0.1$	$p<0.01$	
Statistical significance	$r=4$	$r=7$	$r=14$
(analysis of yes–no data enumeration data)	$p<0.01$	$p<0.05$	n.s.
After prednisone treatment	normal in all cases	normal in all cases	in 6 cases Index value > 0.70

*values 3.15 mg/dl, 24%, 0.70 are equal to $\bar{x} \pm 2SD$ in control neurotics; n.s. = not significant

198

tically significant (in 46 out of 50 patients). The CSF albumin level was slightly higher after prednisone treatment. The lowering of the CSF IgG quotient from 30.6% to 17.8% after therapy was highly significant and occurred in 43 out of 50 patients ($p<0.01$). Mean IgG index value was significantly lower after therapy (1.0 vs 0.80; $p< 0.02$), and the reduction of the IgG index value was observed in 34 out of 50 patients.

Table 3 presents the influence of prednisone medication on CSF IgG spectrum in MS cases characterized initially (before prednisone treatment) by intrathecal IgG production. In this group we have encountered a highly significant lowering of the CSF IgG index value from 1.69 before therapy to 1.13 after treatment ($p<0.001$), a highly significant decline of the CSF IgG quotient ($p<0.01$) as well as a significant drop of the CSF IgG level ($p<0.01$). The lowering of the CSF IgG index, the IgG quotient and IgG level occurred in a statistically significant number of cases. The complete normalization of these parameters occurred in many MS patients of this group. Complete normalization of IgG index occurred in 11 out of 23 cases (48%).

Table 4 presents the influence of prednisone medication on CSF IgG spectrum in MS characterized initially (before therapy) by normal CSF IgG level, normal CSF IgG quotient and normal CSF IgG index. In this group, in contrast to the previous one (Table 3), the difference between mean CSF IgG level and mean IgG index value before and after therapy did not reach statistical significance. It is worth mentioning that mean IgG index value was even higher after therapy, and that in 6 out of 27 cases (22%) the normal IgG index turned to abnormal after prednisone therapy. The CSF IgG quotient was significantly lower after therapy ($p<0.01$) as a result of the lowering of serum IgG quotient (Table 1).

Table 5   The influence of prednisone medication on CSF Ig KL/LL chain ratio in 50 MS cases

	Before treatment (n)	After treatment (n)	
KL/LL ratio normal 0.85–1.18	28	37	As a result of medication derangement of normal starting ratio was noticed in 4 out of 28 cases (14%)
KL/LL ratio abnormal <0.85> 1.18	22	13	Complete normalization of abnormal KK/LL ratio was noticed in 13 out of 22 cases (59%)

Table 5 shows the influence of prednisone therapy on the CSF IgG KL/LL chain ratio in the whole group of 50 MS patients. Before treatment abnormal ratios were found in 22 out of 50 cases. After treatment abnormal ratios were found in 14 out of 50 cases. As a result of such medication complete normalization of the KL/LL ratio was achieved in 13 out of 22 cases (59%). Derangement of the normal KL/LL starting ratio was noticed in 4 out of 28 cases.

DISCUSSION

Some investigators have suggested that the observed decrease of CSF IgG level and CSF IgG quotient after administration of ACTH or corticosteroids might be due to the reduction of the serum IgG level or serum quotient. Our results concerning the significant lowering of serum IgG level and serum IgG quotient partly confirmed this supposition. Undoubtedly, the lowering of CSF IgG level and CSF IgG quotient after prednisone medication results partly from the lowering of serum IgG level and serum IgG quotient. The correct estimation of the local, intrathecal IgG production was achieved by calculating the IgG index value. The statistically significant reduction of the mean IgG index value observed in MS cases characterized by intrathecal IgG production before therapy and in the whole MS group, as well as the normalization of the IgG index value in 11 out of 23 cases (48%) point to a reduction of the intrathecal synthesis of IgG in MS cases subjected to high dose prednisone medication. This conclusion receives a strong support from additional findings that showed a normalization of IgG KL/LL ratio in CSF of 13 out of 22 (59%) MS cases during the high dose prednisone medication. To the best of our knowledge it is the first report dealing with the influence of corticosteroid therapy on the KL/LL chain ratio. Concordant with our observations are those of Trotter *et al*[11] and Tourtellotte *et al*[7] concerning the reduction in intensity or disappearance of oligoclonal bands of CSF IgG caused by ACTH or corticosteroid therapy in a number of MS patients.

The reduction of local IgG synthesis may be related to the beneficial clinical effect of prednisone treatment in MS. However, only negligible changes, i.e. a slight decrease of the CSF IgG level were found in MS patients which demonstrated a normal CSF IgG spectrum before the treatment. The mean IgG index was even slightly higher after therapy in this MS subgroup. Additionally, as a result of this therapy abnormal IgG indices were noticed in a few (6 out of 27) MS cases with a normal IgG index before medication, and abnormal KL/LL ratios were noticed in 4 out of 28 cases with a normal KL/LL ratio before therapy. The obtained results thus seem to indicate that the CSF IgG spectrum could be a valuable test for qualification of MS patients for high dose prednisone therapy and that therapy should be preferentially applied in cases showing a distinct intrathecal synthesis of immunoglobulins.

References

1. Górny, M., Wróblewska, Z., Pleasure, D., Miller, S., Wajgt, A., Koprowski, H. (1983). CSF antibodies to myelin basic protein and oligodendrocytes in multiple sclerosis and other neurological diseases. *Acta Neurol. Scand.,* **67,** 338
2. Kim, S. M., Murray, M. R., Tourtellotte, W. W., Parker, J. A. (1970). Demonstration in tissue culture of myelinotoxicity in cerebrospinal fluid and brain extracts from multiple sclerosis patients. *J. Neuropath. Exp. Neurol.,* **29,** 420
3. Panitch, H. S., Hooper, C. J., Johnson, K. P. (1980). CSF antibody to myelin basic protein: measurement in patients with multiple sclerosis and subacute sclerosing panencephalitis. *Arch. Neurol.,* **37,** 206
4. Tabira, T., Wolfgram, F., Webster, H., Wray, S., McFarlin, D. (1977). Myelinotoxicity of CSF fractions from multiple sclerosis patients tested in an *in vivo* model. *Neurology,* **27,** 374

5. Traugott, U., Raine, C. S. (1981). Anti oligodendrocyte antibodies in cerebrospinal fluid of multiple sclerosis and other neurologic diseases. *Neurology,* **31,** 695
6. Wajgt, A., Bogaczyńska, E. (1980). Oligoclonal CSF immunoglobulin in relation to measles and parainfluenza antibody response in multiple sclerosis. In Bauer, H., Poser, S., Ritter, G. (eds.). *Progress in multiple sclerosis research.* pp. 132–141. (New York: Springer Verlag)
7. Tourtellotte, W. W., Baumhefner, R. W., Potvin, A. R., Ma, B. I., Potvin, J. H., Mendez, M., Syndulko, K. (1980). Multiple sclerosis *de novo* CNS IgG synthesis – effect of ACTH and corticosteroids. *Neurology,* **30,** 1155
8. Rose, A. S., Ellisan, G. W., Myers, L. W., Tourtellotte, W. W. (1976). Criteria for clinical diagnosis of multiple sclerosis in MS – Japan Conference on multiple sclerosis. *Neurology,* **26,** 20
9. Mancini, G., Carbonara, A. O., Heremans, J. R. (1965). Immunochemical quantitation of antigens by single radial immunodiffusion. *Immunochemistry,* **2,** 235
10. Tibbling, G., Link, H., Öhman, S. (1977). Principles of albumin and IgG analysis in neurological disorders. I. Establishment of reference values. *Scand. J. Clin. Lab. Invest.,* **37,** 385
11. Trotter, J. L. and Gorvey, W. F. (1980). Prolonged effects of large dose methyloprednisolone infusion in m.s. *Neurology,* **30,** 702

37
Changes in T-cell subsets according to the course of MS and immunosuppressive treatment

W. SOUKOP, E. SLUGA, H. TSCHABITSCHER and H. LISKA

The determination of T-helper and suppressor cells using monoclonal antibodies gives us information about the immunoregulatory subpopulation of T-cells in peripheral blood. The ratio T-helper : T-suppressor cells constitutes an immunoregulatory index. A disturbance of this ratio, which amounts to 2:1 in normal subjects, has been observed in various diseases of autoaggressive pathogenesis[4].

A decrease of the number of suppressor cells has, for instance, been reported during acute attacks of rheumatoid arthritis. In multiple sclerosis, a disease of still unknown aetiology in which, however, autoimmune disorders play a role, several authors report changes of the ratio helper : suppressor cells which correlate with the course of the disease as well as with MS lesions[1-3,5,6].

The present study investigates changes of the immunoregulatory T-helper/suppressor ratio in correlation with:

(1) clinical course
(2) immunosuppressive treatments and
(3) cerebrospinal fluid findings.

Conclusions as to disease dynamics and therapy follow.

Changes of the T-helper/suppressor ratio (HSR) in comparison with the clinical course were studied in 47 examinations performed on 35 patients, 29 females and 6 males.

"Leu"-antibodies were used for determining the subpopulations. The ratio of T-helper to suppressor cells was expressed as

$$HSR = \frac{\% \text{ helper cells}}{\% \text{ suppressor cells}}$$

The standard ratio found in our laboratory was 2.3.

According to clinical findings patients were divided into six groups:

Group 1: Patients presenting complete remission without any neurological deficits,

Group 2: patients presenting residual neurological symptoms during the interval between recurrent relapses,

Group 3: patients having presented stationary neurological deficits for at least 1 year,

Group 4: patients experiencing continuously progressing deterioration of deficits,

Group 5: patients presenting subacute exacerbations, these are slight new deteriorations of pre-existing deficits without any additional deficits, and

Group 6: patients exhibiting acute obvious symptoms of deficits representing an exacerbation.

Group 1 included seven patients; HSR was increased in two of them (33%); the mean value of HSR was 2.5.

Group 2 included ten patients: HSR was increased in seven of them (71.4%); the mean value was 3.0.

Group 3 included four patients; HSR was increased in one of them (25%); the mean value was 2.3.

Group 4 included eight patients; HSR was increased in six of them (75%); the mean value was 3.12.

Group 5 included nine patients; HSR was increased in six of them (66.7%); the mean value was 2.45.

Group 6 included nine patients; HSR was increased in eight of them (90.7%); the mean value was 4.7.

The mean value of HSR in our patients amounted to 2.99, which is above the standard value. The highest increase of HSR was found in patients suffering from acute neurological deficits in the form of an exacerbation, followed by the group with continuously progressing deterioration. Patients exhibiting remission but continuing deficits have a higher mean value of HSR than those with mild attacks. The highest value in the group with remissions and continuing symptoms was reached by a female patient (HSR = 6.4) who experienced a slight attack 2 weeks later and whose HSR was then 3.4. Patients with stationary symptoms were found to be within the range of normal, and in patients with complete remissions the mean values of HSR were only slightly raised.

According to the course of the disease, the patients in groups 5 and 6 may be differentiated into patients suffering from relapsing multiple sclerosis, and patients suffering from relapsing progressive multiple sclerosis. Patients in group 1 present a relapsing–remitting course, while patients in group 2 exhibit predominantly a relapsing–progressive course. The patients of groups 3 and 4 were primary progressive MS patients. A clear relative decrease of suppressor cells (24–17%) was observed during exacerbations – as described in the literature – independent from duration and course of the disease.

We investigated the effect of immunosuppressive treatment with ACTH and azathioprine on the T-helper : suppressor cell ratio, again expressed by the

HSR. In patients with acute exacerbations who had received at least 2 weeks treatment with ACTH before HSR determination, HSR was clearly reduced (significantly), the mean value being 1.56 and helper cells being relatively reduced (48%). On the other hand, the mean value of HSR amounted to 3.0 in these patients 6 months later if they did not receive ACTH. Patients who did not receive immediate pretreatment exhibited a mean HSR of 4.7 during exacerbations. Patients during remissions with continuing neurological deficits behaved similarly with or without azathioprine treatment. A decrease of HSR correlating with clinical improvement during immunosuppressive therapy was observed in five patients during exacerbations.

Spinal fluid IgG was compared with HSR in 16 patients. Increased HSR correlated with increased spinal fluid IgG in 12 patients, in one case both values were within the range of normal. In three cases increased IgG correlated with normal HSR values, however in two cases the examination took place after ACTH treatment, when subset relations are probably already changed.

In conclusion we may say on the basis of our investigations that the T-sub-populations responsible for immunoregulation, helper and suppressor cells, show changes which correspond to the clinical course, and that the HSR as immunoregulatory index provided information on disease dynamics. Especially, a persisting increased HSR after the attack has subsided appears to correlate with an increased incidence of exacerbations, and thus with the progress of the disease. The highest index value occurs in cases with acute exacerbations, in particular during the initial phase. The high index values were the consequence of a relative reduction of suppressor cells. During ACTH treatment changes in the quantitative relations occurred suggesting the suspicion that helper cell decreased.

The use of other monoclonal antibodies not only against T-cells and macrophage antigens may in the future furnish further information on the behaviour of immunoregulation in multiple sclerosis.

The determination of the immunoregulatory index in the form of HSR in clinical routine provides additional information on the immune status of MS patients, and permits a more specific immunosuppressive and immuno-regulatory treatment.

References

1. Hauser, S. L., Reinherz, E. L., Hoban, C. J., Schlossman, S. F. and Weiner, H. L. (1983). Immunoregulatory T-cells and lymphocytotoxic antibodies in active multiple sclerosis: weekly analysis over a six-month period. *Ann. Neurol.*, **13**, 418–425
2. Hauser, S. L., Bresnan, M. J., Reinherz, E. L. and Weiner, H. L. (1982). Childhood multiple sclerosis: clinical features and demonstration of changes in T-cell subsets with disease activity. *Ann. Neurol.*, **11**, 463–468
3. Huddlestone, J. R. and Oldstone, M. B. A. (1979). T suppressor (Tg) lymphocytes fluctuate in parallel with changes in the clinical course of patients with multiple sclerosis. *J. Immunol.*, **123**, 1615–1618.
4. Reinherz, E. L., Rubenstein, A., Geha, R. S., Strelkauskas, A. J., Rosen, F. S. and Schlossman, S. F. (1979). Abnormalities of immunregulatory T-cells in disorders of immune function. *N. Engl. J. Med.*, **301**, 1018–1022

5. Reinherz, E. L., Weiner, H. L., Hauser, S. L., Cohen, J. A., Distaso, J. A. and Schlossman, S. F. (1980). Loss of suppressor T-cells in active multiple sclerosis: analysis with monoclonal antibodies. *N. Engl. J. Med.*, **303**, 125–129

6. Traugott, U. and Raine, C. (1982). Identification and dynamics of T-cell subsets and B-cells during the development of multiple sclerosis lesions. *J. Neuroimmunol.*, **1**, 17 (abstract)

38
T lymphocyte subsets in the CSF in various stages of MS

A. GUSEO

Immunologic changes within the central nervous system may be more accurately reflected in cerebrospinal fluid (CSF) than in peripheral blood lymphocytes. There are increasing data about the functional difference of early (active), and avid lymphocytes, but their true nature is not yet clear[1]. Some results indicate the suppressor nature of avid cells[2], while others stressed that T-helper cells bind more avidly to sheep red blood cells[1]. Traugott and co-workers[3] showed in experimental allergic encephalomyelitis (EAE) that active or high affinity T-cells decrease dramatically in the periphery with disease activity, and that early T cells are not suppressor cells[4]. Most authors found an increased T-cell number, a decreased active and avid T cell population in active and also in chronic progressive MS cases. The up-to-date results concerning the active, avid and late total lymphocyte populations are summarized in Table 1.

Table 1 Behaviour of T lymphocytes (active, avid and total) in MS periphery (P) and CSF

		Active	*Avid*	*Total*
DECREASE no. of T-cells		Traugott et al (1978)[3] EAE	Kam-Hansen (1980)[9] CSF	Sagar and Allonby (1979)[13] P
		Kam-Hansen (1979)[5] CSF (1980)[6] CSF+P	Oger et al (1975)[10] P Oger and Antel (1982)[11] P	Huddlestone and Oldstone (1979)[14] P Sandberg-Wollheim (1982)[15] P
		Turner et al (1980)[7] P Traugott et al (1982)[8] P		
INCREASE no. of T-cells			Offner et al (1978)[12] P	Naess (1976, 1978)[16,17] CSF Allen et al (1976)[18] CSF Naess and Nyland (1978)[19] CSF Traugott (1978)[20] CSF
				Turner et al (1980)[7] P Oger et al (1981)[21] P Oger et al (1982)[11] P

MATERIAL AND METHODS

CSF samples in 40 MS cases were investigated in various stages of their disease for active (5 minute), avid (the whole surface of the lymphocyte is covered by sheep red blood cells (SRBC)), and late total (24 hour) E rosetting lymphocytes, using a modified method described by Wybran et al[22]. Four periods of immunosuppressive treatment in brain tumour patients were also investigated. Determinations of T cells were performed at first admission, before and after steroid treatment and at regular intervals during immunosuppressive therapy.

RESULTS

The average numbers of all three T cell populations in MS are similar to control cases (Table 2). In cases showing active disease, at the beginning of a bout – as we started the steroid therapy – avid and total T cells decrease, while active cells increased slightly. After steroid treatment the number of active cells falls, but the averages of avid and total T cells increase.

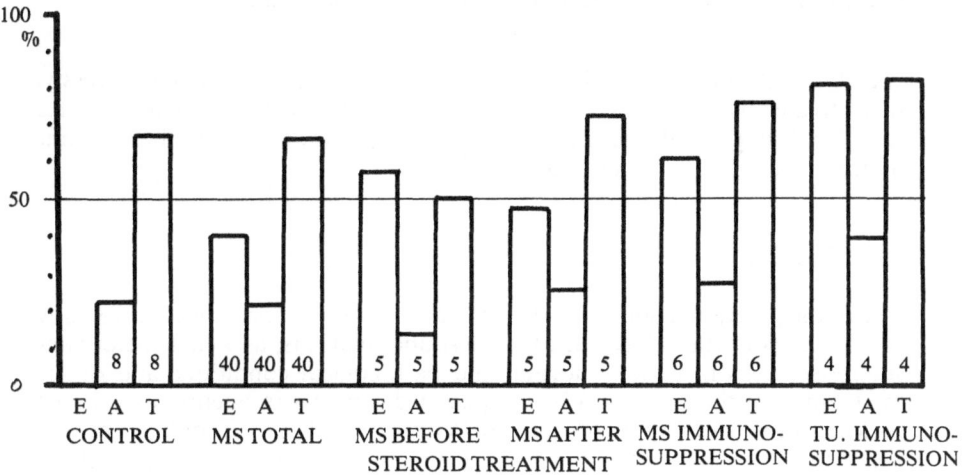

Figure 1   T Lymphocytes in the CSF in MS

The increase of all three populations was more significant after azathioprine therapy. In patients treated for brain gliomas by the scheme of COMP, or for lymphomas by the scheme of COP, the increase of all three T cell populations was the highest. The increase in total T cells was never higher than the increase in avid cells, therefore, the elevation reflects the increase of avid cells. Investigating the action of steroid therapy on CSF T lymphocytes, in almost all cases an elevation of all three cell populations was found (Table 3).

In longterm follow-up of cases, we find somewhat of a fluctuation in T cell populations. Low avid as well as total T cell count was found in exacerbations

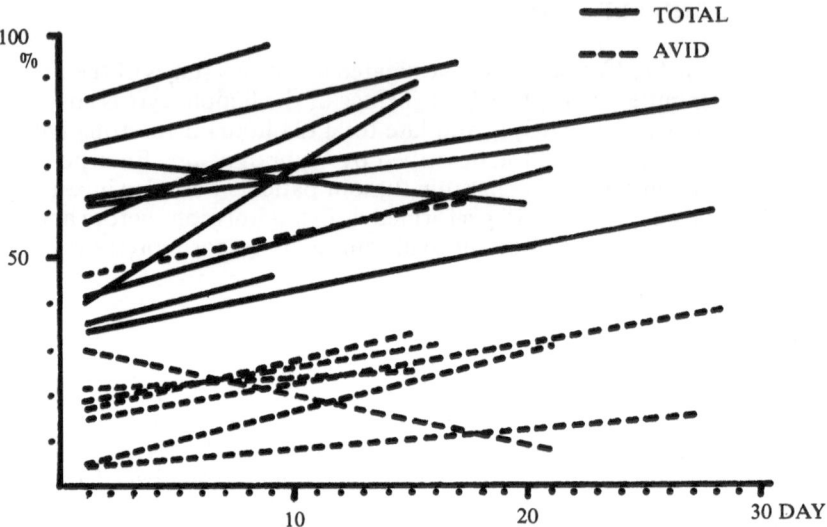

Figure 2 T Lymphocytes in the CSF before and after steroid treatment

and also in chronic progressive cases. The only patient in chronic progressive stage, treated by cyclophosphamide, showed a dramatic drop of avid as well as total T cells in the CSF, despite the high doses of parallel steroid therapy, and showed no change in the clinical course.

DISCUSSION

One of the greatest problems in the evaluation of these results is that we know very little about the behaviour of these subpopulations, as well as helper and suppressor cells in various normal and pathological conditions and on the modulation of their function by various medicaments frequently used in MS patients. Most of the patients have infections, which can modulate not only the course of the disease, but also the actual immunological state, and, therefore, what we actually demonstrate is an aspecific symptom without any specific relevance to MS pathogenesis. Traugott and co-workers[8] demonstrated that early T cells are not suppressor cells. In active disease the number of avid cells decreases. The reduction in the number of total T cells is not higher than the fall of avid cells, therefore we suppose they belong to the suppressor cell population. Similar suggestions were demonstrated by Oger and Antel[2]. If that is true, it is more interesting that steroid treatment, as well as immunosuppression by azathioprine, increases their number in the CSF selectively. Similar results were demonstrated by Naess and Nyland[23] using ACTH and Brinkmann and Hommes[24] after cyclosphophamide treatment.

SUMMARY

In active MS cases the decrease of avid and, in the same portion, the total T lymphocytes in the CSF seems to be characteristic. After stabilization of the clinical picture this level returns to normal. After steroid or immunosuppressive treatment a rapid elevation of avid and, proportionally, of total T cells was found.

Immunosuppressive treatment in non-MS cases caused the same increase in T cell populations. No clear correlation of active T cells and disease activity could be demonstrated.

We suppose that avid cells belong to the suppressor T cell population, and that they react selectively to steroid and azathioprine therapy.

References

1. Dore-Duffy, P. and Zurier, R. B. (1979). *Clin. Immunol. Immunopathol.*, **13**, 261
2. Oger, J. J. and Antel, J. P. (1982). *Workshop on Immunosuppressive Treatment of MS.* Nijmegen
3. Traugott, U., Stone, H. S. and Rain, C. S. (1978). *J. Neurol. Sci.*, **36**, 55
4. Traugott, U., Sheinberg, L. E. and Raine, C. S. (1982). *Ann. Neurol.*, **11**, 182
5. Kam-Hansen, S. (1979). *Neurol.*, **29**, 897
6. Kam-Hansen, S. (1980). *Scand. J. Immunol.*, **12**, 99
7. Turner, A., Cuzner, M. L., Davison, A. N. and Rudge, P. (1980). *J. Neurol. Neurosurg. Psychiatry*, **43**, 305
8. Traugott, U., Shevach, E., Chiba, J., Stone, H. and Raine, C. S. (1982). *Cell. Immunol.*, **70**, 345
9. Kam-Hansen, S. (1980). *Linköpping University Medical Dissertation*, No. 88
10. Oger, J. J., Arnason, B. G. W., Wray, S. H. and Kistler, J. P. (1975). *Neurology*, **25**, 444
11. Oger, J. J., Antel, J. P., Noronha, A. and Arnason, B. G. W. (1982). *Neurology*, **32**, 199
12. Offner, H., Konat, G., Raun, N. E. and Clausen, J. (1978). *Acta Neurol. Scand.*, **57**, 380
13. Sagar, M. and Allonby, H. B. (1979). *J. Neurol. Sci.*, **43**, 133
14. Huddlestone, J. R. and Oldstone, M. B. A. (1979). *J. Immunol.*, **123**, 1615
15. Sandberg-Wollheim, M. (1982). *Jubilee Conference on MS.* Copenhagen, p. 107
16. Naess, A. (1976). *Scand. J. Immunol.*, **5**, 165
17. Naess, A. (1978). *Acta Neurol. Scand.*, (Suppl.) **67**, 243
18. Allen, J. C., Sheremata, W., Cosgrove, J. B. R., Osterland, K. and Shea, M. (1976). *Neurology*, **26**, 579
19. Naess, A. and Nyland, H. (1978). *Eur. Neurol.*, **17**, 61
20. Traugott, U. (1978). *J. Neurol.*, **219**, 185
21. Oger, J. J., Jackevicius, S., Antel, J. P., Rosenkoetter, P. and Arnason, B. G. W. (1981). *Annals Neurol.*, **12**, 82
22. Wybran, J. and Fudenberg, H. H. (1973). *J. Clin. Invest.*, **52**, 1026
23. Naess, A. and Nyland, H. (1981). *Acta Neurol. Scand.*, **63**, 57
24. Brinkman, C. J. J. and Hommes, O. R. (1982). *Workshop on Immunosuppressive Treatment of MS.* Nijmegen.

Section III
Spinal Cord Dysfunctions in Multiple Sclerosis

39
Clinical and paraclinical assessment of spinal cord dysfunction

B. CONRAD and R. BENECKE

Since a casual therapy of spinal cord dysfunction in MS-patients so far does not exist, optimalization of symptomatic treatment is of major importance. Precondition for an effective symptomatic therapy as well as for prospective longterm studies on the feature and course of MS is a precise assessment of clinical deficits on a quantitative basis.

Clinical assessment of spinal cord dysfunction concentrates on information on several motor disabilities, by using large rating scales[1,2] whose general problems will be discussed.

For an objective measurement of the most important aspects of spinal cord involvement, spasticity, ataxia and paresis, analysis of natural complex movements like walking or bicycling has to be achieved, since only those types of movements adequately reflect the functional status of the patient. Those movements were subjected to a detailed analysis by recording electro- and mechanographic activities, angles of the joints, torque, power and rotation rates. It will be shown that there exist highly unspecific (protective) gait disorders, which have to be differentiated from more specific disabilities, due to increased 'spastic' muscle tone or paresis.

The prominent findings in spastic patients were a prolonged recruitment of leg muscle activity. A computerized integration of EMG activity provided an objective measure of spasticity which enabled symptomatic treatment to be optimally adjusted.

References

1. Kurtzke, J. F. (1961). *Neurology*, **11**, 686–694.
2. Poser, S. (1978). *Schriffenrihe Neurologie*. Vol. 20. (Berlin: Springer-Verlag)

40
Functional testing of the spinal cord

P. J. DELWAIDE

Electrophysiological techniques are now available which allow us to measure in man:

(1) Excitability of the motor nucleus (H max/M max ratio),
(2) presynaptic inhibition acting IA afferents (vibratory inhibition of the monosynaptic reflex),
(3) reciprocal inhibition (inhibition of the soleus H reflex induced by peroneal nerve stimulation, and
(4) excitability of the interneuronal network.

Taken together, these techniques permit us to disclose that there are many pathophysiological disturbances in spasticity. Comparisons between various patients indicate that each has his own pathophysiological profile. As some therapeutic means correct specifically one pathophysiological trouble, it is suggested that the choice of therapy could rely on the pathophysiological analysis of spasticity which is currently possible by electrophysiological methods.

41
Increased flexor or reflex and spastic contracture in flexion, mechanisms and management

E. PEDERSEN

Lesions of the spinal cord can affect the pathways controlling the segmental spinal reflexes. This may give rise to facilitation of the reflexes either by an increase of pre-existing facilitation or by a reduction of inhibition.

Such an increase of the reflexes can include the stretch, flexor and bladder reflexes which are involved in many of the clinical manifestations in multiple sclerosis. Impairment of the stretch reflex leads to increased reaction but also to reduction of reciprocal inhibition. Increased bladder reflexes are responsible for the uninhibited neurogenic bladder with the symptoms: frequency of voiding, urgency and urge incontinence. Increased flexor reflex is the basis for flexor spasms and contracture in flexion.

This paper will concentrate on the flexor reflex but also involve its connections with the stretch and bladder reflexes.

The flexor reflex is an exteroceptive reflex as it takes its origin outside the site of reaction. Most wellknown is the flexor reflex elicited by stimulation of the skin of the legs, the resulting withdrawal serves as a protective reaction.

The flexor reflex is a polysynaptic spinal reflex comprising several spinal segments. Such polysegmental activity is necessary in order to obtain coordinated movements of the whole leg, as seen in the withdrawal reaction.

The spinal pathways of the flexor reflex are under suprasegmental tonic inhibition, especially mediated by the dorsal reticulospinal pathways. A lesion of this pathway between the brainstem and the spinal segments leads to a reduction of the tonic inhibition, which in turn results in an increase of the flexor reflex. Increase of the flexor reflex is not exclusively linked to the spinal lesions but also seen following cerebral lesions.

The reflex can be elicited by mechanical, thermic or electrical stimulation of the plantar skin. The reflex reaction is dependent on the intensity of the stimulation which again is dependent on the duration of the stimulation and on the area of the skin stimulated. By stimulation of the skin the receptors are activated but the reflex can also be elicited in another way, namely by stimulation of the afferent nerves mediating the input from the receptors. Such stimulation is possible by electrical stimulation over the posterior tibial nerve behind the medial malleolus, and this type of elicitation of the reflex is more stable with better reproducible results and with less ability to so-called habituation. With intervals of at least 2 minutes between the elicitation of the reflex habituation is very seldom seen. Our standard method is elicitation by a train of five square electrical pulses of a duration of 0.05 ms and separated by 1 ms intervals.

By a threshold stimulation a latency of 70–200 ms is recorded. By increasing stimulation the latency will be reduced to a minimum of about 60 ms when recorded from the tibialis anterior muscle. This minimum latency is equal in spastic patients and normal subjects. Increase of stimulation not only reduces the latency but also increases the reaction. This reaction may be in two parts including a short first component and a second component of longer duration, the latter being responsible for the withdrawal reaction. In spastic patients the reaction of the reflex may be very long and with a tendency to rhythmicity.

The increased flexor reflex caused by cerebral lesions may differ from the increased flexor reflex after spinal lesions by a less marked first component in the EMG reaction, and by the preservation of the reciprocal inhibition which can be demonstrated by alternating activity in the tibialis anterior muscle and the gastrocnemius.

As already mentioned the reflex can be elicited by stimulation of the skin and such stimulation can be intensive, for example in bedridden patients where lesions of the skin of the heels or the sacral region provoke reflex movements, which again stimulate the skin and possibly lead to bed sores, which again give more intensive stimulation that means a vicious circle is in operation. This mechanism can result in contracture in flexion with a spastic leg in flexion, and if insufficiently treated can end in a fixed position due to changes in the tendons and joints. Such contracture may further be facilitated by a wrong positioning of the legs of the bedridden patient.

Many patients with increased flexor reflex develop flexor spasms. Flexor spasms are involuntary flexor movements of the legs with a considerable variation in duration and frequency. They may be painful and in some patients most distressing. It is assumed that the ordinary flexor afferent inflow in the case of increased flexor reflexes more easily activates the motoneurons. Such ordinary inflow from the skin is important as demonstrated by the reduction of flexor spasms by blockade of the relevant nerves.

A recording of the flexor spasms is important in order to study the mechanisms influencing the spasms, and particularly in evaluating appropriate treatment of the spasms.

Equipment for counting the flexor spasms was designed in our laboratory. It consists of an EMG amplifier, a rectifier circuit and a chart recorder, which is able to convert the often complicated electromyogram of the flexor spasms to a single trace which can then be counted electronically or visually. The method is generally used over 6–9 hours during the night. The method cannot differentiate between voluntary movements in normal subjects and flexor spasms in patients.

The co-ordination of flexor and extensor muscles of the legs is important for example in the gait. A unilateral contraction of the flexor and relaxation of the extensor is associated with the contralateral contraction of extensor and relaxation of flexor.

The flexor and stretch reflexes may also be antagonistic, as is shown by the fact that flexor spasms may depress the stretch reflex. This means that there is a possibility of influencing the stretch reflex by flexor reflex afferent input to the spinal cord, and also that not both stretch and flexor reflexes need be influenced in the same way for example by a compound.

The study of the influence of flexor reflex afferent on the stretch reflex is in progress in our laboratory, and differences have been found between normal subjects and spastic patients. We are trying to extend the investigation and to utilize these as a basis for a further elaboration of functional electrical stimulation.

The flexor activity of the leg is linked to the striated sphincters of the pelvic floor, and it is also possible to pick up reaction from pelvic sphincters on ordinary flexor reflex stimulation.

The afferent inflow from the bladder during filling can alter the flexor reflex in two ways. One of them increases the flexor reflex and reduces the mono-synaptic reflexes, whereas the other has the opposite pattern namely reduction of the flexor reflex and increase of the monosynaptic reflexes. The first pattern is combined with difficulty in initiating voiding and a small uroflow, the other with easy initiating of voiding and good uroflow.

In spinal lesion one might expect a general release of flexor and bladder reflexes and also, therefore, a simultaneous reaction in flexor muscles and the pelvic floor. Such simultaneous reactions are found but more frequently the primary reactions are found in the detrusor, and it seems likely that the uninhibited detrusor contractions trigger off the elicitation of the flexor spasms and this is seen in most cases. This means that one should carefully consider the possibility of influencing the flexor spasms by treatment of the uninhibited neurogenic bladder, for example by compounds (anticholinergic, smooth muscle relaxants, α-adrenergic blocking agent) and surgical interventions of the bladder neck or selective sacral neurotomy.

As mentioned the flexor reflex may facilitate a spastic contracture in flexion. It is most important to try to avoid the development of such contracture by suitable positioning of the patient, to try to avoid bed sores, and physical therapy to prevent contractures of the joints.

The methods of treatment may include all possibilities of treatment of spasticity including both increased stretch and flexor reflexes.

The physical methods will include physio- and occupational therapy, cryo-therapy and electrical stimulation, particularly as functional electrical stimulation of the leg.

Many antispastic drugs are available. Among the compounds effective are particularly baclofen, dantrolene sodium and tizanidine. Baclofen is effective in depressing the flexor reflex and has also proved to be effective in reducing flexor spasms. Dantrolene sodium is also effective on spasticity, and with peripheral action on the striated muscle it is supposed to be effective on both stretch and flexor reflexes. In the original animal experiment it was selected due to its effect on the flexor reflex, but not much information is available about the clinical effects on flexor reflexes in patients. Tizanidine will possibly prove to be of value but has not yet found its definite place.

If a contracture has developed intrathecal phenol may be appropriate. This is only acceptable in patients where the legs are unable to support the patient, but in such cases it is a simple technique which under X-ray control can be given without damaging the bladder and/or the bowel, and which can be most helpful in patients with flexor spasms and/or contractures rendering life difficult for the patient and for the nursing staff.

Selected References

Dimitrijevic, M. R. and Nathan, P. W. (1968). Studies of spasticity in man. 3. Analysis of reflex activity evoked by noxious cutaneous stimulation. *Brain*, **91**, 349

Klemar, B., Pedersen, E. and Jensen, N. O. (1983). Influence of Flexor Reflex Stimulation on the T-reflex. In eds. E. Pedersen, J. Clausen and L. Oades. *Actual problems in MS research*, (FADL's Forlag, A. S.)

Pedersen, E. (1969). *Spasticity. Mechanism, Measurement, Management.* (Springfield, Ill: Thomas)

Pedersen, E., Klemar, B. and Tørring, J. (1979). Counting of flexor spasms. *Acta Neurol. Scand.*, **60**, 164

Mai, J. and Pedersen, E. (1976). Central effect of bladder filling and voiding. *J. Neurol. Neurosurg. Psychiatry*, **39**, 171

Shahani, B. T. and Young, R. R. (1971). Human flexor reflexes. *J. Neurol. Neurosurg. Psychiatry*, **34**, 616

Tørring, J. and Pedersen, E. (1981). Standardisation of the electrical elicitation of the human flexor reflex. *J. Neurol. Neurosurg. Psychiatry*, **44**, 129

42
Tizanidine, a new antispastic agent: 6 years clinical experience in 152 MS patients

R. E. GONSETTE, Y. DE SMET and L. DEMONTY

INTRODUCTION

Rational therapy to alleviate spasticity must be based on three factors:

(1) an accurate clinical definition of symptoms and signs with their respective importance,
(2) a reasonable knowledge of the pathophysiologic mechanisms focusing on the primary process at the neuroanatomic level, and
(3) experimental data concerning the pharmacologic action of antispastic drugs.

Unfortunately, in this field facts are far outweighed by hypotheses and presumptions mostly based on animal experiments. Nevertheless, since spasticity is one of the most frequent and most disabling symptoms in patients with multiple sclerosis (MS), we found it interesting to present our clinical experience for 6 years with a new antispastic agent (tizanidine) and to briefly review the putative mechanisms, neuroanatomic substrates, and pharmacology that could explain the efficacy of this drug on certain spastic symptoms in MS.

MATERIAL AND METHODS

In 1976, a preliminary open study was performed in 12 patients. During this clinical evaluation, the efficacy of tizanidine was confirmed by gradual withdrawal of the drug and progressive substitution of a placebo. Once it appeared that tizanidine was effective and well tolerated, a double blind cross-over study was conducted in 30 patients, comparing tizanidine to baclofen. The results of this study are summarized in Table 1.

Table 1 Double blind cross-over study comparing tizanidine to baclofen (30 patients)

Efficacy	Tizanidine (6 mg daily)	Baclofen (60 mg daily)	Placebo
Marked	14%	26%	16%
Moderate	36%	26%	16%
Total	50%	52%	32%

Table 2 Material (1976–1982)

Number of patients treated:	152
Sex: Males:	66
Females:	86
Age: ≤30 years;	11
31–50 years:	69
> 50 years:	72

Table 3 Material (152 patients)

Clinical forms	
Remittent	40
Remittent–progressive	79
Progressive	33
Disability status (Kurtzke scale)	
Mild (0–3)	45
Moderate (4–6)	69
Severe (≥ 7)	38

Using a daily dose of 6 mg, which in fact is a low dose, it appeared that tizanidine was nearly as effective as baclofen and, moreover, that side-effects were definitely less marked. The high placebo response in this group is likely to be due to the extreme suggestibility of MS patients when using short term treatment periods, and it therefore appeared necessary to design a longterm clinical study.

One hundred and fifty-two patients entered this longterm trial, and their distribution according to sex and age is listed in Table 2. Patients were followed by the same investigator. Spasticity was evaluated using the Ashword scale, and disability using the Kurtzke scale.

The distribution according to clinical types and disability of the patients is listed in Table 3. As a matter of fact, in most of the patients, the disability score was mild or moderate and the mean duration of the disease quite long (17 years), as we selected patients with a stable spastic syndrome.

EFFICACY

Multiple sclerosis is characterized by multiple central nervous system lesions, associating in the same patient real spastic symptoms (muscular stiffness and clonus), as well as components of the upper motoneurone syndrome (spasms). We found it interesting, therefore, to evaluate the efficacy of tizanidine against those different symptoms and our results are listed in Table 4.

It appears that hypertonia was most frequently encountered (2/3 of the patients) and that tizanidine is definitely more effective against real spastic symptoms (muscular stiffness and clonus) than against components of the upper motoneurone syndrome (spasms).

The selective antispastic action of tizanidine was confirmed in a group of 70 patients in whom one of the three symptoms was definitely more pronounced and more disabling (Table 5). Thus, in our experience, tizanidine is a real 'antispastic' drug in the neurophysiologic sense of the term, as opposed to baclofen which is more effective in reducing spasms.

To combine the advantages of both antispastic drugs, tizanidine was given in association with low doses of baclofen in 20 patients. This association was perfectly tolerated, and produced an optimal therapeutic effect on muscular stiffness and spasms with a marked reduction of usual side-effects due to baclofen (weakness and tiredness).

Where the dose is concerned, the mean effective daily dosage usually lies between 6 and 12mg. In some cases, when spastic symptoms are particularly marked, higher doses (12–24 mg) must be used. As a matter of fact, in most patients individual efficacy is obtained by gradually increasing an initial dose of 2 mg up to 6 or 8 mg.

Table 4 Efficacy of tizanidine against spasticity and the upper motoneurone syndrome

Symptoms	Number of patients (n = 152)	Efficacy		
		Marked	Moderate	Total
Muscular stiffness	103	53	26	79 (76%)
Clonus	47	26	14	40 (85%)
Spasms	34	2	13	15 (44%)

Table 5 Selective antispastic action of tizanidine

Symptoms	Number of patients (n = 70)	Efficacy		
		Marked	Moderate	Total
Muscular stiffness	49	18	11	29 (59%)
Clonus	17	12	3	15 (88%)
Spasms	4	0	1	1

IMMEDIATE AND LONGTERM TOLERANCE

The clinical use of antispastic agents is frequently limited by adverse reactions. In this respect, tizanidine appears to be particularly well tolerated as side-effects were observed in only 20% of the 152 patients (Table 6). Interestingly enough, weakness was noted in seven cases, which means less than 5% of the patients. The very low negative action of tizanidine on muscular force seems an important advantage of this new antispastic agent when compared to diazepam and baclofen. It is worth pointing out that a dramatic improvement of walking was observed in some patients due to the excellent efficacy of tizanidine against patellar and ankle clonus without inducing any muscular weakness. In our experience, tizanidine definitely is the antispastic drug with the lowest incidence of side-effects.

We were particularly interested in the longterm tolerance of tizanidine. For 6 years, nearly 140 000 tablets have been delivered and out of 152 patients, 44

Table 6

Side-effects	Number of cases
Drowsiness	9
Weakness	7
Tiredness	4
Lowered blood pressure	3
Dry mouth	3
Nausea	2
Headache	1
Painful legs	1
Total	30 (20%)

Total number of patients = 150

Table 7 Reasons for discontinuation of treatment. 152 patients – 6 years

Adverse reactions	30
Uncooperation	24
Inefficacy	23
Intercurrent relapses	13
Working-out efficacy	8
Spontaneous improvement	4
Intercurrent disease or death	6
Total	108 (71%)

Table 8

Duration of treatment (years)	Number of patients
4–5	15
2–3	20
1	9
Total	44

are still treated with this substance. Reasons for discontinuation of treatment in 108 patients are given in Table 7.

Duration of treatment in 44 chronically treated patients is given in Table 8. In addition, a specific longterm safety study was conducted in nine patients for 12 months using daily doses higher than 12 mg. In those patients, no changes were observed in regularly checked vital signs, ECG ophthalmological examination and different laboratory values.

In our clinical experience with tizanidine for 6 years, the longterm safety of this new substance may be considered as excellent.

DISCUSSION

Spasticity is an ill-defined term, used to describe different clinical conditions characterized by an abnormal muscle tone. Spastic hypertonia is related to the pyramidal syndrome while plastic hypertonia is observed in extrapyramidal diseases[1,2].

From a more precise point of view 'spasticity' must be considered as a proprioceptive reflex disinhibition producing a muscular stiffness as well as an increased resistance to passive lengthening. In opposition, flexor spasms and increased flexor tone are due to increased exteroceptive reflexes. Those two symptoms, as well as weakness, should be better considered as related to the upper motoneurone syndrome. In fact, they are not spastic signs, even if they are frequently associated with spasticity, particularly in MS patients.

The exact pathophysiology of spasticity remains to be elucidated, but at least three feedback systems originating from the muscle or its direct synergists are involved: the direct myotatic stretch reflex, the inverse myotatic stretch reflex and finally feedback systems involving secondary endings from muscle spindles as well as tendinous joints and cutaneous afferent fibres.

It must be stressed that spasticity does not result from γ-motoneurones nor muscle spindles dysfunction. In fact, reflex hyperactivity results from hyper-excitability of α-motoneurones due to spinal lesions as well as to lesions of descending cortical spinal pathways.

The exact pharmacological action of centrally acting antispastic drugs remains mostly speculative but, on a theoretical point of view, they possibly act in two different ways[5].

First, antispastic drugs possibly act by enhancing or mimicking the inhibitory mechanisms. It is well known that presynaptic inhibition is mediated by the GABA neurotransmitter. However, its activity is not specific for a particular spinal stretch reflex pathway, and this could explain why diazepam, a substance globally enhancing the GABA neurotransmission, induces weakness as well as spasticity release (myorelaxant action). When the postsynaptic inhibition is concerned, its exact pharmacology remains unknown[6,7]. The inhibitory neurotransmitter released by Renshaw's cells (recurrent inhibition) are still to be discovered, but it seems that substance P experimentally decreases the cholinergic firing at the precedent synapse. Baclofen possibly influences this regulatory mechanism due to its hypothetic antisubstance P activity[8]. Second, antispastic drugs possibly counteract facilitatory volleys to α-motoneurones. Substance P and serotonin are excitatory neurotransmitters released by medulloreticulospinal tracts directly projecting on the anterior horn[11]. It has been suggested that those two neuro-transmitters are possibly inhibited respectively by baclofen and cyproheptadine[9,10]. Polysynaptic excitatory spinal pathways are possibly mediated by substance P and this could also explain the 'spasmolytic' effect of baclofen.

It has been recently suggested that the tonic component of the myotonic stretch reflex results from multiple successive activations of the same phasic monosynaptic stretch reflex in the absence of normally intervening inhibitory mechanisms impaired by MS lesions[3,4]. Preliminary pharmacological studies suggest that tizanidine should restore or mimic those inhibitory mechanisms. In this way, tizanidine should exert a real and quite selective 'myotonolytic' action. This is consistent with our clinical observations that this new substance is mostly effective against clonus and muscular stiffness. Moreover, being a selective antispastic drug, tizanidine does not induce muscular weakness as opposed to less selective substances like baclofen and diazepam[12-17].

CONCLUSIONS

In our experience, tizanidine is particularly useful for the treatment of clonus and muscular stiffness, and less effective in controlling flexor and extensor spasms. The clinical antispastic action of tizanidine is quite similar to that of diazepam, but adverse reactions and particularly muscular weakness and tiredness are definitely less marked.

In opposition, baclofen is more effective than tizanidine in reducing spasms in MS patients but again useful doses frequently produce muscular weakness.

Tizanidine appears, therefore, to be a real antispastic drug exerting a 'myotonolytic' action as opposed to the 'myorelaxant' action of diazepam and the 'spasmolytic' action of baclofen.

In addition to its exceptional tolerance, this selective myotonolytic action of tizanidine is a definite advance in the relief of spasticity in MS patients. Moreover, in association with low doses of baclofen, tizanidine produces an optimal therapeutic response, with a marked reduction of side-effects and particularly of weakness and tiredness in patients experiencing complex spastic syndromes.

SUMMARY

Tizanidine is a new centrally acting antispastic drug. Its efficacy and tolerance have been observed in 152 patients treated for 6 years. Tizanidine is mostly effective against muscular stiffness and clonus, and less effective against spasms.

The immediate as well as the longterm tolerance is excellent. Muscular weakness and tiredness, the most usual side-effects after administration of other antispastic drugs, were very rarely observed.

Tizanidine can be used in association with other antispastic drugs permitting a better control of complex spastic syndromes, with lower doses and less side-effects.

Where the pharmacological action of tizanidine is concerned, it appears from neurophysiologic experiments and clinical use, that this new substance acts in an original way, different from that of baclofen and diazepam.

References

1. Clemente, C.D. (1978). Neurophysiologic mechanisms and neuroanatomic substrates related to spasticity. *Neurology,* **28,** 40
2. Young, R.R. and Delwaide, P.J. (1981). Drug therapy. Spasticity. *N. Engl. J. Med.,* **304,** 28–96
3. Berardelli, A., Hallett, M., Kaufman, C., Fine, E., Berenberg, W. and Simon, S.R. (1982). Stretch reflexes of triceps surae in normal man. *J. Neurol. Neurosurg. Psych.,* **45,** 513
4. Berardelli, A., Sabra, E.F., Hallet, M., Berenberg, W. and Simon, S.R. (1983). Stretch reflexes of triceps surae in patients with upper motor neuron syndromes. *J. Neurol. Neurosurg. Psych.,* **46,** 54
5. Davidoff, R.A. (1978). Pharmacology of spasticity. *Neurology,* **28,** 46
6. Mai, J. and Pedersen, E. (1976). Clonus depression by popranolol. *Acta Neurol. Scand.,* **53,** 395
7. Hall, P.V., Smith, J.E., Lane, J., Mote, T. and Campbell, R. (1979). Glycine and experimental spinal spasticity. *Neurology,* **29,** 262
8. Duncan, G.W., Shahani, B.T. and Young, R.R. (1976). An evaluation of Baclofen treatment of certain symptoms in patients with spinal cord lesions. *Neurology,* **26,** 441
9. Barbeau, M., Richards, C.L. and Bedard, P.J. (1982). Action of cyproheptadine in spastic paraparetic patients. *J. Neurol. Neurosurg. Psych.,* **45,** 923
10. Silverglat, M.J. (1981). Baclofen and tricyclic antidepressants: possible interaction. *JAMA,* **246,** 1659

11. Botney, M. and Fields, H. L. (1983). Amitriptyline potentiates morphine analgesia by a direct action on the central nervous system. *Ann. Neurol.,* **13,** 160

12. Hennies, O. L. (1981). A new skeletal muscle relaxant (DS 103–282) compared to Diazepam in the treatment of muscle spasms of local origin. *J. Int. Med. Res.,* **9,** 62

13. Gerstenbrand, F., Lorinez, A., Lupin, H. P. and Ringwald, E. (1979). Langzeit-behändlung mit dem Insidazolinderivat DS 103–282. *Neverenarzt,* **50,** 806

14. Rinne, U. K. (1980). Tizanidine treatment of spasticity in multiple sclerosis and chronic myelopathy. *Cur. Ther. Res.,* **28,** 827

15. Hassan, N. and McLellan, D. L. (1980). Double-blind comparison of single doses of DS 103–282, Baclofen and placebo for suppression of spasticity. *J. Neurol. Neurosurg. Psych.,* **43,** 1132

16. Corston, R. N., Johnson, F. and Godwin-Austen, R. B. (1981). The assessment of drug treatment of spastic gait. *J. Neurol. Neurosurg. Psych.,* **44,** 1035

17. Knutsson, E., Martensson, A. and Gransberg, L. (1982). Antiparetic and antispastic effects induced by tizanidine in patients with spastic paresis. *J. Neurol. Sci.,* **53,** 187

43
Objective assessment of the myorelaxant properties of tizanidine

R. BENECKE, B. CONRAD and K. LÜNSER

An open clinical study was carried out in MS patients with myelopathy ($n = 27$) to investigate the antispastic efficacy and tolerance of tizanidine, a new muscle relaxant, whose mechanism of action is still under investigation. The treatment periods were 1–2 months. Clinical assessment of spasticity was carried out according to Kurtzke's scale. Furthermore, objective functionally relevant measurement of spasticity were performed by means of analyses of bicycling on a common ergometer machine. Bipolar recordings of the electromyographic activity of the main leg muscles were performed with surface electrodes.

The e.m.g. in each muscle was rectified and averaged within eight rotations. The kinesiological characteristics of spasticity during bicycling are broadening of the muscle recruitment period within the rotation. Using this method, the effects of tizanidine were tested after acute administration (0.1 mg/20 kg) as well as under chronic application (8–20 mg/day), as used in the clinical study.

With tizanidine chronically applied up to 1 year about 50% of the patients showed various degrees of improvement in spasticity. With the dosages used, the tolerance of the tizanidine was good, drowsiness often combined with an intermittent fall in blood pressure was the only clinically important side effect. In most patients the clinically appearing beneficial effect of tizanidine could be confirmed by the objective kinesiological investigation.

44
Is electrical stimulation of the spinal cord useful in MS patients?

J. GYBELS and D. VAN ROOST

INTRODUCTION

In view of the rather empirical basis on which spinal cord stimulation (SCS) was introduced in the treatment of neurological sequelae and of possible placebo-effects, we were very much impressed by a patient we observed recently. This 31-year-old man who presented a MS-related paraparesis until the age of 30, and since then a complete tetraplegia as well as an anaesthesia underneath the C4 level, became able to move his arms actively during the 2 hours that followed a tonic–clonic seizure, provoked by a metrizamide myelography. Nature here gave a demonstration that longstanding extremely strongly impaired motor control could be partially restored, *in casu* at the occasion of a tonic–clonic seizure, and that the restoration outlasted the restoration provoking factor by several hours.

In a recent literature review[1], we tried to answer the following questions:

(1) What is the effect of SCS on the symptoms and signs of dystonic motor disorders?
(2) Is there a difference between the effect of SCS in MS patients, who have a fluctuating clinical course, and other conditions, such as cerebral palsy, trauma, cerebellar atrophies etc. where the clinical course is either stabilized or progressive?
(3) Is there a difference of results between SCS in the cervical and in the thoracic medulla?
(4) Is there a difference of results between SCS at low (<150 Hz) and high (>1000 Hz) frequency?
(5) What can be learned from the clinical results of SCS about possible mechanisms underlying the eventual modifications provoked by SCS?

HISTORICAL REVIEW

The application of spinal cord stimulation for the modification of dystonic or hyperkinetic conditions arose in 1973 from a fortunate fortuity[2,3]. Cook and Weinstein[3] at least described as such their findings in the course of treating a woman for pain who was affected by multiple sclerosis.

The technique of 'dorsal column stimulation', since 1967 known to be useful for pain relief was employed in this patient, and led not only to an immediate alleviation of her distressing low back ache, but also, with a delay of a few days, to a regained ability of raising her legs off the bed, which had been impossible before. As the favourable effect on motor impairment was reproducible in the same patient after stimulation deprivation, and also in four additional MS patients, Cook applied SCS in 70 other MS patients and reported a substantial motor improvement in some 90% of the patients treated, including micturitional ameliorations.

Similar to those in the field of intractable pain therapy, the first SCS for the modification of dystonic conditions (MDC) were performed by surgical implantation through a laminectomy in the thoracic area, of bipolar electrodes extra-, endo- or intradurally, fairly close together, over the posterior midline of the spinal cord. Connections were made with a radio receiver device implanted subcutaneously, mostly in the subcostal or subclavicular region. The electrodes were energized through a radio frequency linked system by placing the transmitter's coil antenna over the skin that covers the receiver. An external miniaturized battery-powered transmitter generated the electric pulses, and allowed the various pulse parameters within a certain range to be changed.

Soon, the more elegant percutaneous insertion of one or two wire electrodes into the epidural space by means of a puncture needle (Tuohy-Huber or Hustead type) replaced the surgical mode, whether as a preliminary selection procedure or as a permanently aimed one, the latter having to deal with the frequent problem of electrode displacement.

The early used voltage, frequency and pulse width parameters for the modification of dystonic conditions were those of SCS for pain therapy, namely 1–10 V, 20–200 Hz and 100–500 μs. For the specific purpose of controlling ataxia however, the initiator of SCS in MS, Cook, mentioned in 1976 the usefulness of higher frequency stimulation, without further specifications[2]. On the other hand Waltz et al emphasized in 1980 the necessity of extending the used frequencies from 100 to 1400 Hz, as they found these frequencies to be individually critical[4].

The level or site of stimulation chosen in MDC from the beginning has been the mid or upper thoracic area, whereas for pain treatment this level is chosen in such a way that stimulation produces paraesthesias in the painful area. Although mid or upper thoracic SCS is still used by several authors, others now prefer the cervical area for stimulation, which according to Waltz[4] would present a higher therapeutic effect, especially between C2 and C4.

METHODS AND MATERIAL

Of the 95 articles published from 1973 up to June 1982 and which we went through[1], 39 papers from 19 different authors or teams, gave clinical data and results, covering a total number of 1008 patients who were treated with SCS for the modification of dystonic conditions. They were scrutinized and listed. The results in terms of overall improvement, motor function improvement, spasticity improvement and bladder improvement, were classified into four appreciative categories, namely 'no', 'fair' (F), 'good' (G) and 'very good' (VG). No, F, G and VG referred respectively to:

(1) no improvement at all, or deterioration;
(2) a slight improvement which is real but does not interfere with the pre-existing level of functioning, and which often can only be perceived by neurological assessment;
(3) an improvement that raises the pre-existing level of functioning in a way that it is useful in daily life activities, and therefore can be perceived by untrained eyes; and
(4) a similar improvement which leads to a spectacular gain of function

It served our purpose to differentiate and to list, as far as possible, the spasticity improvement separately from the improvement in motor function, even if undoubtedly the latter is influenced by the first. However, the assumed obviousness of this relationship might be the reason why many times the words 'spasticity' and 'motor impairment' were found to be used miscellaneously in the literature about SCS. Yet, can a reduction in spasticity in one case result in an improvement of motility, whereas in another case it deprives the patient of his last bit of support? This example illustrates why those publications are of special interest that describe an obtained improvement in terms of a score in a reproducible objective test, as a parameter of a well-defined neurological function (muscle strength, muscle tonus, coordination, etc.). The basic assessment approach throughout the studies of SCS for MDC has been, of course, the clinical neurological examination, with the evaluation of the myotatic reflexes etc., extended eventually to video-taping, to a psychological appreciation, and to a clinical disability rating, as provided for instance by the Kurtzke, Karnofsky and Pedersen scales. Beyond this first category of assessment, several other tests with more technical, and for that reason quantifiable character, have been used in various amounts. In more than one third of the articles concerning SCS for MDC, findings were based upon clinical observations of the above-mentioned first category alone. Only 13% of the papers used four or more additional tests, covering 86 patients, that is 8.5% of the total number of patients figuring in our review.

RESULTS

The amount of improvement yielded by SCS in MDC differs, often quite largely, from one author to another. Figures of a somewhat more practical interest perhaps were obtained when for all the papers the sums of only 'good' and 'very good' improvement percentages were averaged, thus representing the means of percentages of dystonic patients who reached under SCS a life style-changing improvement: 47% overall improvement, 37% motor function improvement, 40% spasticity improvement and 48% bladder function improvement. A 'very good' overall improvement was obtained in an average of 17% of all the scrutinized cases, a 'very good' motor function improvement also in 17%, a 'very good' spasticity improvement in 15%, and a 'very good' bladder function improvement in 28% of all the cases.

These total means are summarized in Table 1 under 'T' (middle columns), together with figures obtained by averaging analogously the results of the most critically elaborated series (left-side columns 'C') and of the largest series (right-side columns 'L'). As largest series we considered those with patient numbers of at least 30, and as most critically elaborated series we elected those that, beyond a clinical examination, were assessed by at least four additional technical tests. In Table 1, the figures of spasticity, and especially those of bladder function improvement, distinguish themselves by higher percentages in the 'very good' row, even when the critically assessed series alone are considered. Moreover, the bladder improvement scores show a statistical highly significant mutual agreement within each of the four appreciative categories. Such a mutual agreement among the percentages is lacking as far as motor and spasticity improvement are concerned, and is present only at a lower significance grade for the percentages of overall improvement. In other words, with SCS, bladder function improves in a higher percentage of MDC patients than spasticity or motor function do, the latter even significantly less. This bladder function improvement is skewed towards the 'very good' rank, and is reported in a pretty unanimous way by the different authors.

Table 1 Mean improvement

	Overall			Motor			Spasticity			Bladder		
	C	T	L	C	T	L	C	T	L	C	T	L
Very good	10	17	19.3	0	17	18	21.6	15	18	26	28	27
Good	18	30	26.3	16	20	20	0	25	22	21	20	11.6
Fair	12	15	14.3	16	14	17.5	34.6	24	21	17	17	24.6
No	60	38	40	68	49	44.5	43.6	36	39	36	35	36.6

Mean improvement expressed as percentages of numbers of patients, derived from the most critical series only (C), from all the series (T) and from the largest series only (L)

It is precisely the impaired bladder function and its recovery that can be assessed in a very objective way by using a battery of urodynamic and electrophysiological tests. These, however, have been employed exhaustively by only very few authors in the field of SCS for MDC.

What about the possibility of false positive interpretations arising from the interference of a spontaneously fluctuating course in MS? We believe we have ruled them out by separating and matching the results in MS patients and those in patients affected by disorders with a stabilized or progressively deteriorating clinical course. Table 2 lists these paired scores on the understanding that they originate respectively from the observations of a common investigator.

Statistical analysis fails to discern, at a high level of significance, the scores of both groups and belonging to different populations.

Table 2

| | Improvement | | | | | | | |
| | MS | | | | Stabilized or progressive deteriorating disorders | | | |
	No	F	G	VG	No	F	G	VG
Dooley[5], 1977	36		64		36		64	
(n = 42)					(n = 14)			
	15	—	27	—	5	—	9	—
Dooley and Sharkey[6], 1981	36.2	14.5	13	36.2	32	—	12	56
(n = 69)					(n = 25)			
	25	10	9	25	8	—	3	14
Siegfried[7], 1980	—	14	86	—	25	50	25	—
(n = 7)					(n = 4)			
	—	1	6	—	1	2	1	—
Campos et al[8], 1981	8	33	42	17	—	8	75	17
(n = 12)					(n = 12)			
	1	4	5	2	—	1	19	2
Davis et al[9], 1981	36	—	57	7	16	53	31	—
(n = 69)					(n = 32)			
	25	—	39	5	5	17	10	—
Lazorthes et al[10], 1981	67	12	19	2	72		28	
(n = 111)					(n = 46)			
	75	13	21	2	33	—	13	—
Reynolds and Oakley[11], 1982	50	—	—	50	25	—	50	25
(n = 2)					(n = 4)			
	1	—	—	1	1	—	2	1
Waltz[12], 1982	30		70		23	11	35	31
(n = 27)					(n = 193)			
	8	—	19	—	44	22	68	59

Improvement expressed both in percentages (upper rows) and in absolute numbers (lower rows) of patients, n indicating the total number of each series

The available literature does not provide sufficient comparable material in order to perform a similar numerical analysis as above, concerning the controversial superiority of cervical over thoracic SCS and concerning the need of stimulation trials at high frequency. Especially our requirement of using detailed data from a control group, evaluated by the same author, was not fulfilled in this case.

DISCUSSION AND CONCLUSION

Summarizing, it must be stated that SCS for MDC in MS really works to a certain extent. For, whenever placebo effects may exist, they alone cannot explain the importance of the improvement which is observed in the bladder, an objectively assessable organ. Subjected to the most critical analysis some 12.5% of the cases remain, in whom the improvement of bladder function can not be denied[1]. Being less critical, a useful relief of disability in terms of bladder function should be accepted in 40–50% of the cases (Table 1). Limb spasticity does not respond to SCS as well as the impaired bladder does. It is questionable if motor function, other than that one impaired by spasticity, can be significantly improved by SCS. The concerning scores indeed show poor mutual agreement, and moreover there is not one single 'very good' case reported among the most critically assessed series.

In the literature on SCS we found some 30 different hypotheses proposed to explain the working mechanism in the modification of dystonic conditions[1]. Out of these 30, the biochemical hypothesis, or the one of functional and anatomical reorganization through plastic properties of the synaptic zone at the level of the lesion, should be taken into consideration with respect to the observed chronological characteristics of the SCS-effects. Observations of skin temperature increase and of the healing of arteriosclerotic ulcers, together with the conclusions of refined bladder function assessment under SCS therapy, suggest an involvement of the autonomic nervous system in the sense of a reduced sympathetic tone, although a reduced sympathetic tone has also been proposed as an effect secondary to a bladder function improvement. The observations of favourable effects well above and below the stimulated segment on the other hand, seem to point beyond local events to some supra-segmental mechanism with a descending inhibitory influence on the central overreactivity. There are no data however, either clinical or experimental, to clearly indicate which might be the working mechanisms of SCS in MDC, and one is left at the moment with rather vague theories, which at best can be described as 'good neurologizing'.

ACKNOWLEDGEMENT

The authors are indebted to Mrs Feytons-Heeren for expert technical assistance.

References

1. Gybels, J. and Van Roost, D. (1983). Spinal cord stimulation for the modification of dystonic and hyperkinetic conditions: A critical review. In *Monograph on Recent Achievements in Restorative Neurology*. Raven Press (in press)
2. Cook, A. W. (1976). Electrical stimulation in multiple sclerosis. *Hosp. Pract.*, **11**, 51
3. Cook, A. W. and Weinstein, S. P. (1973). Chronic dorsal column stimulation in multiple sclerosis. *NY State J. Med.*, **73**, 2868
4. Waltz, J. M., Reynolds, L. O. and Riklan, M. (1981). Multi-lead spinal cord stimulation for control of motor disorders. *Appl. Neurophysiol.*, **44**, 244
5. Dooley, D. M. (1977). Demyelinating, degenerative and vascular disease. *Neurosurgery*, **1**, 220
6. Dooley, D. M. and Sharkey, J. (1981). Electrical stimulation of the spinal cord in patients with demyelinating and degenerative diseases of the central nervous system. *Appl. Neurophysiol.*, **44**, 218
7. Siegfried, J. (1980). Treatment of spasticity by dorsal cord stimulation. *Int. Rehab. Med.*, **2**, 31
8. Campos, R. J., Dimitrijevic, M. M., Faganel, J. and Sharkey, P. C. (1981). Clinical evaluation of the effect of spinal cord stimulation on motor performance in patients with upper motor neuron lesions. *Appl. Neurophysiol.*, **44**, 141

9. Davis, R., Gray, E. and Kudzma, J. (1981). Beneficial augmentation following dorsal column stimulation in some neurological diseases. *Appl. Neurophysiol.*, **44**, 37
10. Lazorthes, Y., Siegfried, J. and Broggi, G. (1981). Electrical spinal cord stimulation for spastic motor disorders in demyelinating diseases – A cooperative study. In Corbin, T. and Hosobuchi, Y. (eds.). *Indications for spinal cord stimulation,* pp. 48–57. (Princeton: Excerpta Medica)
11. Reynolds, F. A. and Oakley, J. C. (1982). High frequency cervical epidural stimulation for spasticity. *Appl. Neurophysiol.*, **45**, 93
12. Waltz, J. M. (1982). Computerized percutaneous multi-level spinal cord stimulation in motor disorders. *Appl. Neurophysiol.*, **45**, 73

Section IV
Monitoring of the Disease

45
A silica gel radioimmunoassay determination of cerebrospinal fluid myelin basic protein levels of various demyelinating disease syndromes associated with multiple sclerosis

K. G. WARREN, I. CATZ and T. A. McPHERSON

Myelin basic protein is a hairpin shaped molecule 170 amino-acids long, located within the major dense line of myelin. The protein is located within the cerebrospinal fluid in increased quantities in patients with active multiple sclerosis. The purpose of this project was to determine the amount of myelin basic protein that could be anticipated by the physician looking after patients with various multiple sclerosis syndromes. A silica gel radioimmunoassay was developed for this project.

METHODS

Myelin basic protein was prepared from normal brain where its concentration is approximately 100–200 mg per 100 gram of tissue. The procedure is carried out at 5 °C in order to minimize proteolytic enzymes. The brain tissue was delipidated with chloroform–methanol. After drying with acetone, the residue is washed, and then approximately 90% of the myelin basic protein is solubilized at pH 3 in the crude acid extract. Purification consists of chromatography on CM-52 at pH 11.6, where the nonbasic proteins are removed due to their low affinity to CM-52 at this high pH. After washing with salt solutions to remove additional weakly bound proteins and a couple of water washes, the CM-52 is resuspended at pH 2.5. This is a critical step that eliminates fast running breakdown products, the lysine rich F1 histone, as well as a trace of myelin basic protein. A pH greater than 2.5 does not eliminate any of the above products, and a pH less than 2.5 eliminates too much myelin basic protein, and subsequently a poor yield occurs. The myelin basic protein is then solubilized in

0.1 N hydrochloric acid and further dialyzed and lyophilized. Further purification can be achieved by gel filtration of sephadex G 150 and elution with 0.1 N hydrochloric acid. The final product shows one peak on SDS-PAGE electrophoresis. The myelin basic protein obtained in this way can be used as standard and as starting product for iodination (^{125}I) and for immunization to prepare antimyelin basic protein in rabbits.

Cerebrospinal fluid from patients containing questionable quantities of myelin basic protein is incubated with antimyelin basic protein. After 18–24 hours radiolabelled myelin basic protein is added. Incubation for another 18–20 hours occurs. Silica gel is then used to separate the free myelin basic protein from the bound myelin basic protein to the antibody, and the latter fraction is then counted.

A typical standard curve for the silica gel radioimmunoassay results. The sensitivity of the assay is 1 ng/ml MBP and the cross reaction with lysozyme and histones is negligible.

The assay was validated by recovery and dilution studies, and all curves were identical. The recovery studies were performed by starting with a cerebrospinal fluid with a low value of myelin basic protein and subsequently adding known amounts of myelin basic protein. Dilution studies were performed by starting with cerebrospinal fluid containing high myelin basic protein levels and serially diluting the specimen with normal cerebrospinal fluid not containing myelin basic protein.

Having developed the assay we studied several clinical groups. Cerebrospinal fluids from 151 children and young adults with leukaemia were used as normal control specimens. Twenty five patients with acute optic neuritis, seven with acute internuclear ophthalmoplegia, 32 patients with chronic progressive multiple sclerosis, 21 with monosymptomatic exacerbations of multiple sclerosis, and 29 patients with polysymptomatic exacerbations of multiple sclerosis were studied.

In the normal control population the mean cerebrospinal fluid myelin basic protein level was 3.9 ng/ml. Two standard deviations above the mean was 6.2 ng/ml.

Nineteen of the 25 patients with optic neuritis had mildly elevated levels of cerebrospinal fluid myelin basic protein. The mean value was 7.6 and the range was from 4 to 15 ng/ml. Six of the seven patients with acute internuclear ophthalmoplegia had mildly elevated levels of cerebrospinal fluid myelin basic protein. The mean value was 6.8 and the range was from 4 to 14 ng/ml. Fifty percent of the 32 patients with chronic progressive multiple sclerosis had elevated levels of cerebrospinal fluid myelin basic protein. The mean value was 6.7 and the range was from 2 to 18 ng/ml. Sixteen of the 21 patients experiencing monosymptomatic exacerbations of multiple sclerosis had elevated levels of cerebrospinal fluid myelin basic protein. The mean value was 8.2 and the range was from 2 to 16 ng/ml. Twenty eight of the 29 patients experiencing more severe attacks of multiple sclerosis in the form of polysymptomatic exacerbations had increased levels of cerebrospinal fluid myelin basic protein. The mean value in this group was much higher than in the other clinical groups. The mean value was 22.3 ng/ml, the standard deviation was 18.5, and the range was from 2 to over 100 ng/ml.

Cerebrospinal fluid myelin basic protein levels can be used as a diagnostic aid, assisting in various clinical situations. The assay can also be utilized to monitor disease activity, response to putative therapies, and guide other research projects.

46
T-lymphocyte subpopulations in patients with MS: a study of 84 cases

N. GENETET, B. POULLOT, M. MADIGAND, O. SABOURAUD
and B. GENETET

INTRODUCTION

Abnormal immune responses have been described in multiple sclerosis, and suggest that a defect of immunoregulation could contribute to the pathogenesis of the disease[1,2]. To determine whether abnormalities of immunoregulatory T cells are associated with multiple sclerosis, we analysed peripheral blood lymphocytes in MS patients during the active and inactive stages of the disease with monoclonal antibodies specific for T helper and suppressor/cytotoxic subpopulations.

PATIENTS

120 blood samples in 84 patients with MS were studied. The patients were classified as having either active (42) or inactive (52) MS. Patients with inactive MS had been stable for at least 6 months before sampling. They had no new functional deficits during this period. Active forms of the disease include: progressive worsening, with progressive functional impairment, but without clear exacerbations (18 cases), remittent courses, with acute exacerbations (34 cases). These last cases were studied either during the acute relapse, defined as the development within 2 weeks before sampling of new deficits; or during the regression of an attack, i.e. from the 3rd week to the 2nd month after an exacerbation.

Regarding the severity of the disease, 42 patients are considered moderate cases, being K3 or less after 10 years of disease – 42 patients are considered severe forms, being K4 at 10 years of duration of MS; in this group of severe forms have also been included some earlier cases whose progression clearly indicates that they will reach K4 before the term of 10 years.

Some patients received immunosuppressive drugs (azathioprine).

METHODS

Peripheral blood mononuclear cells were isolated from heparinized venous blood by means of Ficoll-Hypaque gradient-density centrifugation. T cell subpopulation typing was performed by indirect immunofluorescence with monoclonal antibodies (OKT – Ortho pharmaceutical) specific for T helper (OKT 4 positive) and T suppressor/cytotoxic (OKT 8 positive) subpopulations. The data are expressed as relative values and by the T4/T8 cell ratio, which defines the balance between helper and cytotoxic/suppressor cells and eliminates the interference of non-T cells in the cellular suspensions.

RESULTS

Generally, the relative values of T helper cells (T4 positive) – Figure 1 – were lower in MS patients than in the control group. No difference was observed between patients in remission, with or without immunosuppressive treatment, with severe or moderate disease. The figures were still lower in progressive forms. The values are very scattered in patients with exacerbations.

The distribution of T suppressor/cytotoxic cells (T8 positive) is identical in progressive forms and controls – Figure 2. There is a decrease in T8 positive cells in patients with inactive disease and active forms with exacerbations. The values are nevertheless widely unsteady in the course of exacerbations.

Figure 1 T helper subpopulations in MS with (○) and without (•) immunosuppressive treatment

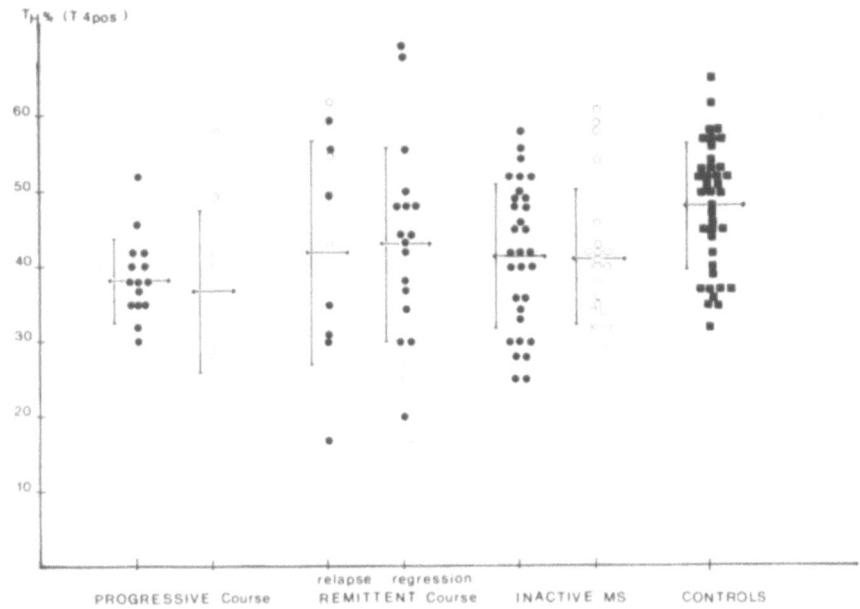

Figure 2 T suppressor cytotoxic subpopulations in MS with (○) and without (•) immuno-suppressive treatment

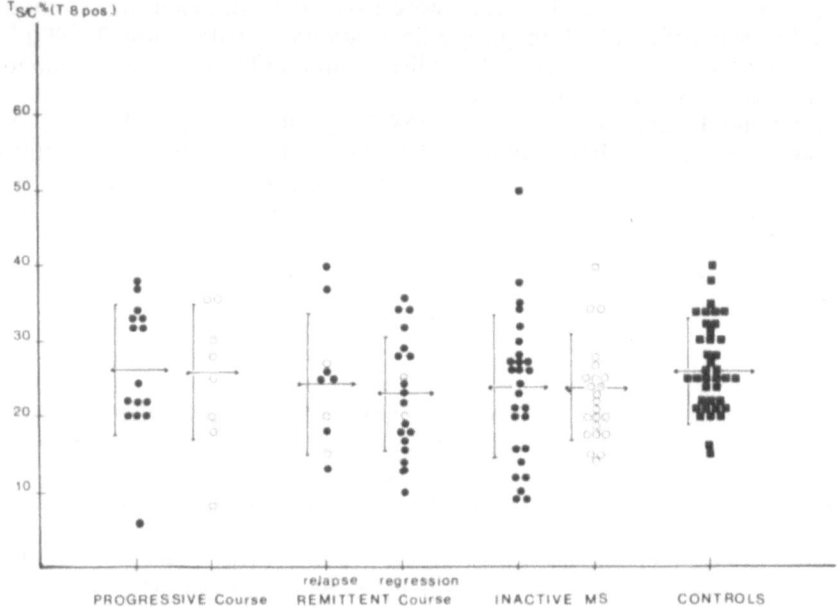

Figure 3 T helper–T suppressor cytotoxic ratio in MS with (○) and without (•) immuno-suppressive treatment

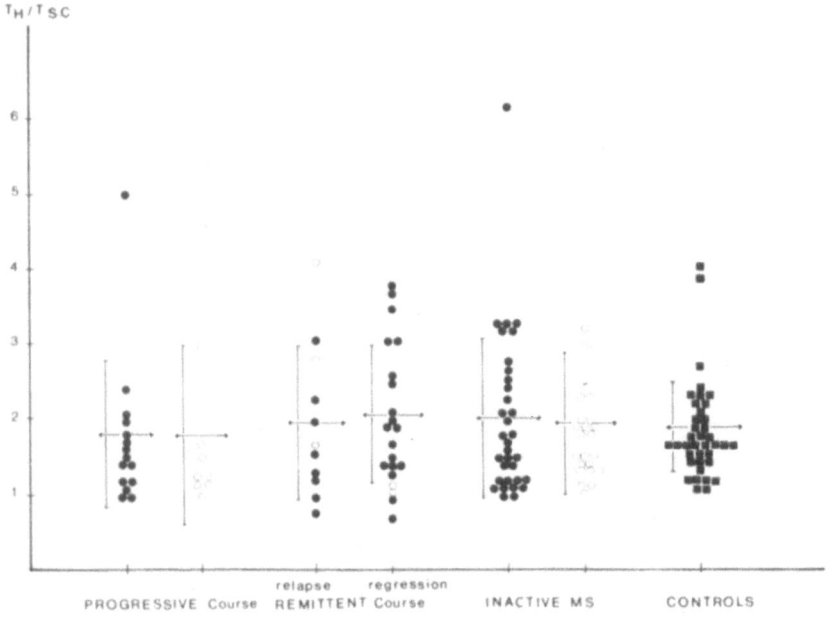

The T helper/suppressor cytotoxic ratio – Figure 3 – doesn't appear different in patients with inactive and progressive disease and in controls. In patients with recent attacks and during the period of regression of an attack, the ratio reflects the dispersion of T helper and suppressor cell values.

Although the T subpopulation distribution does not appear different in patients with or without immunosuppressive therapy, we excluded from the statistical analysis all the patients with immunosuppressive therapy or any other drug during the 2 months before lymphocyte analysis, in order to avoid the possible influence of such therapeutic agents in altering lymphocyte distribution in peripheral blood of patients with MS.

Student's *t* test was used to compare mean values in each group of patients classified as previously described with age and sex matched controls.

Table 1 illustrates the data of T lymphocyte subpopulation characterization in inactive MS. The mean value of T helper cells in 31 patients is significantly decreased ($p<0.01$), as compared with controls. The mean values of T suppressor cells and T_h/T_s cells ratios are not different between the groups.

Table 1 Inactive MS

Patients	Samples (n)	Age (mean)	T Lymphocytes % TH (T4 pos.)	TS/C (T8 pos.)	TH/TS.C Ratio
11 Severe	13	44.09 ± 7.84	45.18 ± 10.24	22.45 ± 11.35	2.25 ± 1.44
20 Moderate	20	36.90 ± 8.78	39.40 ± 8.89	23.85 ± 8.28	1.84 ± 0.76
31 Patients	33	39.45 ± 9.03	41.45 ± 9.64	23.43 ± 9.47	2.01 ± 1.08
			$p<0.01$		
31 Controls	31	39.39 ± 9.40	48.77 ± 7.89	26.00 ± 5.55	1.95 ± 0.63

Table 2 Active MS – remittent course

Patients	Samples (n)	Age (mean)	T Lymphocytes % TH (T4 pos.)	TS/C (T8 pos.)	TH/TS.C Ratio
7 Recent exacerbation	7	28.57 ± 7.68	39.43 ± 15.24	26.29 ± 9.59	1.65 ± 0.85
19 Regressive	20	35.22 ± 8.99	44.83 ± 12.93	23.06 ± 7.97	2.14 ± 0.94
26 Patients	27	33.36 ± 9.02	43.32 ± 13.45	23.96 ± 8.38	2.00 ± 0.92
26 Controls	26	34.35 ± 8.74	46.36 ± 8.74	26.15 ± 4.94	1.87 ± 0.59

In patients with active remittent forms of the disease, seven patients examined during the 2 weeks following an exacerbation and 19 MS tested during the period of regression of an attack (Table 2), the distribution of T lymphocyte subpopulations is not significantly different from control distribution. The mean value of T helper cells looks lower in patients whose samples were examined during the 2 weeks following an acute attack.

In 11 patients (15 samples) with severe disease, following a gradually progressive course (Table 3) the mean value of T helper cells is significantly decreased ($p<0.01$) as compared with matched control group.

In Table 4 are combined the cases with disease in activity: remittent course with recent exacerbation and progressive aggravative course. The T helper cells were significantly decreased ($p<0.01$), while T suppressor/cytotoxic cells were not affected. Changes in T lymphocyte distribution were not important enough to modify significantly the T helper/suppressor cell ratio.

Table 3 Active MS – progressive course

Patients	Samples (n)	Age (mean)	T Lymphocytes % TH (T4 pos.)	TS/C (T8 pos.)	TH/TS.C Ratio
11 MS	15	39.27 ± 6.23	38.67 ± 5.49 ‡ p<0.01	26.33 ± 8.69	1.77 ± 0.98
11 Controls	11	38.82 ± 7.93	48.27 ± 9.74	26.36 ± 6.77	1.97 ± 0.98

Table 4 Active MS

	n	Age (mean)	T Lymphocytes % TH (T4 pos.)	TS/C (T8 pos.)	TH/TS.C Ratio
With recent exacerbation	7	28.57 ± 7.68	39.43 ± 15.25	26.29 ± 9.59	1.65 ± 0.85
Progressive forms	11	39.27 ± 6.29	38.67 ± 5.49 p<0.01	26.33 ± 8.69	1.77 ± 0.98
Total	18	35.61 ± 9.82	38.91 ± 9.30 ‡ p<0.01	26.32 ± 8.75	1.73 ± 0.92
Controls	18	35.39 ± 8.84	48.39 ± 9.61	25.44 ± 5.59	2.00 ± 0.67

CONCLUSION

In contrast to other authors[3,4] we do not find an evident selective defect in T suppressor cells in peripheral blood of patients with active MS. Conversely, our results show a decrease in T helper cell subpopulation in MS. This abnormality, which represents a minor but significant change, especially in patients with active forms of the disease, could be discussed in view of recently published data about the identification of T lymphocyte subsets in the cerebro-spinal fluid and in the perivascular infiltrates in demyelinating lesions of MS. Several preliminary studies[5-7] agree with the fact that the lymphocytes in the central nervous system are predominantly T helper cells. In this regard, abnormalities in T lymphocyte distribution in peripheral blood of MS could be considered as the reflection of a preferential migration of T helper cells towards the central nervous system rather than as the indication of an immune dysregulation associated with clinical exacerbations in multiple sclerosis. These data lend support to the recognition of active progressive course as a type or a period in the evolution of MS.

References

1. Antel, J.P., Arnason, G.W. and Medof, M.E. (1979). Suppressor cell function in multiple sclerosis: correlation with clinical disease activity. *Ann. Neurol.,* **5,** 338
2. Gonzalez, R.L., Dau, P.C. and Spitler, L.E. (1979). Altered regulation of mitogen responsiveness by suppressor cells in multiple sclerosis. *Clin. Exp. Immunol.,* **36,** 78
3. Reinherz, E.L., Weiner, H.L., Hauser, S.L., Cohen, J.A., Distaso, J.A., and Schlossman, S.F. (1980). Loss of suppressor T cells in active multiple sclerosis. Analysis with monoclonal antibodies. *N. Engl. J. Med.,* **303,** 125
4. Bach, A.M., Phan-Dinh-Tuy, F., Tournier, E., Chatenoud, L. and Bach, J.F. (1980). Deficit of suppressor T cells in active multiple sclerosis. *Lancet,* **2,** 1221

5. Panitch, H. S. and Francis, G. S. (1982). T lymphocyte subsets in cerebrospinal fluid in multiple sclerosis. *N. Engl. J. Med., 307,* 560
6. Nyland, H., Matre, R., Mork, S., Bjerke, J. R. and Naess, A. (1982). T lymphocytes subpopulations in multiple sclerosis lesions. *N. Engl. J. Med., 307,* 1643
7. Brinkman, J. J., Terlaak, H. J., Hommes, O. R., Poppema, S. and Delmotte, P. (1982). T lymphocytes subpopulations in multiple sclerosis lesions. *N. Engl. J. Med., 307,* 1644

47
Multiple sclerosis cerebrospinal fluid lymphocytes secretion *in vitro*: effect on myelinated cultures

J. J. HAUW, O. de BRUNIER, J. M. BOUTRY, E. SCHULLER,
E. ROULLET, R. MARTEAU, F. LHERMITTE and O. LYON-CAEN

INTRODUCTION

It has been demonstrated in various conditions that sera, cerebrospinal fluid (CSF) and lymphoid cells demyelinate and inhibit the myelination of cultured central and peripheral nervous tissues[1,2].

Sera from about 60–70% of patients with multiple sclerosis (MS) destroy myelin of the central nervous system (CNS) in culture. On the contrary, the peripheral myelin of the same cultures is spared[1,3]. The specificity of these data has been challenged since Ulrich and Lardi[4] have shown that sera from high percentages of patients with other neurological diseases (OND) have similar effects. The mechanism of demyelination induced by MS serum is unknown. This contrasts with data obtained in experimental autoimmune encephalomyelitis (EAE), where demyelination is due to immunological factors: the demyelinating activity is complement-dependent, linked to IgG and, in the guinea pig, to the IgG2 serum fraction[5]. Galactocerebrosides seem to be a major target, as shown by absorption studies[6]. On the contrary, in MS, although demyelination activity of serum is complement-dependent, results of absorption studies favour the presence of a non γ-globulin demyelinating factor – which could be an enzyme[1,2]. However, in the *in vivo* system tadpole optic nerve, the IgG fraction of sera from MS patients induces more myelin lesions than that from controls[7]. These results, obtained with a small number of patients on a particularly vulnerable model, need confirmation. It may be added that no myelination-inhibiting activity has been found in MS sera[4], in contrast with the data obtained with EAE[2].

Few results have been, as yet, obtained with CSF. Kim *et al*[8] have reported that pooled CSF concentrated approximately 200 times (to bring the level of globulin up to or beyond that in serum) demyelinate mouse cerebellum in culture. The demyelinating activity appears linked to IgG preparations isolated by protein A-sepharose column chromatography, as shown with the tadpole optic nerve system. On the other hand, it has been shown by Sandberg-Wollheim and her team[9,10] (1969–1974) that cells from the CSF synthesize immunoglobulins in cell cultures. These results prompted us to search for CSF cell secretion in MS and for the myelinotoxicity of the culture supernatant.

PATIENTS, MATERIAL AND METHODS

Patients

Forty definite MS patients, 20 in relapsing–remitting forms, 20 in chronic progressive forms, were studied. They fulfilled the clinical criteria of diagnosis from McAlpine et al[11].

Twelve OND were used as controls; 11 were classified as inflammatory diseases (two subacute sclerosing panencephalitis, one neuro-Behçet, eight viral meningitis); the last one was a meningioma.

In every case, electrophoresis and Laurel's immuno-electrophoresis of CSF were performed.

CSF lymphoid cell cultures

After the cell count of an aliquot, recently obtained CSF was centrifuged for 7 minutes at $140\,g$, washed and cultured for 3 days in Iscove and Melchers' modification of Dulbecco's medium (Flow laboratories) supplemented with 5% of newborn calf serum, IgG depleted (Gibco laboratories). The cultures were then centrifuged 7 minutes at $140\,g$. Aliquots of the supernatant were used for immunodiffusion determination of IgG level (Laurel's immuno-electrophoresis), the pellet for cell count and for cytocentrifugation; the remnant was stored at $-80\,°C$ until demyelination test. The cell secretion was expressed by the ratio:

$$2 \times \frac{\text{Total IgG of the supernatant}}{\text{Initial number of cells} + \text{Final number of cells}}$$

Myelinated cultures: newborn rat cerebellum or 28 day gestation guinea pig spinal cord ganglia were cultivated on collagen-coated coverslips in Leighton tubes[13]. Culture medium was the following: Eagle's MEM 35%, Hanks' BSS 35%, decomplemented fetal calf serum (Gibco laboratories) 30%, supplemented with glucose $600\,mg/100\,ml$.

Demyelination assays were performed from 12th to 20th days *in vitro*. Two to four test cultures and two to four control cultures (concentrated medium and complement) were used for each test.

Individual CSF cell culture tests were performed after 10 to 20 times concentration of lymphoid cell culture supernatants added in 10% concentration (+ 10% complement) to myelinated culture medium (7–660 ng IgG/culture).

Pooled CSF cell culture tests were performed after 30 times concentration of respectively 14 and 20 lymphoid cell cultures supernatants (+ 10% complement added in 30% concentration to myelinated cultures medium) (2.2 μg IgG/culture).

Demyelination was judged upon bright field examination of living cultures and of Sudan black B stained preparations.

Statistical analysis was performed by the Mann and Whitney test.

RESULTS

These are given in Tables 1 and 2. The main value of the secretion of CSF lymphocytes obtained during exacerbations (seven cases) was 0.18 ng IgG/cell. In the five cases where the lumbar puncture was done at a distance from an exacerbation, it was 0.07 ng IgG/cell.

Table 1 Immunoglobulin secretion by CSF cultures

	Number		Secretion mean value ± SE (ng IgG/cell)	No secretion
Definite MS	40			
Relapsing–remitting	12		0.13 ± 0.04	8
Chronic progressive	14		0.36 ± 0.13	6
OND	12	SSPE 2	0.08 ⎫ 0.044	
Inflammatory	5 {			6
		Meningitis 3	0.02 ⎭	
Non-inflammatory	1		0.002	—

Table 2 Demyelination *in vitro*

Individual MS CSF supernatants in culture (7–660 ng IgG/culture)	No demyelination	4 OND
		13 MS (4 chronic progressive, 9 relapsing–remitting)
Pooled MS CSF supernatants in culture (2.2 μg IgG/culture)	No demyelination	1 assay
	Demyelination	1 assay

DISCUSSION

We found no correlation between IgG synthesis *in vitro* and CSF IgG content in patients, and with the presence or absence of oligoclonal pattern, with the age of the patient or the duration of the disease. On the contrary, although the total CSF secretion was sometimes higher in pleiocytic inflammatory OND, the mean value of IgG secretion by CSF lymphoid cells (expressed in ng Ig/cell) was higher in MS than in inflammatory OND ($p<0.05$) and in chronic progressive forms than in relapsing–remitting forms of the disease. However, this last result was not statistically significant (perhaps on account of the small size of classes). Although the main value of CSF lymphocytes secretion during exacerbations was higher than that of remissions, the difference was not statistically significant, probably for the same reason. It can be recalled that Sandberg-Wollheim[10] has already shown that the amount of synthesized IgG was greater during exacerbations than during remissions.

As far as demyelination of nervous tissue cultures by supernatants of lymphoid cells *in vitro* is concerned, we could not find any myelin morphological change in individual assays. The results of the tests with pooled and concentrated supernatants were less clear-cut: in the first assay, no demyelination was obvious, on the contrary mild morphological changes were observed in the second test. These results could be related to the differences in concentrations: the culture medium with pooled supernatants contained 3.5 times more immunoglobulins than that of the individual tests. However, we have no explanation for the variable results that we obtained with pooled supernatant. Further experiments are in progress.

ACKNOWLEDGEMENTS

Supported by a grant from the Association pour la Recherche sur la Sclérose en Plaques (ARSEP) and from the Société Médicale des Hopitaux de Paris. We thank G. Deloche for the statistical analysis of results and A. Lhermitte for typing the manuscript.

References

1. Bornstein, M. B. (1981). Tissue culture techniques applied to demyelinating disease. *TINS*, **4**, 238
2. Seil, F. J. (1982). Demyelination. In Fedoroff, S. and Hertz, L. (eds.). *Advances in Cellular Neurobiology*. Vol. 3, pp. 235–274. (NY: Academic Press)
3. Bornstein, M. B. and Raine, C. S. (1977). Multiple sclerosis and experimental allergic encephalomyelitis: specific demyelination of CNS in culture. *Neuropathol. Appl. Neurobiol.*, **3**, 359
4. Ulrich, J. and Lardi, H. (1978). Multiple sclerosis: demyelination and myelination inhibition of organotypic tissue cultures of the spinal cord by sera of patients with multiple sclerosis and other neurological diseases. *J. Neurol.*, **218**, 7
5. Lebar, R., Boutry, J. M., Vincent, C. *et al.* (1976). Studies on auto-immune encephalomyelitis in the guinea-pig. Part 2 (an *in vitro* investigation on the nature, properties and specificity of the serum-demyelinating factor). *J. Immunol.*, **116**, 1439
6. Raine, C. S., Johnson, A. B., Marcus, D. M. *et al.* (1981). Demyelination *in vitro*. Absorption studies demonstrate that galactocerebroside is a major target. *J. Neurol. Sci.*, **52**, 117
7. Stendahl-Brodin, L., Kristensson, K. and Link, H. (1981). Myelinotoxic activity on tadpole optic nerve of IgG isolated from CSF and serum of patients with multiple sclerosis. *Neurology*, **31**, 100
8. Kim, S. U., Murray, M. R. and Tourtelotte, W. W. (1970). Demonstration in tissue culture of myelinotoxicity in cerebrospinal fluid and brain extracts from multiple sclerosis patients. *J. Neuropathol. Exp. Neurol.*, **29**, 420
9. Sandberg-Wollheim, M., Zettervall, O. and Muller, R. (1969). *In vitro* synthesis of IgG by cells from the cerebrospinal fluid in a patient with multiple sclerosis. *Clin. Exp. Immunol.*, **4**, 401
10. Sandberg-Wollheim, M. (1974). Immoglobulin synthesis *in vitro* by cerebrospinal fluid cells in patients with multiple sclerosis. *Scand. J. Immunol.*, **3**, 717
11. McAlpine, D., Lumsden, C. and Acheson, E. (1972). *Multiple Sclerosis: a Reappraisal*. (Edinburgh: Churchill Livingstone)
12. Iscove, N. N. and Melchers, F. (1978). Complete replacement of serum by albumin, transferrin and soybean lipid in cultures of lipopolysaccharide-reactive B lymphocytes. *J. Exp. Med.*, **147**, 923
13. Hauw, J. J., Novikoff, A. B., Novikoff, P. M., Boutry, J. M. and Robineaux, R. (1972). Culture of nervous tissue on collagen in Leighton tubes. *Brain Res.*, **37**, 301

48
Isotopic cisternography in multiple sclerosis: possible correlations with disease course

D. INZITARI, R. CAPPARELLI, D. SITÀ, F. BARONTINI, P. MARINI and
L. AMADUCCI

INTRODUCTION

Previously reported data[1] indicated an abnormal isotopic cisternography (IC) pattern in about 47% of a group of 38 multiple sclerosis (MS) patients studied by means of this technique. The presence of an abnormal IC was significantly correlated with higher values of both the Link's[2] and Tourtellotte's[3] indices. Since then a further 27 MS patients have been submitted to IC. Here we are reporting the correlations between cisternographic patterns, clinical features and CSF findings in the larger group of definite MS cases.

MATERIAL AND METHODS

Method of IC and classification criteria for cisternographic pictures are given in the above quoted paper. Out of the 65 patients 33 were men and 32 women. In comparing subgroups of patients with and without abnormal IC the following variables were considered:

(1) Clinical: sex, age, duration of disease, disability score, stage of activity, type and severity of course. Disability was assessed at the time of IC examination by means of the Kurtzke scale[4]; the clinical course was defined as remitting or chronic–progressive according to the McAlpine's criteria[5]. Among the total group, 25 patients were selected, due to the possibility of assessing the severity of disease course using the criteria indicated by Brodin and Link[6]: out of the 25, 10 showed no or little disability after 10 years of disease, while 15 were moderately to severely disabled after 5 years.

(2) CSF: cell count per mm^3; CSF/blood albumin ratio; IgG index according to Tibbling and Link[2]; agar-gel electrophoresis IgG pattern[7].

RESULTS

In 25 (38.5%) of the 65 MS patients there was an abnormal IC finding. In 24, the pattern was defined as 'mixed': the tracer filled the ventricular system 2–6 h after lumbar injection. At 24 h there was little or no activity within the ventricles; the flow over the convexities was normal but the reabsorption at the vault was slower than in normal pictures. In one case the ventricular influx was very early and transient, while the reabsorption at the vault was markedly slower. The comparison between subgroups with and without abnormal IC showed no significant difference in relation to sex ratio, mean age and duration of disease (Table 1). An abnormal IC was significantly more frequent among patients with chronic–progressive and 'malignant' course and among those with a higher disability score (Table 2). In considering the CSF findings (Table

Table 1 Comparison between normal and abnormal IC groups by sex, age and duration of disease

	IC		
	normal	abnormal	p
Sex (M/F)	21/19	12/13	n.s.
Age (years)	37 ± 10	40 ± 10	n.s.
Duration of disease (years)	8.2 ± 6	12 ± 7	n.s.

n.s. = not significant

Table 2 Comparison between MS patients with or without abnormal IC by clinical course, stage, disability score and severity of disease

	IC		
	normal (n = 40)	abnormal (n = 25)	p
Clinical course			
remitting	19/40	2/25	<0.001
chronic–progressive	21/40	23/25	
Stage			
active	26/40	20/25	
inactive	16/40	5/25	n.s.
Disability score	3.9 ± 2.2	5.6 ± 1.7	<0.005
Severity*			
benign form	8/14	2/11	<0.05
malignant form	6/14	9/11	

*Benign form: slight or no disability after 10 years.
Malignant form: moderate to severe disability within 5 years after onset (Brodin and Link, 1980[6])

Table 3 CSF findings in normal vs abnormal IC groups

	IC		
	normal (n = 40)	abnormal (n = 25)	p
Cell count per mm³	8.3 ± 11	7.8 ± 10	n.s.
CSF/blood albumin ratio	6.2 ± 2	7.0 ± 3.4	n.s.
IgG index (Link)	0.9 ± 0.4	1.3 ± 0.6	<0.02
Oligoclonal IgG pattern	16 (40%)	12 (48%)	n.s.

3) an abnormal IC pattern was significantly correlated only with higher mean values of the Link's IgG index.

DISCUSSION

Although no definite physiopathological significance can be attributed, up to now, to the modifications of the IC pattern, the finding of an abnormal picture with a fairly high percentage in MS appears of interest. The pathological processes that may be involved in the modification of the CSF dynamics in MS are: (1) cerebral atrophy; (2) chronic phlogosis of leptomeninges with partial subarachnoid block; (3) periventricular tissue modification with increased transependymal flow. Possible physical–chemical mechanisms deserve further investigation. The significance of the increased autochthonous CSF IgG levels in cases with abnormal IC is not clear: elevated concentrations in CSF of high molecular weight proteins such as IgG may affect the diffusion of the tracer as well as the CSF dynamics; on the other hand the accumulation of IgG within the subarachnoid space may be the consequence of slower CSF flow and/or re-absorption. Until now no correlation has been provided between CSF IgG levels and the type of course and severity of disease. The abnormal IC pattern appeared to be significantly linked with the chronic–progressive and the more severely evolutive forms. This finding may be simply an expression of the severity of the above indicated pathological alterations, but the possible role of CSF dynamics alteration in influencing some morphological features of MS (i.e. ventricular enlargement, periventricular tissue modifications), as well as the clinical picture and course, should not be excluded.

Some of the patients with a malignant course have been studied very early by means of IC: the picture was abnormal in spite of the initial stage of disease. Based on the above reported data and following this last observation, the possible prognostic value of IC in MS should also be taken into consideration.

References

1. Bartolini, S., Inzitari, D., Castagnoli, A. and Amaducci, L. (1982). Correlation of isotopic cisternographic patterns in multiple sclerosis with CSF IgG values. *Ann. Neurol.*, **12**, 486
2. Tibbling, G., Link, H. and Ohman, S. (1977). Principles of albumin and IgG analyses in neurological disorders. I. Establishment of reference values. *Scand. J. Clin. Lab. Invest.*, **37**, 385
3. Tourtellotte, W. W. and Booe, I. M. (1978). Multiple sclerosis: The blood–brain barrier and the measurement of *de novo* central nervous system IgG synthesis. *Neurology*, **28**, 76
4. Kurtzke, J. F. (1965). Further notes on disability evaluation in multiple sclerosis, with scale modifications. *Neurology*, **15**, 654
5. McAlpine, D., Lumsen, C. E. and Acheson, E. D. (1972). *Multiple sclerosis. A reappraisal*. 2nd Edn. (Edinburgh, London: Churchill Livingstone)
6. Brodin, L. S. and Link, H. (1980). Relation between benign course of multiple sclerosis and low-grade humoral immune response in cerebrospinal fluid. *J. Neurol. Neurosurg. Psych.*, **43**, 102
7. Lowenthal, A., Van Sande, M. and Karcher, D. (1960). The differential diagnosis of neurological diseases by fractionating electrophoretically the CSF proteins. *J. Neurochem.*, **6**, 51

49
Management of acute multiple sclerosis by a long acting intrathecally administered corticosteroid

I. S. NEU, N. H. KOENIG and W. GUENTHER

ABSTRACT

There are a number of relative or absolute contra-indications to the conventional cortisone therapy of the acute episode of multiple sclerosis. Furthermore, chronic progressive spinal types of MS present a particular therapeutic problem. As an alternative to systemic corticosteroid therapy, intrathecal application of a depot corticosteroid is available. The advantage of this treatment and controversial opinions are discussed. In contrast to systemic application, our own investigations of the endogenous serum cortisol levels after a single administration of 40 mg triamcinolone acetonide revealed no suggestion of suppression of the suprarenal cortex. Clinical application showed good tolerance with a satisfactory therapeutic action.

INTRODUCTION

Glucocorticoids have been used in the treatment of the acute episode of multiple sclerosis since the 1950s, introduced under the conception of inflammatory inhibition and antioedematous action. In this connection both the principle of adrenal cortex stimulation by ACTH and also of the synthetic corticosteroids are applied without being able to produce evidence of a clear superiority of one of the two principles over the other. The therapeutic result to be expected is, however, restricted only to a shortening of the episode, possibly accompanied by changes in the cerebrospinal fluid in the sense of a rapid return to normal. An influence on the entire course of the disease, such as a reduction of the frequency of the episodes, could not be achieved.

Without wishing to enter into the results of corticosteroid therapy in detail, let it be said that the greater success of this treatment is to be seen in the acute episodic remittent type with supraspinal involvement. On the other hand, the success is less in patients who experience a further degeneration in the course of a chronic progressive spinal type of the disease.

Even if the conventional therapy with systemically applied corticosteroids lasting 4–6 weeks is relatively well tolerated in general, a number of known undesirable effects are to be expected. Furthermore, concomitant diseases such as subclinical or manifest diabetes mellitus, pre-existing florid gastric ulcers, intercurrent infections or rarer diseases such as a cortisone-induced glaucoma or a corresponding cataract, are relative or even absolute contra-indications to this therapy. Moreover, systemic corticoid therapy in female MS patients is a particular problem if an episodic deterioration in need of treatment occurs during early pregnancy, because with systemic corticoid administration a teratogenic effect on the fetus must be expected. In order to keep these undesirable effects as low as possible the following theoretical considerations and reports from the literature have induced us to carry out intrathecal corticosteroid therapy:

(1)   High levels of the active substance in the vertebral canal can be expected after intrathecal application. In that way a direct anti-oedematous action on the plaques in this region seems possible.

(2)   After intracisternal administration of corticosteroids Lehrer[1] was able to show that the white matter of the nervous system showed higher concentrations of active substance than the grey matter, and that, moreover, systemic administration required a dosage 5–10 times greater than the intrathecal dose in order to attain the same concentrations of the active substance in the CNS.

(3)   After intrathecal administration of corticosteroid, Massaro[2] was able to establish, in MS patients, both an improvement in the clinical condition and an almost always identical decline in the IgG of the CSF, which was statistically significant.

However, intrathecal corticosteroid therapy is a matter of controversial discussion to various authors, and is sometimes even emphatically rejected[3,4]. But if the objections are considered critically, then serious side-effects attributable to the substance itself must be differentiated from those due to the technique of administration. The latter include inoculation meningitis which is avoidable by consistent sterile work, among other things, and therefore does not constitute a contra-indication.

Among substance-induced side-effects are aseptic meningitis and adhesive arachnitis with corresponding neurological sequelae, especially paraplegias and bladder disorders are often quoted. Disagreement is rife on whether cortisone itself or the adjuvants technically necessary for the preparation, particularly benzyl alcohol or polyethylene glycol, are to be incriminated here. In these reports it is, however, striking that prednisolone acetate has always been used. Rejection of intrathecal therapy is also sometimes based, for example, on the fact that the whole course of the disease was not influenced, something which is not even to be expected, since intrathecal corticosteroid therapy compared with systemic therapy is not a basically different form of treatment but only a modification of it. It also appears, for example, not convincing pathophysiologically that, with undisturbed CSF dynamics, the intraventricular detection of corresponding substances is to be expected after lumbar application of drugs.

In the selection of the corticosteroid for intrathecal use we were prompted by the following criteria to administer triamcinolone acetonide:

(1) This substance is a crystalline depot corticosteroid which, in contrast to the rapidly diffusing free corticosteroids, can liberate the active agent into the subarachnoid space continuously over a long period, so that a constantly high intravenous concentration of active substance can be expected without repeated administrations being necessary. The high concentration of the drug can be expected to persist for at least 14 days.

(2) The side-effects, given in the literature as serious, practically all relate to prednisolone acetate. There are no corresponding reports on triamcinolone acetonide.

(3) Scanning electron optical studies of the different available crystalline depot corticosteroids show that triamcinolone acetonide has the most uniform and roundest crystal shape, in contrast to the sharp-edged crystals of other types. The comparison of the picture also leads one to suppose that irregularly shaped crystals, such as those of prednisolone acetate, may have caused the side-effects described by other authors.

RESULTS

With reference to our own investigations, we first measured the effect of systemic administration of corticosteroid on the endogenous cortisol levels in comparison to that of intrathecal depot corticosteroid administration. For this purpose the endogenous cortisol levels were measured as blank values at 8.00 a.m. on 3 consecutive days in 15 hospitals. Immediately after the third withdrawal of blood 40 mg triamcinolone acetonide was injected intrathecally once. The cortisol levels were measured again on the 1st, 3rd, 5th, 10th and 15th days after injection in each case.

This showed that after intrathecal administration of corticosteroid on the first day a slight depression of the endogenous cortisol level occurred, which, however, still remained within the normal range, and in the measurements on the following days produced no statistically significant changes compared with the initial level. In comparison with this, a control group of patients showed a marked fall in the endogenous cortisol levels to below the reference range after a single intramuscular administration of 40 mg triamcinolone acetonide. This investigation, therefore, showed that intrathecal application of cortisone does not suppress the adrenal cortex, in contrast to intramuscular injection[5].

Thereafter, we first treated 31 multiple sclerosis patients with 40 mg triamcinolone acetonide after a CSE puncture. 10 of these patients distinctly improved, principally the spastic, but also the neurogenic, bladder disorders being influenced. The CSF monitoring puncture made 4–6 weeks later in four patients with previous pathological findings showed a regression of the pleocytosis and γ-globulins on electrophoresis. In nine patients there was only slight improvement of all findings while 12 remained unchanged[6].

Side-effects were seen only in a few cases, and consisted of more marked complaints following puncture. Even in this group we saw, in agreement with a few authors, none of the side-effects described elsewhere as serious, in particular no aseptic meningitis or adhesive arachnitis. Since that time we perform intrathecal steroid therapy as a potential routine treatment for MS in suitable cases.

In now over 200 applications we have so far seen no serious side-effects. Only in one female patient who had also received intrathecal treatment with triamcinolone acetate in the course of another neurological disease, persistent paraesthesias lasting several hours occurred in the cauda equinal region, which, however, then completely receded.

CONCLUSION

(1) The intrathecal administration of corticosteroids is not a fundamentally different form of therapy compared with the systemic administration of corticosteroids. It is, however, a possible alternative, especially in relative or absolute contra-indications for systemic corticosteroid administration.

(2) We see the indication for therapy of MS with administration of intrathecal corticosteroids particularly in the spinal forms, especially after acute or subacute degeneration. A special indication can be the treatment of female patients with episodic aggravations during pregnancy.

(3) A prerequisite for a well tolerated application of the drug is absolute sterility in the individual lumbar puncture.

(4) In our view, at the moment there exists a contra-indication to the treatment when an irritation of the root apparently occurs in connection with the lumbar puncture. In such cases, after withdrawal of the CSF for diagnostic purposes, the application of depot corticosteroids is dispensed with.

(5) Under the conditions stated, the intrathecal administration of triamcinolone acetonide is well tolerated by MS patients.

(6) If a further intrathecal application after the first, or in association with a later episode, does not produce an improvement of the clinical picture, further intrathecal applications are dispensed with.

References

1. Lehrer, G. M., Maker, H. S. and Weissbarth. (1973). Brain, uptake of methylprednisolone acetate from the cerebrospinal fluid and systemic sites. *Arch. Neurol.*, **28**, 324
2. Massaro, A. R. (1978). Modifications of the cerebrospinal fluid IgG concentrations in patients with multiple sclerosis treated with intrathecal steroids. *J. Neurol.*, **219**, 221
3. Bernat, J. L. (1981). Intraspinal steroid therapy. *Neurology*, **31**, 168
4. Nelson, D. A., Vates, T. S. and Thomas, R. B. (1973). Complications from intrathecal steroid therapy in patients with multiple sclerosis. *Acta Neurol. Scand.*, **49**, 176
5. Neu, I., Reusche, E. and Rodiek, S. (1978). Endogener Cortisolspiegel nach intrathekaler Gabe von Triamcinolon Acetonid bei neurologischen Erkrankungen. *Dtsch. Med. Wschr.*, **103**, 1368
6. Rodiek, S. O. and Neu, I. (1979). Klinische Erfahrung mit intrathekaler Gabe von Triamcinolon-Acetonid bei neurologischen Erkrankungen. *Therapiewoche*, **29**, 1123

50
Diagnostic value of α_2-macroglobulin crossed immunoelectrophoresis in multiple sclerosis

B. YORDANOV, E. TZVETANOVA and O. GRIGOROVA

INTRODUCTION

We have conducted this study for the following reasons:

(1) An increased activity of the acid and neutral proteinases is claimed to cause degradation of myelin basic protein and demyelination[1-3].
(2) α_2-Macroglobulin (α_2-M) is known to be one of the major proteinase inhibitors in the blood[4].
(3) The conclusion of Rastogi, Clausen and Fog, that 'the serum α_2-M abnormality traced by crossed immunoelectrophoresis may be useful in the diagnosis of MS'.

MATERIAL AND METHODS

Patients

Serum samples from 342 patients were studied: 105 with multiple sclerosis (MS) – 79 with definite diagnosis, 17 with probable and 9 with possible; 159 with other neurological diseases (OND); 68 mentally ill patients (MIP) and 10 normal subjects (Table 1).

Table 1 MS – patients

Patient material	Total number	Age Mean	Age Range	Sex Male	Sex Female	Duration Mean	Duration Range
MS – Definite	79	34	17–36	38	41	6.0 y	6 mon–19 y
MS – Probable	17	39	6–53	10	7	2.0 y	2 d–9 y
MS – Possible	9	42	27–69	4	5	6.4 y	7 mon–24 y
MS – Total	105	38	6–69	52	53	5.4 y	2 d–24 y

Methods

The following techniques were used in this study:

(1) Crossed immunoelectrophoresis (CI) after Clarke and Freeman[6], with some modifications to demonstrate serum α_2-M.

(2) CSF studies (cells, total protein, agarose electrophoresis, IgG after Mancini[7], albumin after Laurell[8], IgG/total protein and IgG/albumin).

RESULTS

The CI pattern of serum α_2-M of a normal subject is represented by an arc with sharp top and without any humps and spurs (Figure 1a).

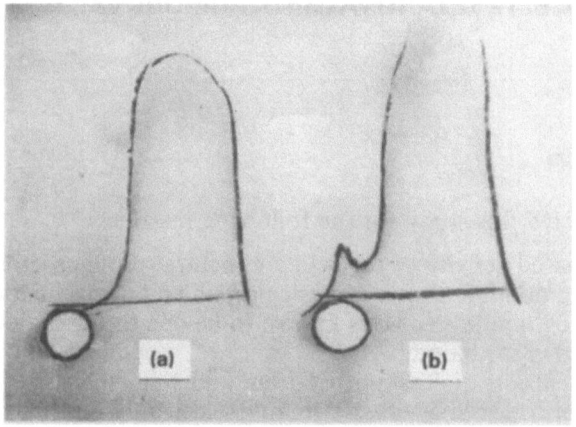

Figure 1a   Normal α_2-M CI-pattern;   **1b**   MH as a double arc near the start

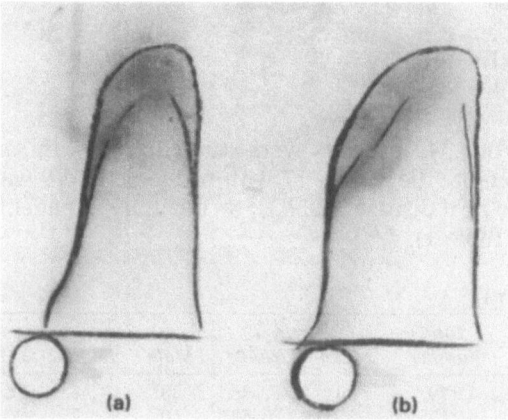

Figure 2   MH as a hump near the start;   **2b**   MH is near to the top of the immunoprecipitation arc

258

The abnormal immunoprecipitation arcs are represented by a double arc, or a hump, or a spur on one side or on the top of the arc, and a flattened top – microheterogeneity (MH) of α_2-M (Figure 1b,2,3,4).

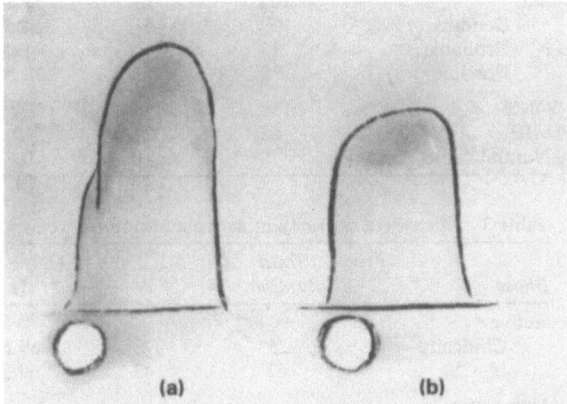

Figure 3a   MH is in the middle on the cathode side;   **3b**   MH as a flattened arc top

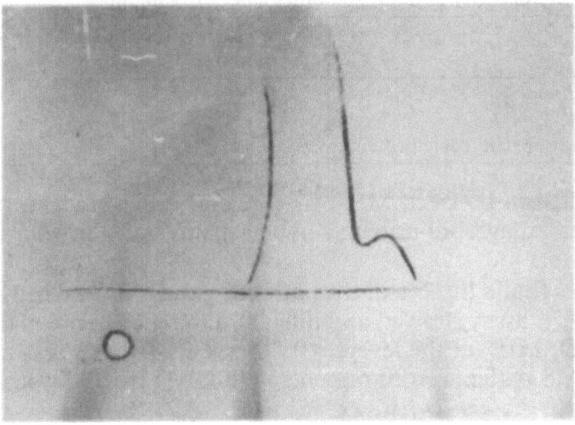

Figure 4   MH is on the anode side

The abnormality was demonstrated on the cathode side in 97% of MS patients and only in 3% on the anode side. The humps were found near the start in 67%, in the middle of the ascending part of the cathode side in 19%, or near the top in 10%.

The α_2-M abnormality was found in 57.1% of MS patients: 64.5% in patients with definite MS diagnosis, 41.2% in patients with probable MS and only in 33.3% with possible MS (Table 2). The MH of α_2-M was seen more often in the patients with findings for the active process of demyelination (in 69%), than in patients with non-active MS (41%) – Table 3.

Table 2 Microheterogeneity of α_2-M in different groups

Patient material	Total number	With MH N	%
MS	105	61	58.1
Definite	79	51	64.5
Probable	17	7	41.2
Possible	9	3	33.3
OND	159	59	37
MIP	68	21	31
Normal subjects	10	0	0

Table 3 Microheterogeneity in active and non-active MS

Phase	Total number	α_2-M MH N	%
Active			
Clinically	23	16	69.6
by CSF	62	43	69.3
Non-active			
Clinically	102	53	51.9
by CSF	17	7	41.0

Table 4 Microheterogeneity of α_2-M and other laboratory findings

Studies	Total number	Patients with pathol. findings N	%
α_2-M CI	105	61	58.1
CSF	84	66	78.6
Hypersensitivity to myelin basic protein	53	29	54.7

Some parallelism between MH of α_2-M and other laboratory data (oligo-clonal hypergammaglobulinrachia, hypersensitivity to myelin basic protein) was found (Table 4).

The MH was found in 37% of the patients with OND and in 31% among the MIP (Table 2). χ^2 assay showed a significant difference between the two groups (MS and OND, MIP) at the level $p < 0.001$ ($\chi^2 = 10.45$). It was not possible to discriminate MS patients from patients with OND by α_2-M patterns.

DISCUSSION

In general our results are in agreement with those in the literature[5], but they differ in some details. They suggest that the immunoprecipitation arc of the α_2-M in MS is not so typical that it can be used as a criterion for discrimination of MS from other neurological diseases. We found MH in 65% out of 79 patients with definite MS and in 37% out of 159 patients with OND. Rastogi *et al* found it in 85% out of 26 patients with MS and only in 29% out of 24 patients with OND. It is difficult to say what is the cause of these discrepancies. Probably it is due to the different number of patients studied and to different criteria used for microheterogeneity.

There is nothing astonishing in the fact that the α_2-M abnormality was found in such a great proportion of the patients with OND. If the hypothesis that the proteinases contribute to the demyelination process, and that the α_2-M binds the proteinases is correct, then we have to expect that in all CNS pathological processes accompanied by myelin breakdown the α_2-M will be abnormal. Our results are in good accordance with this speculation.

The α_2-M MH might be characteristic but a non-specific feature for MS. The diagnostic value of α_2-M MH is less than that of CSF abnormalities (IgG, oligoclonal bands), but the former is the more practicable and non-traumatic procedure comparing CSF investigations.

The cause of α_2-M MH in serum is still unknown. The presence of MH indicates that two major types of α_2-M with different electrophoretic mobilities, but with partial or total identical antigenic properties, are present in the serum. This may be due to the formation of α_2-M complexes with the proteinases and peptide fragments or other substances liberated by leukocytes.

CONCLUSIONS

Crossed immunoelectrophoresis is a valuable method for the demonstration of some antigenic and electrophoretic properties of α_2-M. α_2-M microheterogeneity is a characteristic but not specific feature for MS. There is not a specific α_2-M pattern in MS, and the cause of the MH in MS is still unknown.

References

1. Einstein, E.R., Dalal, K.B. and Csejtey, J. (1970). Increased proteinase activity and changes in myelin basic protein and lipids in multiple sclerosis plaques. *J. Neurol. Sci.,* **11**, 109
2. Govindrajan, K.R., Rauch, H.C., Clausen, J. and Einstein, E.R. (1974). Changes in cathepsin B-1 and D, neutral proteinase, and 2', 3'-cyclic nucleotide-3'-phosphohydrolase activity in monkey brain with experimental allergic encephalomyelitis. *J. Neurol. Sci.,* **23**, 295
3. Husch, H.E. and Parks, M.E. (1979). A thiol proteinase highly elevated in and around the plaques of multiple sclerosis. *J. Neurochem.,* **32**, 505
4. Barrett, A.J. and Starkey, P.M. (1973). The interaction of χ_2-macroglobulin with proteinases. Characteristics and specificity of the reactivity and a hypothesis concerning its molecular mechanism. *Biochem. J.,* **133**, 709
5. Rastogi, S.C., Clausen, J. and Fog, T. (1981). Abnormal serum χ_2-macroglobulin in multiple sclerosis. *Eur. Neurol.,* **20**, 33
6. Clarke, H.G. and Freeman, T. (1968). Quantitative immunoelectrophoresis of human serum proteins. *Clin. Sci.,* **35**, 403
7. Mancini, G., Carbonara, A.O. and Heremans, J.F. (1965). Immunochemical quantitation of antigens by single radial immunodiffusion. *Immunochemistry,* **2**, 235
8. Luarell, C.B. (1966). Quantitative estimation of proteins by electrophoresis in agarose gel containing antibodies. *Anal. Biochem.,* **15**, 45

51
The IgG index and the diagnosis of MS: a Bayesian approach

H. K. van WALBEEK, E. A. H. HISCHE and H. J. van der HELM

Having determined immunoglobulin G (IgG) and albumin concentrations in 1100 cerebrospinal fluid and serum samples, we calculated the IgG index. Likelihood ratios for MS were calculated by using a training set consisting of 100 patients with definite MS, and one consisting of 97 patients suffering from diseases from which MS must be differentiated.

Predictive values for the IgG index are given in a graphical representation of Bayes theorem.

The following statements will be discussed and shown to be wrong.

(1) When the diagnosis MS is considered, an IgG index which is above normal always increases the probability of MS.
(2) A clearly elevated index makes the diagnosis MS probable.
(3) When the diagnosis MS is probable, a low IgG index does not change my opinion since in MS the IgG index is not always elevated.

52
Neuro–urological problems in MS: diagnosis and treatment

H. van POPPEL, P. KETELAER and R. L. VEREECKEN

Diagnosis and treatment of voiding and sexual dysfunctions take an important place in the total care of the MS patient. In considering neurogenic disorders not only bladder activity but also urethral activity is important[1]. Both can be normal, over- or underactive. In the urethral closure mechanism we distinguish the proximal urethral structures and the external urethral sphincter (Figure 1). At the Danish Jubilee Conference on MS in June 1982, we presented a review of the urological problems of 500 MS patients[2]. Some 32% of them had a documented neurogenic bladder and/or urethral dysfunction.

Figure 1 Anatomy of the urethral closure mechanism in males and females[1]

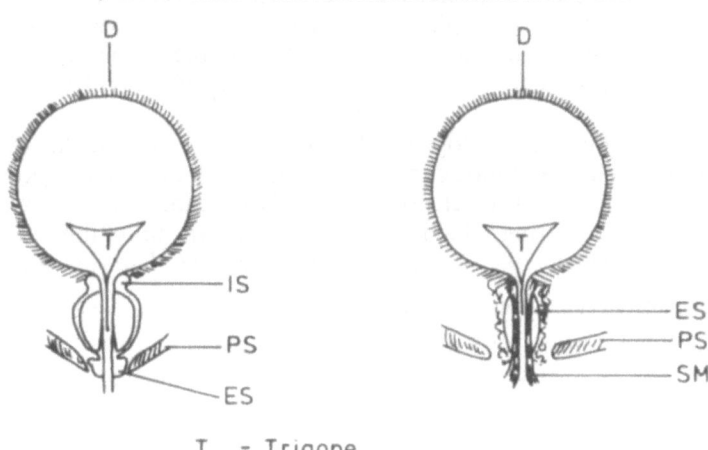

```
T  = Trigone
D  = Detrusor
IS = Internal Sphincter (smooth)
PS = Peri-urethral Sphincter
ES = External Sphincter (striated)
SM = Smooth muscle
```

Proper diagnosis will result from intravenous urography (IVU) and urethrography and from urodynamic workup with uroflowmetry, cystometry and pelvic floor electromyography (EMG). We discussed the technical aspects and the value of these examinations in Copenhagen. We now want to discuss recent diagnostic and therapeutic procedures.

In cases where a discrepancy exists between the clinical findings and the routine cystometry, a prolonged recording of bladder pressure in particular circumstances is required[3]. Since patient's mobility is hindered during classical cystometry, tele-cystometric measurements are indicated. For this proposal a pressure transducer is introduced in the bladder suprapubically, and a second one in the rectum. Urine loss is monitored by a Urilos napkin connected to an amplifier. A telemetric three channel system will record pressure variations and urine loss during, for example, 24 hours while the patient is doing his physiotherapy, is sleeping or voiding. There is no disturbance by transurethral catheters or by non-physiologic bladder filling as done in classical cystometry. The mean indications in MS are all kinds of intermittent voiding disorders, for example urgency or incontinence occurring by night or recurring periodically.

A few new examinations were started in co-operation with the Department of Physical Medicine and Rehabilitation at our institution. In this way we are studying the correlation between clinical urologic disorders and evoked potentials[4,5]. Stimulation is effectuated on the tibial nerve, the penis or the bladder neck; recording of the potentials and their latency can be done in the sphincters, the medulla or the cortex. Averaged somato-sensory potentials were recorded from the conus medullaris at $T_{12}-L_1$ and from the cerebral cortex at vertex. We stimulate the posterior tibial nerve classically, and the pudendal nerve by two annular electrodes around the penis. We try to find the correlation between both. Moreover, we attempt to confirm the possible existence of a clinical–electrophysiological correlation between supra- and infranuclear bladder dysfunctions, or over- and underactive bladder function, and abnormal or prolonged sensory conduction time of cortical and medullar evoked potentials.

There is a well known aetiological relationship between muscular spasticity and uninhibited bladder contraction. Everyone also knows that urethral and anal sphincter activity can be clearly different, as demonstrated by a routine fine needle EMG during classical cystometry. An uninhibited bladder contraction can be provoked by or provoke a peripheral spasm, and thus a

Figure 2 Possible aetiological interaction between skeletal, sphincter and bladder spasticity

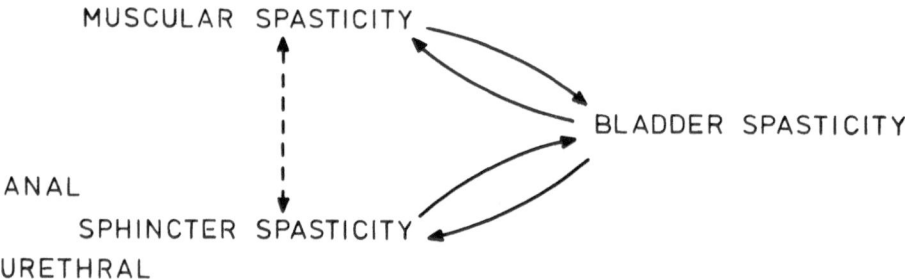

pelvic floor spasm (Figure 2). We try to differentiate pelvic floor spasticity and spasticity of the legs by also recording adductor EMG during cystometry. In this way we recognized real dyssynergia between bladder contraction and pelvic floor spasticity, and false dyssynergia where a non-inhibited bladder contraction induces a so-called mass spasm that also interferes with normal micturition (Figure 3).

Figure 3a Striated muscle spasm inducing and preceding bladder contraction
Figure 3b Bladder spasm inducing sphincter and skeletal muscle spasm
Figure 3c Bladder contraction inducing pure sphincter dyssynergia without skeletal muscle spasm

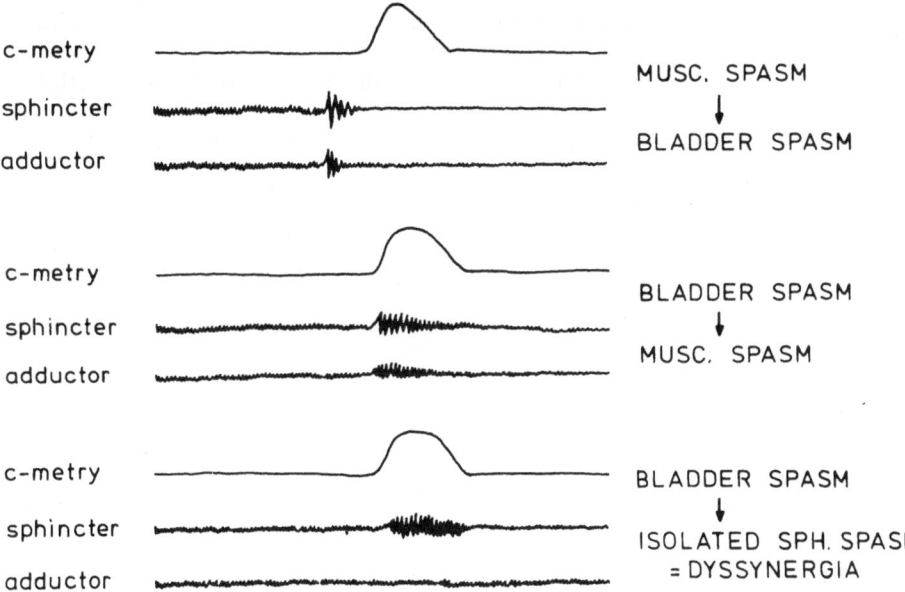

In treating voiding dysfunctions in MS, as incontinence, great attention is paid to alternative solutions for the indwelling transurethral catheter. Leaving a patient with an indwelling catheter is indeed not readily accepted by most urologists, because of the well-known complications. Everyone knows about infection, stone formation, kidney function loss, urethroprostatitis, epididymitis, and the patent hole urethra in females. In order to prevent these complications we effectuated bladder instillations with commercialized acid solutions such as Subi G or Solutio R. The results are disappointing. In patients where an indwelling catheter is inevitable we now only effectuate a bladder washing through a rigid cystoscope every 2 or 3 months, in order to evacuate urinary egg-shell concrements left behind after each catheter change; it is effectuated every 2 weeks for latex and every month for silicone catheters.

Because of all the mentioned complications we certainly prefer suprapubic cystostomy, which is very easily effectuated under local anaesthesia with the commercialized 'Cystofix': a pig tail catheter with several drainage openings is inserted in the bladder through a needle hole of varying diameter. In preventing urine loss this procedure proved excellent in men, but is disappointing in females because of the often enlarged diameter of the urethra by large sized catheters inserted in order to avoid micturition. Some authors effectuated operative bladder neck closure for this proposal; perhaps periurethral teflon injections will have a place in these cases.

Patients with bladder atonia or functional urethral obstruction will do excellently with intermittent catheterization. In the hospital it is performed by the nurse under aseptic conditions and with an antibiotic cover; at home it can be effectuated by the family of the patient without observing all rules of asepsia. This is the 'clean' catheterization. In patients with non-invalidated upper limbs, auto-catheterization is an elegant and self-independence confirming procedure. Since the mirror catheter allows the female patient to inspect her external genitals and to do a good direct catheterization, infections are very rare when the catheterizations are done at least 3 times a day (Figure 4). A lot of male and female patients have successfully learned this method in the last 2 years.

Figure 4   Mirror-catheter 'Bruynen Boer'

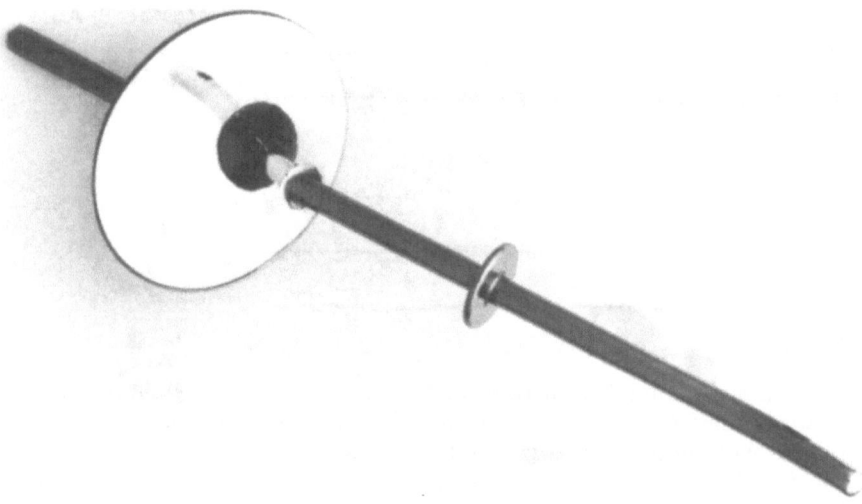

In medical therapies the use of propantheline bromide, flavoxate, betanechol and imipramine is well-known. Phenoxybenzamine (Dibenyline® and Dibenzyran®) is a new drug we have prescribed in a large number of patients. Our study with longterm results was presented at the World Congress of Urology in San Francisco last year[6]. Dibenzyran is an α-blocking agent; α-receptors are predominant in the bladder neck region; the main indications are bladder neck dysfunctions. Since the mentioned study, however, we also started administration in uninhibited bladders with good results in cases where bladder neck spasticity is probably the aetiological factor of the bladder over-activity. In several patients, however, treatment had to be discontinued because of orthostatic hypotension and dizziness, compromising general re-habilitation and re-education exercises.

Medical therapy of external urethral sphincter dyssynergia by systemic administration of spasmolytic agents (Valium®, Lioresal®, Dantrium®) also often gives general fatigue. In these cases a local sphincter infiltration is effectuated with a surprising success rate. Indeed infiltration gives dis-appearing of sphincter activity on EMG with perfect relaxation at micturition, and better emptying of the bladder. But also uninhibited bladder contrac-tions caused by pelvic floor spasticity are not induced, leading to better continence. The mechanism of effect of this treatment is not yet totally understood, nor why this infiltration with a fast-acting product as lidocaine is effective during weeks or even months. The infiltration can easily be repeated when uroflowmetry worsens or incontinence increases. Since we experienced the beneficial effect of sphincter infiltration we left the previously effectuated more delicate and technically more difficult pudendal infiltration. This technique markedly reduced the number of endoscopic external sphinc-terotomies.

Some patients with an overactive bladder do not respond to high doses and various anticholinergic medication, probably due to malabsorption. We attempted to influence this bladder dysfunction by the application of inter-ferential therapy, a relative recent therapy in physical medicine[7]. Interferential therapy generates a sinusoidal alternating current with a variable frequency of 0–100 c/s produced by the interference of two sinusoidal currents of median frequency range (4000–4100 c/s). This permits a deep field electrical stimulation without pain and negligible superficial sensory effect (Figure 5). In

Figure 5 Principle of interferential current therapy

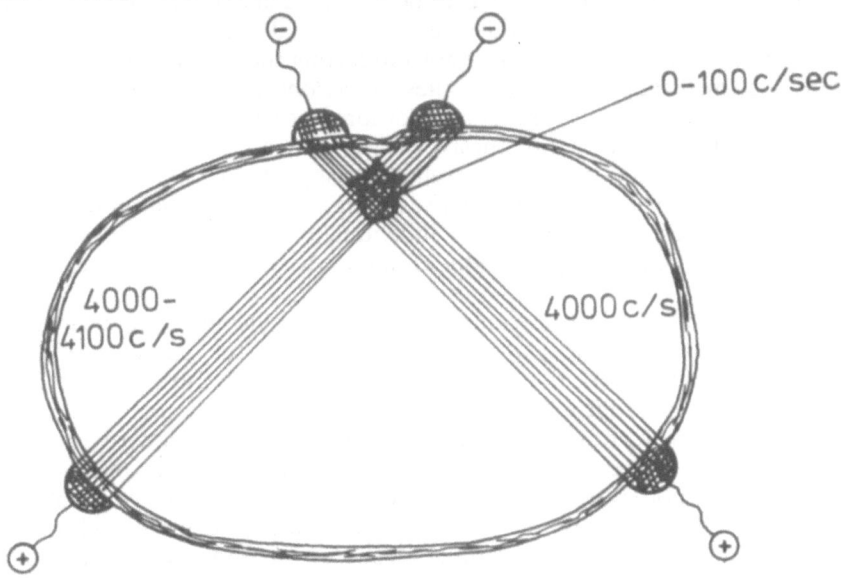

Figure 6 Nocturnal electronic erection monitoring by Hg loop electrodes

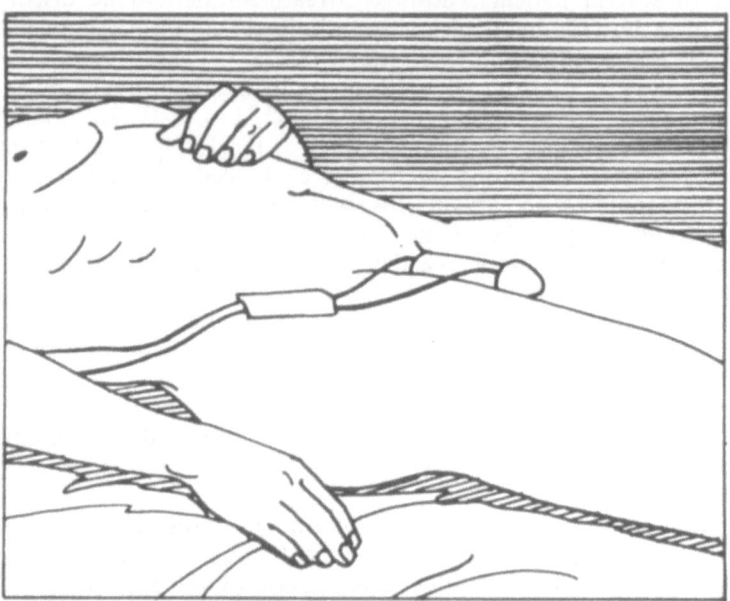

a number of patients we experienced a subjective and objective improvement of frequency, bladder capacity and continence, but this is only a preliminary result.

All the above mentioned treatments are quite simple, conservative and reversible. Indeed, bladder pathology can change during MS evolution. So medical treatment, if effective, has to be preferred above, e.g. a transurethral resection of a dyssynergic bladder neck or external urethral sphincter, which we reserve for patients resistant or not supporting the therapy by the previous mentioned medications. Moreover, these resections do not always succeed and if they succeed the results are mostly not longlasting.

An external collector prosthesis will not be applied without previous urodynamic work-up showing a well emptying bladder that could not be treated by other measures. An ideal prosthesis has not been manufactured and each patient has to be considered individually before prescribing his best prosthesis. In females application of an external prosthesis is until now inefficient.

The results of surgical implantation of internal incontinence devices were initially frustrating. The Rosen prosthesis, where the bulbous urethra is clamped between a fork that is filled or emptied by an intrascrotal balloon, gave too many complications such as urethral pressure necrosis. The newer Scott prosthesis with an intra-abdominal pressure regulation reservoir is a better solution. These devices are very expensive and longlasting results are not yet available; moreover, manipulation requires normal upper limb validity.

Urinary diversion must be considered as a last outcome for chronically infected bladders where re-education is unsuccessful, and where renal function is in danger; we effectuated ileal or colonic loops; the latter is preferred because of the surgical possibility of making an antireflux procedure avoiding late kidney damage, well-known in ileal loop derivations.

Finally, sexual dysfunction as a loss of erection, occurring mostly very early in MS patients, can be objectively and properly diagnosed. For some patients in the initial stage of the disease, or in a rather low grade stabilized MS this can be the main problem. Nocturnal erection monitoring can be done very easily by stamps or another erectiometer applied around the penis in the evening. The following day the occurrence of erection during the night can be easily controlled. An electronic recording by an annular mercury loop electrode permits graphic registration (Figure 6). On the other hand, penile or bladder neck stimulation and evoked potentials recorded in the anal and urethral sphincter can show normal or increased latency[8].

Besides sophisticated inflatable prostheses of both corpora cavernosa, a silicone silver prosthesis (Jonas type) can be inserted very easily through a subglandular incision. The penis can be manipulated in an erect or flexed position.

As we have seen, urologists have a big armoury to help MS patients. We must realize, however, that perfect results for urological treatment are rare, and that treatment is mostly symptomatic. In most patients however, an important subjective and/or objective improvement is obtainable.

References

1. Gosling, J. (1979). The structure of the bladder and urethra in relation to function. *Urol. Clin. N. Am.*, **6**, 31
2. Van Poppel, H., Vereecken, R. and Leruitte, A. (1982). Introduction to neuro–muscular dysfunction of the lower urinary tract in MS. *Proceedings Jubilee Conference on M.S.*, 6–9 June. Copenhagen, Denmark (In press)
3. Vereecken, R. L., Puers, B. and Das, J. (1983). Continuous telemetric monitoring of bladder function. *Urol. Res.*, **11**, 15
4. Haldeman, S., Bradley, E. E. and Bhatia, N. (1982). Evoked responses from the pudendal nerve. *J. Urol.*, **128**, 974
5. Kaneko, S., Park, Y. C., Yachiku, S. and Kurita, T. (1983). Evoked central somato-sensory potentials after penile stimulation in man. *Urology*, **21**, 58
6. Vereecken, R., van Poppel, H., Leruitte, A. and Boeckx, G. (1982). Long-term α-blocking therapy in detrusor–urethra dyssynergia. *Abstr. Soc. Int. Urol.*, **22**, *XIX Intern. Congress*, San Francisco, 5–10 September
7. Ganne, J. M. (1976). Interferential therapy. *Austr. J. Physiol.*, **22**, 101
8. Vereecken, R. L. *et al* (1982). Electrophysiological exploration of the sacral conus. *J. Neurol.*, **227**, 135

Section V
Ophthalmological Aspects of Multiple Sclerosis

Section V
Ophthalmological Aspects of Multiple Sclerosis

53
Central nervous system involvement in clinically pure optic neuritis (a pilot study in 25 patients)

E. A. C. M. SANDERS, J. P. H. REULEN and L. A. H. HOGENHUIS

SUMMARY

Twenty-five pure ON patients were investigated by visual evoked response (VER), auditory brainstem evoked response (ABER), somato-sensory evoked response (SSER), blink reflex, ENG and CT-scan investigations. All patients but one recently developed a unilateral ON. One patient had a bilateral relapse. Electrophysiological tests revealed VER P_{100} peak increased delays in all patients (100%), ABER abnormalities in eight (32%), SSER abnormalities in six (24%), blink reflex disorders in three (12%), ENG abnormalities in eight (32%) and CT-scan hyperdense lesions in five (20%) of the patients.

Electronystagmographic investigation was done by a new procedure of horizontal saccadic and smooth pursuit eye-movement recording. In the total group of 25 patients an overall number of 12 showed one or more 'silent' CNS abnormalities, demonstrated by the above described methods (excl. VER). In these 12 patients there is probably more than a pure ON alone. In seven of the 12 cases intrathecal IgG synthesis was found by CSF isoelectric focusing. So in seven of the 25 patients (28%), multiple CNS white matter involvement, in combination with intrathecal IgG synthesis was supposed. In these seven, but probably 12, patients the ON could be regarded as a single clinical symptom of a systemic MS. Whether these patients have a higher risk for developing clinical MS in the near future than the other 13 patients, can only be proved by a prospective study of all 25 patients.

INTRODUCTION

Ever since the first clinical and pathological reports on multiple sclerosis, there have been observations of the involvement of the optic nerve by the demyelinating process[1,2]. Most multiple sclerosis patients suffer an optic neuritis in the course of their disease[3]. Optic neuritis occurs not only during the course of the disease, but is often also the presenting complaint. Optic neuritis may be the initial symptom in 15–34% of multiple sclerosis patients[4,5]. Of patients whose initial presentation is due to optic neuritis, 8–80% may develop multiple sclerosis within a period of follow-up from 1 to 20 years. The longer the period of follow-up, the higher the incidence of multiple sclerosis. However, studies on this subject revealed the highest incidence of multiple sclerosis within a period of 6 months after the initial optic neuritis attack[6].

In clinically manifest optic neuritis, there is no way to predict whether multiple sclerosis will be detected in the near future or not. In prospective studies of optic neuritis patients, no definite conclusion has been made about the predictive value of cerebrospinal fluid data[7-9].

Several reports on HLA-typing in multiple sclerosis and optic neuritis suggested that they resembled two different clinical pictures of one and the same disease[10,11].

In the past few decades, there have been set up new methods to improve diagnostic certainty about MS. Among them evoked response, electro-myographic, electronystagmographic and CT-scan techniques. They are able to demonstrate non-symptomatic lesions within the central nervous system.

With this knowledge, we were interested in the possibility of demonstrating subclinical lesions in patients with monosymptomatic optic neuritis.

MATERIALS AND METHODS

In twenty-five clinically pure optic neuritis cases, we performed electro-physiological (VER, ABER, SSER, blink reflex, ENG), CT-scan and CSF iso-electric focusing investigations. All patients were investigated within 1–6 months after the development of first complaints of visual loss.

RESULTS

The Visual Evoked Responses

These were recorded with Halliday's pattern reversal checkerboard method. All patients showed an increased latency of the P_{100} peak in the affected eye. Abnormal wave forms were mostly seen during the acute stages of the optic neuritis attack. In seven (28%) patients, there was an increased latency also in the non-affected eye. We have no good explanation for this phenomenon.

The Auditory Brainstem Evoked Responses

We recorded these responses with a monaural 'click' stimulation method. Responses were recorded bilaterally. In eight (32%) patients, abnormal ABERs were recorded, mostly showing an increase of the delay between the third and fifth spike. Abnormal wave forms were not counted as abnormal evoked responses.

The Somato-Sensory Evoked Responses

These were recorded with bilateral stimulation of the median nerve at the level of the wrist. The delay time between the N_{14} and N_{20} peak was the only parameter studied. This is because of the difficult interpretation and poor reproducibility of other components (i.e. amplitudes). An increased delay time (N_{14}–N_{20}) was found in six (24%) patients.

Blink reflexes

We recorded these with needle electrodes stimulating the supra-orbital nerves separately and recording electrodes in the orbicularis oculi muscles. In three (12%) patients the records showed an abnormal delay of the first (R_1) or second (R_2) response or combinations (R_1 and R_2).

Horizontal saccadic and smooth pursuit eye-movements (ENG)

These recordings showed an increased saccadic latency in eight (32%) patients. One patient showed an internuclear ophthalmoplegia[12].

CT-scan

CT-scan with a special slice through the orbits revealed a broadened optic nerve in two (8%) patients. The phenomenon of a broadened optic nerve was only once before reported by Mikol[13] in a patient with a clinical state of definite multiple sclerosis, who was suffering acute visual loss at the time of investigation.

Five (20%) patients, including those with optic nerve asymmetry, showed hyperdense contrast enhanced lesions in one or both hemispheres. One patient, who had a recurrence of optic neuritis in the contralateral eye, was investigated by the CT-scan on four different occasions; his hyperdense contrast enhanced lesions were located in different areas of the brain at each of the four examinations.

The combination of electrophysiological investigations revealed non-symptomatic lesions in eleven (44%) of the optic neuritis patients. These lesions were mostly located in the brainstem (Figure 1).

The sum total of electrophysiological and CT-scan investigations detected non-symptomatic lesions in twelve (48%) of the twenty-five optic neuritis patients (Figure 2).

As in the reports of previous workers, the cerebrospinal fluid was investigated in search of intrathecal IgG synthesis. By using the isoelectric focusing technique, intrathecal IgG synthesis was detected in nine (36%) patients (Figure 2).

In a statistical analysis, there was found a significant association between the total of electrophysiologically revealed central nervous system abnormalities (excluding the visual evoked response) and a proven intrathecal immuno-

Figure 1   The combination of electrophysiological investigations (ABER, SSER, blink reflex, ENG) detected subclinical CNS lesions in eleven (44%) of 25 clinically pure optic neuritis patients.

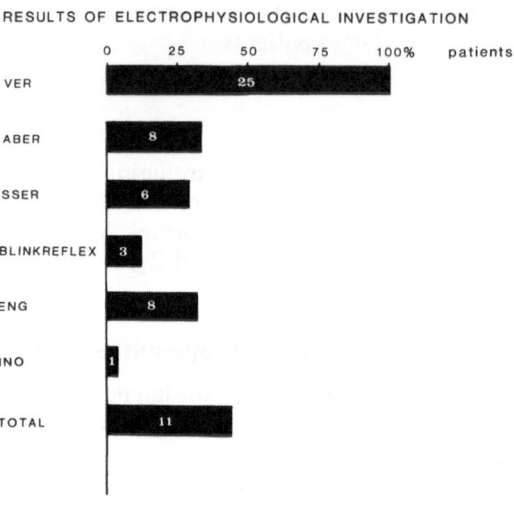

Figure 2   The overall data of CSF, electrophysiological (ABER, SSER, blink reflex, ENG) and CT-scan data revealed: (1) intrathecal IgG synthesis in two (8%) patients, (2) subclinical CNS lesions in five (20%) patients, (3) both subclinical lesions and intrathecal IgG synthesis in seven (28%) patients. Fourteen (56%) of the 25 ON patients showed one or more abnormalities besides the delayed VER P_{100} peak.

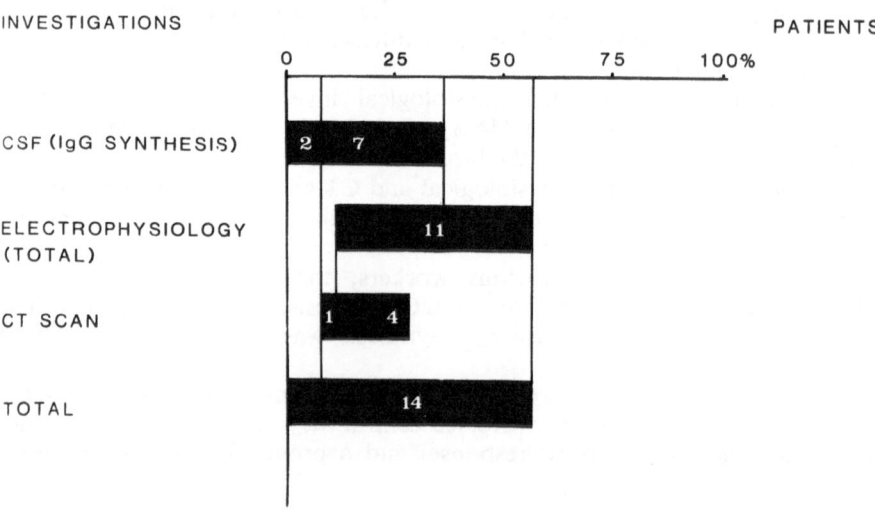

globulin synthesis ($p<0.005$). This association remains when the CT-scan data are included amongst the indicators of non-symptomatic central nervous system lesions.

No pattern was found to relate the various types of visual evoked response disorders with intrathecal immunoglobulin synthesis (χ^2-test).

In an overall combination of results, there were seven (28%) patients, who showed both non-symptomatic central nervous system lesions and intrathecal immunoglobulin synthesis. One could infer that at least these seven, but probably twelve, patients had a subclinical form of multiple sclerosis at the time of the optic neuritis attack.

From the data in this pilot study, the following conclusions can be drawn:

(1) In nearly half of the clinically pure optic neuritis patients, there are more lesions than in the optic nerve alone, at the time of the attack.

(2) The measurement of visual evoked response is not capable of discriminating between pure optic neuritis and optic neuritis as part of a multiple sclerosis syndrome.

(3) There is a statistically significant relation between non-symptomatic central nervous system lesions and intrathecal immunoglobulin synthesis in pure optic neuritis patients.

(4) Only a prospective study of these, and greater numbers of patients can more precisely determine the predictive power of these tests.

References

1. Parinaud, H. H. (1884). Troubles oculaires de la sclérose en plaque. *Prog. Méd. (Paris),* **12,** 641

2. Uhthoff, W. (1889). Untersuchungen über die bei der Multiple Herd Sklerose vorkomenden Augenstörungen. *Arch. Psychiat. Nervenkr.,* **21,** 303

3. McAlpine, D., Lumsden, C. E. and Acheson, E. D. (1965). *Multiple Sclerosis. A Reappraisal.* (Edinburgh, London: Churchill Livingstone)

4. *Leibowitz, U., Alter, M. and Halpern, L. (1966). Clinical study of Multiple Sclerosis in Israel. IV: optic neuropathy and MS. Arch. Neurol.,* **14,** 459

5. Wikstrom, J., Poser, S. and Ritter, G. (1980). Optic neuritis as an initial symptom in Multiple Sclerosis. *Acta Neurol. Scand.,* **61,** 178

6. Cohen, M. M., Lessel, S. and Wole, P. A. (1979). A prospective study of the risk of developing Multiple Sclerosis in uncomplicated optic neuritis. *Neurology (Minneap.),* **29,** 208

7. Sandberg-Wollheim, M. (1975). Optic neuritis: studies on the cerebrospinal fluid in relation to clinical course in 61 patients. *Acta Neurol. Scand.,* **52,** 167

8. Hutchinson, W. M. (1976). Acute optic neuritis and the prognosis for Multiple Sclerosis. *J. Neurol. Neurosurg. Psychiat.,* **39,** 283

9. Nikoskelainen, E., Frey, H. and Salm, A. (1981). Prognosis of optic neuritis with special reference to cerebrospinal fluid immunoglobulin and measles virus antibodies. *Ann. Neurol.,* **9,** 545

10. Platz, P., Ryder, L. P., Staub Nielsen, L., Svejgaard, A., Thompson, M. and Wollheim, M. S. (1975). HLA and idiopathic optic neuritis. *Lancet,* **i,** 520

11. Stendahl, L., Link, H., Moller, E. and Norrby, E. (1976). Relation between genetic markers and oligoclonal IgG in CSF in optic neuritis. *J. Neurol. Sci.,* **27,** 93

12. Reulen, J. P. H., Sanders, E. A. C. M. and Hogenhuis, L. A. H. (1983). Eye-movement disorders in Multiple Sclerosis and optic neuritis. *Brain,* **106,** 121

13. Mikol, F., Bouchareine, A., Aubin, M. L. and Vignaud, J. (1980). La tomodensitométrie dans la sclérose en plaques. *Rev. Neurol. (Paris),* **136,** 481

54
Prognostic value of CSF IgG in monosymptomatic optic neuritis

H. I. SCHIPPER, S. POSER, H. WUZÉL and W. BEHRENS-BAUMANN

The frequency with which patients with monosymptomatic optic neuritis develop multiple sclerosis (MS) is still under discussion. On the basis of clinical examinations, figures vary from 11.5 to 85%[1]. Various attempts have been made to study parameters which might influence the risk. As far as the prognostic value of CSF IgG alterations is concerned, divergent opinions exist which might be influenced in part by methodical problems[2-4].

In order to study this question, we are currently monitoring a group of patients with initially isolated optic neuritis. Only patients with no indication of possible MS bouts prior to the optic neuritis attack are included. This is a preliminary report of 39 cases after a follow-up period between 1 and 7 years with a mean of 3.2 years. Patients were re-examined ophthalmologically, neurologically and, when consenting, by lumbar puncture.

Initially, a central scotoma had been found in all patients. At re-examination, ophthalmological deficits were mild. Only one patient still had reduction of visual acuity, few reported painful motility or showed pupillar abnormalities. About 45% had partial optic nerve atrophy. A surprisingly high percentage (55%) displayed concentric red field defects on perimetry. This finding is probably in accord with other authors reporting defective colour vision[5]. There was no correlation between ophthalmological changes and MS risk or CSF alterations.

At the time of re-examination, 16 (41%) of our 39 patients had developed definite or probable MS. There are some uncertainties in this figure, since on the one hand in some patients the observation period is not yet long enough, and on the other hand patients not developing MS apparently appeared in a lower percentage for re-examination.

It has previously been reported that the course of MS developing after monosymptomatic optic neuritis is strikingly benign[1,3,4]. In our group this might best be illustrated by the fact that none of the patients was severely disabled and in five cases the disease had not even been diagnosed previously. There was no fixed interval between optic neuritis and MS manifestation. Most of those who developed MS did so within the first year. So far we did not observe any manifestations after the third year.

At CSF examination during the acute attack of optic neuritis, mononuclear pleocytosis was observed in only 22 cases, with no apparent correlation of prognostic value. At re-examination five patients without and 11 patients with MS had pleocytosis. Out of these 11, only four could be regarded as being in a state of clinical activity.

CNS local IgG production is best demonstrated in two different ways:

(1) *Quantitatively* by comparing the CSF/serum-quotients of IgG with the respective quotients of albumin which is synthetized only extracerebrally. Therefore, different schemes have been developed. We are applying the evaluation graph described by Reiber[6]. In this scheme the two quotients are plotted against each other. It permits easy recognition of normal values, pathological IgG production, blood–CSF barrier dysfunction, and a combination of both.

(2) *Qualitatively* by determination of oligoclonal IgG subfractions in CSF by means of isoelectric focusing in polyacrylamide gels (pH 3.5–9.5, LKB). This technique is more sensitive and permits the demonstration of intrathecal IgG production even when other parameters are still within the normal range.

The *diagnostic* value of the two different methods for determining IgG production – quantitatively *vs* qualitatively – is compared in Figure 1 which shows the results of 27 patients during the initial acute attack of optic neuritis. There is a first group of 16 patients with clearly elevated IgG quotients and oligoclonal IgG in CSF. A second group of 10 patients (1/3!) has normal IgG levels, and can be identified only by the presence of oligoclonal IgG. The third

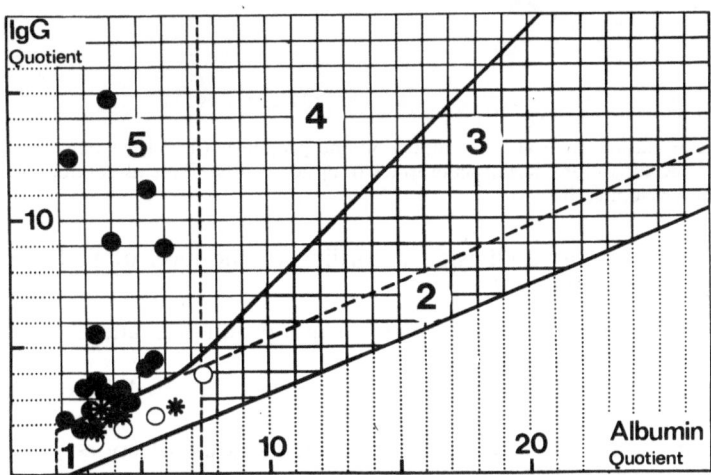

Figure 1   IgG production during acute attack of optic neuritis ($n = 27$). 1 Normal range. 2 + 3 Blood/CSF barrier dysfunction. 4 Combination of blood/CSF barrier dysfunction and intrathecal IgG production. 5 Intrathecal IgG production. Oligoclonal IgG: present = ●, weakly present = *, not detectable = ○

group of four patients has no detectable inflammatory IgG production with either method. Even if a fifth patient is included in whom only quantitative measurements were possible, the latter group is surprisingly small. This can only in part be explained by the exclusion of misdiagnosed cases at re-examination.

As far as the *prognostic* value of IgG determination is concerned we have first to state that the low number of patients without inflammatory IgG production ($n = 5$) does not yet permit any definite conclusions. It may, however, be said that no patient out of this group so far developed MS[7]. These patients, therefore, are not included in Figure 2 which shows only those 34 patients who displayed detectable IgG alterations during the acute stage of optic neuritis. If three patients with blood–CSF barrier dysfunctions are disregarded, two groups can be identified: one with normal or slightly elevated IgG levels and a second group with a very high amount of autochthonously produced IgG, at an IgG quotient > 6. All these eight patients developed MS.

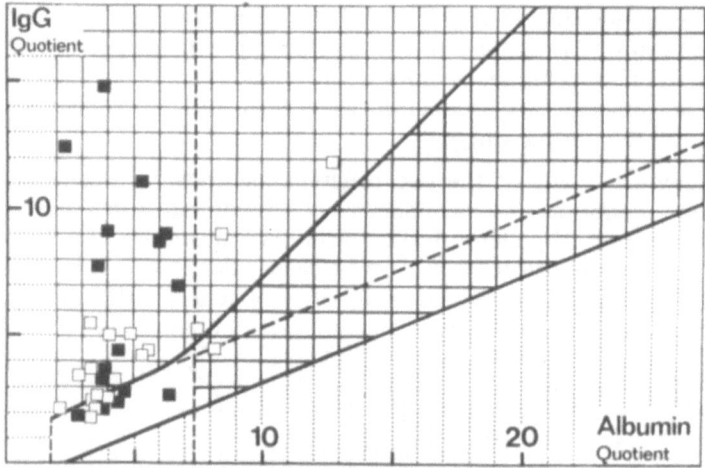

Figure 2 Correlation of local IgG production and prognosis ($n = 34$) (patients with inflammatory CSF IgG alterations during acute attack of optic neuritis). Patients developing: MS : ■, patients not developing MS : □

In other words, a subdivision according to the level of CNS local IgG production appears possible:

(1) those without demonstrable local IgG production and a very low MS risk (small group),

(2) those with oligoclonal IgG and normal or slightly elevated IgG quotients and an intermediate MS risk,

(3) and those with very high IgG quotients (plus, of course, oligoclonal IgG) and a very high MS risk.

Our follow-up CSF examination gives further evidence that the amount of autochthonously produced IgG remains fairly constant: none of the optic neuritis patients without any CSF IgG alterations had oligoclonal IgG or

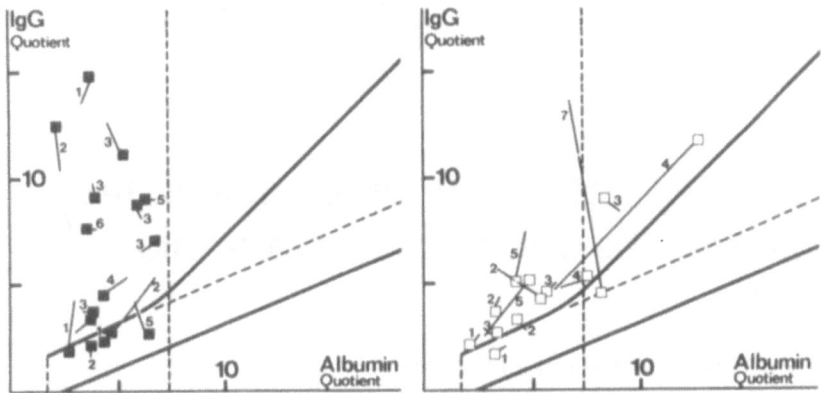

Figure 3 IgG production changes at re-examination ($n = 34$) (patients with inflammatory CSF IgG alterations during acute attack of optic neuritis). Patients developing MS (left side) = ■ , patients not developing MS (right side) = □ . Time interval (in years) is marked by numbers, difference in measurements by bars

elevated IgG levels at re-examination. On the other hand, all patients who had had inflammatory IgG production during the acute attack of optic neuritis, still had these abnormalities at re-examination, regardless of whether they had developed MS or not. There is strikingly little change in the amount of auto-chthonously produced IgG even when patients were controlled after several years (Figure 3). The relevance of this continuous IgG production is not yet known. It must be doubted that all of it can be attributed to clinically silent plaques. Our results certainly suggest that clinical symptoms are not the only parameter for the activity of the underlying immune process.

References

1. Cohen, M. M., Simmons Lessell, M. D. and Wolf, P. A. (1979). A prospective study of the risk of developing multiple sclerosis in uncomplicated optic neuritis. *Neurology, 29*, 208
2. Haller, P. (1981). *Die Opticusneuritis.* (Stuttgart: Thieme)
3. Nikoskalainen, E., Frey, H. and Salmi, A. (1981). Prognosis of optic neuritis with special reference to cerebrospinal fluid immunoglobulins and measles virus antibodies. *Ann. Neurol., 9*, 545
4. Sandberg-Wollheim, M. (1975). Optic neuritis: Studies on the cerebrospinal fluid in relation to clinical course in 61 patients. *Acta Neurol. Scand., 52*, 167
5. Zeller, R. W. (1967). Ocular findings in the remission phase of multiple sclerosis. *Am. J. Ophthalmol., 64*, 767
6. Reiber, H. (1980). The discrimination between different blood/CSF barrier dysfunctions and inflammatory reactions of the CNS by a recent evaluation graph for the protein profile of cerebrospinal fluid. *J. Neurol., 224*, 89
7. Lennerstrand, G. and Stendahl-Brodin, L. (1982). Pattern VEP in two immunochemical subtypes of optic neuritis. *Acta Ophthalmol., 60*, 313

55
Cerebrospinal fluid findings in isolated optic neuritis compared to multiple sclerosis

U. WURSTER, U. PATZOLD and J. HAAS

INTRODUCTION

The close relationship between multiple sclerosis (MS) and optic neuritis (ON) is undisputed. While ON is the first symptom in about 17% of all MS cases[1], involvement of the optic nerve during the course of the disease may reach up to 96%, as demonstrated by visually evoked potentials which also detect sub-clinical lesions[2]. Post mortem examinations have revealed pathological changes in optic nerve or chiasm in every one of 36 unselected consecutive MS cases[3]. Immunological abnormalities of the same kind as in MS have been encountered in patients with ON but usually at a considerably lower incidence rate[4,5].

Given the close association between ON and MS the question arises whether cerebrospinal fluid (CSF) findings could be used to predict the subsequent development of MS. Earlier reports on this issue are inconclusive, and have apparently been hampered by insufficiencies in methodology[6]. Several patients developed MS despite a normal CSF, and disturbing phenomena like transient bands have been described after separation by agar-gel electrophoresis[7]. It may be hoped that more discriminating electrophoretic methods like iso-electrofocusing will yield less ambiguous results, and that calculation of intracerebral IgG synthesis with the help of one of the specially devised formulas available nowadays will likewise render more reliable values.

METHODS

During the last $3\frac{1}{2}$ years we have studied 63 patients with isolated optic neuritis. Visual disturbances of an infectious, vascular, compressive, metabolic, hereditary or toxic nature were excluded, as were those with additional neurological signs and symptoms. Thirteen cases with bilateral loss of vision and a history of heavy alcohol and/or tobacco consumption were

Table 1 Comparison of CSF parameters in multiple sclerosis and optic neuritis

	Multiple sclerosis		*Optic neuritis*		$p \leqslant$
CSF oligoclonal bands present		120		37	
Sex	(n = 120)	78♀, 42♂	(n = 37)	30♀, 7♂	n.s.
Age	(n = 120)	36.2 ± 11.5 years	(n = 37)	30.5 ± 9.4 years	0.001
CNS IgG syn (mg/day)	(n = 120)	18.1 ± 20.3	(n = 37)	8.6 ± 12.1	0.01
Total protein (mg/l)	(n = 120)	343 ± 109	(n = 37)	308 ± 80	n.s.
Cells/μl	(n = 120)	12.5 ± 17.2	(n = 37)	13.1 ± 14.7	n.s.
ANAE positive cells	(n = 103)	81.8 ± 8.1%	(n = 35)	83.8 ± 8.5%	n.s.
CSF oligoclonal bands absent		9/129 = 7.0%		26/63 = 41.3%	0.001

Means ± standard deviations are given. Statistical significances have been tested with the χ^2-test for different frequencies, otherwise the *t*-test has been used; n.s. = not significant

assembled in a separate group. The results were compared to a set of 129 clinically probable (with proven oligoclonal bands) or definite MS patients with a disease duration of less than 5 years. Lumbar fluid from patients with optic neuritis was collected mostly within 2 weeks, but not later than 6 months after the initial attack.

Laboratory studies included total CSF cell count, differential count after acid α-naphthylacetatesterase (ANAE) staining, determination by radial immunodiffusion of IgG and albumin in the CSF and serum and calculation of the IgG synthesis rate by Tourtelotte's formula[8]. IgG oligoclonal bands of un-concentrated CSF were separated on ready made (LKB) isoelectric focusing polyacrylamide gels pH 3.5–9.5 followed by silver staining[9]. Means ± SD are given in all Tables and Figures.

RESULTS

In Table 1 the data obtained for both groups of patients are summarized. Only 7.0% of all MS patients do not possess oligoclonal bands, whereas in optic neuritis a far higher percentage of 41.3% lacks this characteristic sign. Further comments will deal mainly with the cases with proven oligoclonal bands, since in their absence other causes of disease cannot be entirely ruled out.

As expected patients with ON are younger by almost 6 years. Although a female preponderance of 4:1 may be noted in ON, this difference is not statistically different from the MS group where a sex ratio of 2:1 prevails. Likewise, no differences have been found for the total protein concentration, the total CSF cell count and the number of ANAE positive cells. On the other hand a very clearcut difference exists in local IgG synthesis with ON patients attaining less than half the production rate of patients with MS.

The histograms in Figure 1a,b reveal that synthesis rates over 54 mg/day were not observed in ON. Moreover, 15 of the 37 ON cases (40.5%) stay below the upper limit of normal of 4 mg/day compared to 25 of the 120 MS patients (20.8%) ($p<0.02$). Blood–brain barrier disturbances seem to be similar both in frequency and distribution in the two forms of the disease (Figure 1).

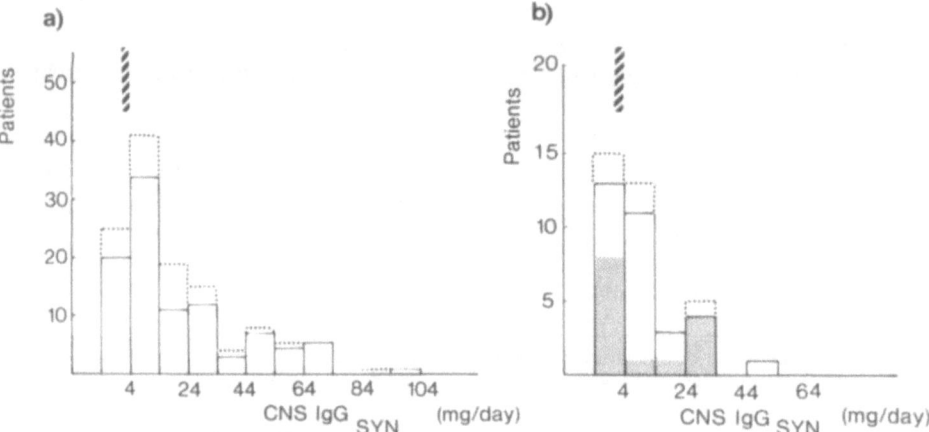

Figure 1 Frequency distribution of intracerebral IgG synthesis in (a) 120 patients with multiple sclerosis; (b) 37 patients with optic neuritis. The dotted lines indicate a disturbed blood–brain barrier (albumin CSF/serum >0.0074). The upper value of the normal IgG synthesis rate of 4 mg/day has been marked by a bar. The shaded area in (b) comprises those cases of optic neuritis which have progressed to multiple sclerosis

The considerable number (41%) without local IgG elevation can only be recognized as producers of pathological IgG by the demonstration of an oligoclonal pattern. Although clearly discernible from normal in most cases, the oligoclonal bands in the CSF of ON patients generally are fewer in number and less pronounced than those from MS patients as can be recognized from Figure 2 and 3. This observation suggested a dependence of the number of bands on the intracerebral IgG synthesis rate. The logarithmic relationship found is shown in Figure 3.

The ANAE stain is a simple method to evaluate the number of T-lymphocytes in the CSF. Percentages of ANAE+ cells were increased to $81.8 \pm 8.1\%$ (means ± SD) in 103 MS cases and to $83.8 \pm 8.5\%$ in 35 ON, which is significantly different from a group of 35 normal controls (neurological patients, whose complaints turned out to be of a psychoneuritic nature) with $64.9 \pm 7.4\%$ (Figure 4). Even in the absence of oligoclonal banding, in 10 out of 26 ON patients the proportion of T-cells exceeded 75%, the highest value of the normal population. In contrast, only $38.1 \pm 6\%$ T-lymphocytes have been counted for the so-called toxic form of ON. The missing cells were made up by monocytes. Expression of the results on a relative basis is to be preferred, because the enormous fluctuation in total cell count leads to high standard deviations if absolute values are calculated (Figure 4).

Preliminary results of the follow-up studies are presented in Table 2. Within an average observation time of 14 months, 14 of the ON patients with oligo-

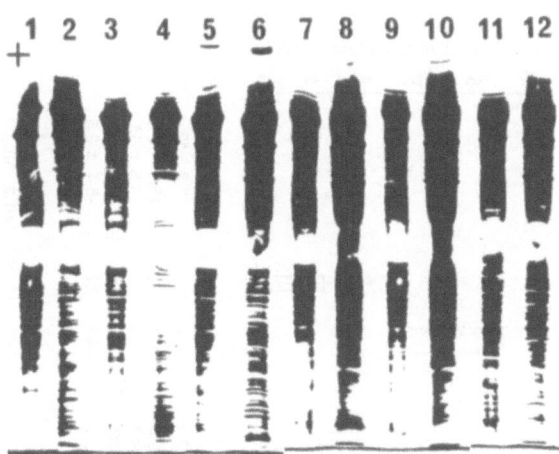

Figure 2 Oligoclonal IgG bands after staining with silver. 30 μl of either serum (left, odd numbers) or CSF (right, even numbers) diluted to 0.02 g/l IgG were separated on isoelectric focusing gels pH 3.5–9.5. IgG synthesis rates amounted to 10.6, 25.4, 2.3 mg IgG/day for the three CSFs from MS patients in lanes 2, 4, 6 respectively. Two patients with ON synthesized − 5.7 (lane 8) and 1.6 (lane 12) mg/day. A normal pattern was found in a case of non-Hodgkin lymphoma with − 9·6 mg/day (lane 10)

clonal bands in their CSF – all of them were women – suffered new neurological symptoms and signs allowing the diagnosis of MS. Five of these 14 who had another spinal fluid tap were all unchanged in regard of concentration and appearance of IgG. In the group without oligoclonal bands, only one patient developed MS. This particular patient has been repunctured twice in the meantime without any alterations in her CSF IgG. On every occasion however, she displayed abnormal T-lymphocyte values without pleocytosis.

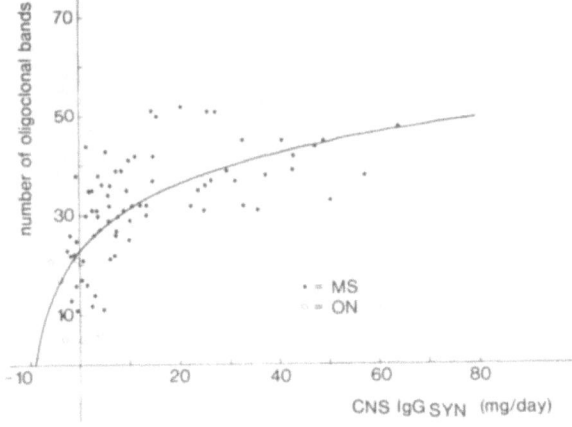

Figure 3 Relationship between intracerebral IgG synthesis and number of oligoclonal bands. The number of abnormal bands visible after silver staining has been counted by an arbitrary scoring system to account for differences in intensity. A minimum of four separate bands was required for a positive rating. The regression line was calculated for 76 MS and 10 ON patients as $y = 3.74 + 11.90 \ln (x + 10)$ with $r = 0.67$

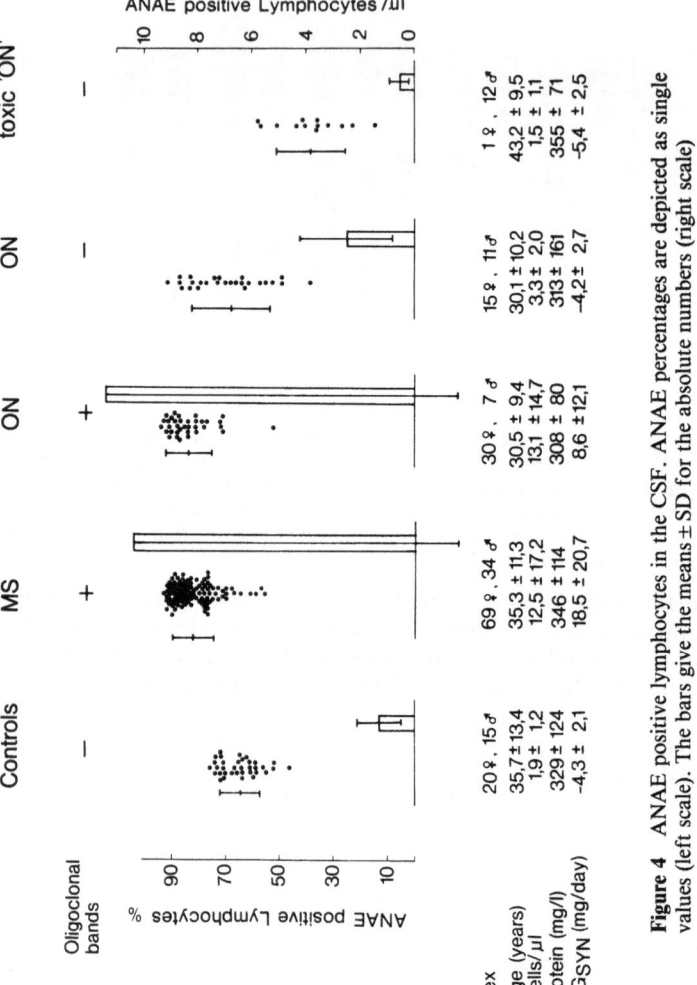

Figure 4 ANAE positive lymphocytes in the CSF. ANAE percentages are depicted as single values (left scale). The bars give the means ± SD for the absolute numbers (right scale).

Table 2 Future development of patients with optic neuritis

Oligoclonal bands	Present	Absent
Total	30♀, 7♂ = 37	15♀, 11♂ = 26
Follow-up	21♀, 3♂ = 24	7♀, 5♂ = 12
Mean observation time (months)	13.5 ± 11.5 (3–47)	14.3 ± 9.3 (3–32)
Patients with MS symptoms appearing within 1, 2, 3, 4 years	9, 3, 1, 1	0, 1, 0, 0

DISCUSSION

McAlpine et al[10] have expressed the view that demyelinating disease is the only common cause of unilateral optic neuritis. In possible MS – and ON may be regarded as such – evoked potentials and CSF examinations may contribute to proper classification and earlier diagnosis than can be achieved on clinical grounds alone.

Formally, the existence of immunological abnormalities in the CSF would then be equivalent to the occurrence of clinically silent lesions in other regions of the CNS as demonstrable, e.g. by somatosensory evoked potentials. By contrast, the latency delay observed in visually evoked potentials (VEP) in cases with ophthalmologically certified ON is merely confirmatory[11]. Moreover, pathological VEPs can also result from compressions, refractive errors or inadequate patient cooperation[12], apart from the fact that they may normalize after a certain time[13]. The inflammatory origin of the optic neuropathy however, can readily be demonstrated via inspection of the CSF.

Several investigators have addressed the question whether CSF findings have any prognostic value regarding the progression of ON to (fully established) MS. Of Link's[14] 21 patients with oligoclonal bands three developed MS, but none of the 20 (including some with tobacco/alcohol 'ON') without this sign. Sandberg-Wollheim[7] found a slightly higher risk for ON patients with proven oligoclonal bands, but progression to MS was also observed in patients with an initially normal CSF. In these latter patients, however, CSF findings frequently became pathological after the clinical diagnosis of MS had been made. In a recent update of her earlier work Nikoskelainen et al[15] likewise reported a higher proportion of subsequent MS cases among the ON patients with initially elevated CSF leukocyte count, relative IgG increase and abnormal bands on cellulose-acetate-electrophoresis.

Nowadays more sensitive methods like differentiating stains for lymphocyte subsets, special formulas for IgG calculation and isoelectric focusing for the demonstration of IgG oligoclonal bands in native CSF are available. Our results show that even when employing these methods CSF alterations in ON are lower both in frequency and magnitude compared to MS.

As pointed out before by Link's group[16,17] CSF parameters are not independent of one another. A similar association evolved from the present study. Increased IgG synthesis was always accompanied by oligoclonal banding, and in the presence of this sign pleocytosis occurred more frequently. Of the 120 MS and the 37 ON patients with oligoclonal bands 74 (61.7%) and 27 (73%) respectively, also displayed pleocytosis, but only 1/9 (11.1%) and 4/26 (15.4%) of the cases with no bands. Our value of 61.7% pleocytosis in MS might appear high, compared to reports in the literature[4], but this effect can probably be attributed to the dominance of 'active' cases in our group of MS patients with a disease duration of less than 5 years. It might be argued that the MS reference group should have been confined to 'active' cases only, since acute ON clearly demarcates an active phase, but we felt that the varying course of ON justifies a broader composition.

As would have been expected the group with the toxic (alcohol/tobacco) form of 'ON' showed normal IgG synthesis rates, no oligoclonal bands and normal cell counts. However, the percentage of ANAE+ cells (38.1 ± 12.6) was significantly diminished compared to normal controls (64.9 ± 7.4%, Figure 4). This observation underlines the value of differential counts also in the absence of pleocytosis. Atypical lymphocytes and plasma cells believed to be pathognomic for MS have been found by Thompson et al[18] despite normal cell counts and Kam-Hansen et al[19] report active T-cells in the CSF to be decreased uniformly after ON, irrespective of mononuclear pleocytosis.

We used the unspecific esterase method for the simultaneous staining of lymphocytes (dot-like or negative) and monocytes (diffuse) in CSF cytocentrifuge preparations. The ANAE stain identifies T-lymphocytes and can therefore be regarded as a simple and inexpensive alternative to either rosetting procedures or pan T monoclonal antibodies.

Initially, specificity of the ANAE stain was claimed for T-helper lymphocytes[20] because of the preferential staining of cells with an Fc receptor for IgM. These so called T_M cells are now believed to represent quite a heterogeneous population and when T-lymphocytes were defined by monoclonal antibodies both suppressor and helper T-cells reacted with ANAE. While Pichler et al[2] found 88% of the OKT 4 (helper) and 73% of the OKT 8 (suppressor) enriched lymphocytes positive in the ANAE stain, Bernard and Dufer[22] arrive at 76% and 24% respectively. Using monoclonal antibodies of the LEU series Armitage et al[23] observed a dot-like reaction in 82% of the helper and 50% of the suppressor cells. Thus, according to these studies carried out in peripheral blood cells, ANAE positivity characterizes a mature resting T-lymphocyte preferably of the helper variety.

The first reports enumerating CSF cells of MS patients by monoclonal antibodies have revealed 80–90% T-lymphocytes, most of which belonged to the helper subset[24,25]. Earlier communications using rosetting assays had also shown a preponderance of T-lympocytes in the CSF of a small number of patients with ON[16,26,27]. Our high values of 81.8% ANAE positive cells in the CSF of MS patients and 83.8% for ON correspond well with these findings and confirm the results of Czlonkowska et al[28], who had also used the ANAE stain in their MS patients. ANAE positivity of CSF cells seems to be a more sensitive indicator of an inflammatory reaction than pleocytosis alone. 30/35 (86%) of our ON patients with proven oligoclonal bands had ANAE+ cells against 27/37 (73%) with pleocytosis. For MS the following figures were found: 83/103 (80.5%) ANAE+ cells against 74/120 (61.7%) with pleocytosis. Even in the ON group with missing oligoclonal bands 10 of 26 CSFs presented elevated ANAE+ counts, whereas the total mononuclear cell count was raised in only four.

Application of corticosteroids is a common therapy for acute ON. Such a treatment may influence the number of ANAE+ cells in the CSF[29]. Three of the five ON patients with normal ANAE+ count had received corticosteroids but none of the 20 MS patients. There are indications that this latter group find themselves in a more stable phase of the disease. Despite these limitations one gains the impression that the CSF cells are among the first (from the parameters tested) to respond to the unknown insult in ON, a view shared by Prange[30]. At this stage the process may either be abrogated or proceed further, extending first to qualitative alterations of intrathecal IgG (oligoclones) and then also to quantitative augmentation.

This argument is supported by the findings of Schipper et al[31] who concluded that the ON patients with the highest amount of intrathecal IgG also run the greatest risk of developing MS. A similar observation was made for possible MS patients who progressed to definite MS significantly more often if the initial IgG index surpassed 1.0[32]. Our own results do not coincide with these reports. Of the 14 patients who developed MS so far, eight had normal IgG synthesis and only six were elevated (Figure 1b). MS became manifest also in one ON patient (of the 12 followed, Table 2), whose only abnormality consisted of an augmentation of ANAE+ cells, but this had to be expected in the light of the fact that also 7% of the definite MS cases lack the typical CSF alterations.

It seems remarkable that so far only women ($p<0.05$) have developed MS in our population, which may, however, not be truly representative, because we did not include all cases of ON in our geographical area. According to a recent review[4] the female sex indeed has a higher susceptibility for ON and also a higher progression rate. Under these circumstances the often quoted figure of 13% (for the lower range of the progression rate) established by Kurland et al[33] for US Army service men is clearly misleading.

The present investigation has shown a more restricted immune response (in the CSF) in ON compared to MS. Such a behaviour would be understandable in view of the small area affected in ON, but with spreading of the plaques beyond the optic nerve a scale-up in CSF indicators should ensue. The stability of both the oligoclonal pattern and the level of intrathecal IgG – in admittedly a limited number of ON cases – apparently do not reinforce these assumptions. Further longitudinal studies are needed to resolve this question, although the same phenomena have also been noticed in MS.

In conclusion one may state that an examination of the CSF certainly is of high value for the differential diagnosis of ON, provided that modern sensitive methods are employed. The immunological reaction apparent in the CSF of patients with ON is not uniform. Instead a graded response seems to be possible. Some patients lack CSF alterations altogether – and it is this group where an intensified search for non-inflammatory causes of the disease may be indicated – in others they are confined to an elevation of T-lymphocytes, yet a majority of 60% develops oligoclonal bands, often with a concomitant increase in intracerebral IgG synthesis. Persons with CSF abnormalities suffer a much higher risk of developing MS, although their absence does not guarantee that MS will never occur.

NOTE ADDED IN PROOF

In their latest report Stendahl-Brodin and Link[34] also arrive at the conclusion that the occurrence of oligoclonal bands in the CSF of a patient with ON significantly increases the risk of the future development of MS.

ACKNOWLEDGEMENT

We thank the Hertie Foundation, Frankfurt, for financial support.

References

1. Wikström, J., Poser, S. and Ritter, G. (1980). Optic neuritis as an initial symptom in multiple sclerosis. *Acta Neurol. Scand.,* **61**, 178
2. McDonald, W. I. and Halliday, A. M. (1977). Diagnosis and classification of multiple sclerosis. *Br. Med. Bull.,* **33**, 4
3. Lumsden, C. E. (1970). The neuropathology of multiple sclerosis. In Vinken, P. J. and Bruyn, G. W. (eds.). *Handbook of Clinical Neurology.* Vol. 9, pp. 217–309 (Amsterdam: North Holland)
4. Perkin, G. D. and Rose, C. (1979). *Optic neuritis and its differential diagnosis.* (Oxford, New York, Toronto: Oxford University Press)
5. Frick, E. and Stickl, H. (1980). Optic neuritis and multiple sclerosis. An immunological study. *Eur. Neurol.,* **19**, 185
6. Perkin, G. D. (1979). Optic neuritis and multiple sclerosis: An immunological comparison. In Rose, F. C. (ed.). *Clinical Neuroimmunology.* pp. 312–328 (Oxford, London, Edinburgh, Melbourne: Blackwell Scientific Publications)
7. Sandberg-Wollheim, M. (1979). Optic neuritis. Cerebrospinal fluid findings and clinical course. *Proceedings Ophthalmology Congress XXIII.* Vol. 1, Kyoto. pp. 347–350 (Amsterdam, Oxford: Excerpta Medica)
8. Tourtelotte, W. W. and Booe, I. M. (1978). Multiple sclerosis: The blood–brain barrier and the measurement of *de novo* central nervous system IgG synthesis. *Neurology,* **28**, 76
9. Wurster, U. (1983). Demonstration of oligoclonal IgG in the unconcentrated CSF by silver stain. In Stathakos, D. (ed.). *Electrophoresis 1982,* pp. 250–259. (Berlin, New York: Walter de Gruyter)
10. McAlpine, D., Lumsden, C. E. and Acheson, E. D. (1965). *Multiple Sclerosis. A Reappraisal.* (Edinburgh and London: Churchill Livingstone)
11. Matthews, W. B., Wattam-Bell, J. R. B. and Pountney, E. (1982). Evoked potentials in the diagnosis of multiple sclerosis: A follow-up study. *J. Neurol. Neurosurg. Psych.,* **45**, 303
12. Nikoskelainen, E. and Falck, B. (1982). Do visual evoked potentials give relevant information to the neuro-ophthalmological examination in optic nerve lesions? *Acta Neurol. Scand.,* **66**, 42
13. Bynke, H., Rosen, M. and Sandberg-Wollheim, M. (1980). Correlation of visual evoked potentials, ophthalmological and neurological findings after unilateral optic neuritis. *Acta Ophthal.,* **58**, 673
14. Link, H. Discussion to Tourtelotte, W. W. (1975). What is multiple sclerosis? Laboratory criteria for diagnosis. In Davison, A. N., Humphrey, J. H., Liversedge, A. L., McDonald, W. I. and Porterfield, J. S. (eds.). *Multiple Sclerosis Research,* pp. 32–34 (Amsterdam, New York: Elsevier)
15. Nikoskelainen, E., Frey, H. and Salmi, A. (1981). Prognosis of optic neuritis with special reference to cerebrospinal fluid immunoglobulins and measles virus antibodies. *Ann. Neurol.,* **9**, 545
16. Kam-Hansen, S., Fryden, A. and Link, H. (1978). B and T lymphocytes in CSF and blood in MS, ON and mumps meningitis. *Acta Neurol. Scand.,* **58**, 95
17. Stendahl-Brodin, L. (1982). Studies on humoral immunity and HLA antigens in multiple sclerosis, optic neuritis and hereditary optic atrophy. *Acta Ophthal. (Suppl.),* **149**, 41–62
18. Thompson, E. J., Kaufmann, P., Shortman, R. C., Rudge, P. and McDonald, W. I. (1979). Oligoclonal immunoglobulins and plasma cells in spinal fluid of patients with multiple sclerosis. *Br. Med. J.,* **1**, 16
19. Kam-Hansen, S., Rostrōm, B. and Link, H. (1980). Active T cells and humoral immune variables in blood and CSF in patients after acute unilateral idiopathic optic neuritis. *Acta Neurol. Scand.,* **61**, 298
20. Grossi, C. E., Webb, S. R., Zicca, A., Lydyard, P. M., Moretta, L., Mingari, M. C. and

Cooper, M. D. (1978). Morphological and histochemical analyses of two human T-cell subpopulations bearing receptors for IgM or IgG. *J. Exp. Med.,* **147,** 1405

21. Pichler, W. J., Lange, M. L., Birke, C. and Peter, H. H. (1982). Relationship of Fc-IgG and Fc-IgM receptors to the antigens defined by OKT antibodies and the acid α-naphthyl-acetate esterase spot within human T cells. *Immunobiol.,* **160,** 424

22. Bernard, J. and Dufer, J. (1983). Cytochemistry of human lymphocyte subpopulations delineated by monoclonal antibodies. *Br. J. Haematol.,* **53,** 351

23. Armitage, R. J., Linch, D. C., Worman, C. P. and Cawley, J. C. (1982). The morphology and cytochemistry of human T-cell subpopulations defined by monoclonal antibodies and Fc receptors. *Br. J. Haematol.,* **51,** 605

24. Brinkmann, C. J. J., Nillesen, W. M. and Hommes, O. R. (1983). T cell subpopulations in blood and cerebrospinal fluid of multiple sclerosis patients: effect of cyclophosphamide. *Clin. Immunol. Immunopathol.,* (in press)

25. Panitch, H. S. and Francis, G. S. (1982). T-lymphocyte subsets in cerebrospinal fluid in multiple sclerosis. *N. Engl. J. Med.,* **307,** 560

26. Traugott, U. (1978). T and B lymphocytes in the CSF of various neurological diseases. *J. Neurol.,* **219,** 185

27. Nyland, H., Naess, A. and Slagsvold, J. E. (1980). Lymphocyte subpopulations in peripheral blood and CSF from patients with acute optic neuritis. *Acta Ophthal.,* **58,** 411

28. Czlonkowska, A., Poltorak, M., Cendrowski, W. and Korlak, J. (1980). Lymphocyte subpopulations in the cerebrospinal fluid and peripheral blood in multiple sclerosis. *Acta Neurol. Scand.,* **62,** 55

29. Wurster, U. and Patzold, U. (1983). Long-term treatment of multiple sclerosis with azathioprine. Effects on cerebrospinal fluid parameters. In Hommes, O. R. (ed.). *Immuno-suppressive treatment in multiple sclerosis* (in press.)

30. Prange, H. (1980). CSF findings in patients with multiple sclerosis and optic neuritis. In Bauer, H. J., Poser, S. and Ritter, G. (eds.). *Progress in Multiple Sclerosis Research*, pp. 129–131. (Berlin, Heidelberg, New York: Springer-Verlag)

31. Schipper, H. I., Poser, S., Wurzel, H. and Behrens-Baumann, W. (1983). Prognostic value of CSF IgG in monosymptomatic optic neuritis. In Gonsette, R. E. and Delmotte, P. (eds.). *Immunological and Clinical Aspects of Multiple Sclerosis,* Chap. 54. (Lancaster: MTP Press)

32. Böttcher, J. and Trojaburg, W. (1982). Follow-up of patients with suspected MS: A clinical and electrophysiological study. *J. Neurol. Neurosurg. Psych.,* **45,** 809

33. Kurland, L. T., Beebe, G. W., Kurtzke, J. F., Nogler, B., Auth, T. L., Lesell, S. and Metzger, M. D. (1966). Studies on the natural history of multiple sclerosis. 2. The progression of optic neuritis to multiple sclerosis. *Acta Neurol. Scand. (Suppl.),* **19,** 157

34. Stendahl-Brodin, L. and Link, H. (1983). Optic neuritis: oligoclonal bands increase the risk of multiple sclerosis. *Acta. Neurol-Scand.,* **67,** 303

56
Ophthalmological manifestations in multiple sclerosis
A statistical review of 1728 cases (1180 confirmed cases)

S. BERVOETS and H. A. De LAET

METHOD

This study concerns only those patients hospitalized at the National Center of Multiple Sclerosis (MS), from 1960 to 1981. In their majority these patients present the 'chronic' form of the disease, of many years duration.

They enter the clinic, as a rule, for medical check-up, but also for social reasons or for revalidation. Many of these patients show a severe MS. For them, the subjective part of the medical examination is tiring and difficult. Therefore, in spite of an obvious goodwill, their co-operation is poor and the results obtained by interrogation, such as visual acuity, quantitative perimetry, power of convergence, etc, have only a relative value.

Our 1728 cases of ophthalmological examinations have been ranged according to the criteria of Schumacher et al[1]. Therefore, we range our cases in four groups:

(1) 1180 cases of positive MS
(2)   270 cases of probable MS
(3)   53 cases of questionable MS
(4)   225 cases of neurologic disorders other than MS.

The ocular signs concerned in this study are:

(1) Sheathing of retinal veins
(2) Optic atrophy
(3) Anterior internuclear ophthalmoplegia
(4) Convergence paresis or palsy
(5) Claude Bernard-Horner's syndrome
(6) Nystagmus
(7) Perimetric defects.

SHEATHING OF THE RETINAL VEINS (SRV)

The search and observation of the SRV is always made after pupillary dilatation. From 1960 to 1971 we used the red-free light (green filter) of the ophthalmoscope (Visuskop Oculus) and since then, the blue filter of the ophthalmoscope of Amalric, intensity 5 (Luneau and Coffineau).

First, as in any other fundus examination, we have to remember the fact that, when observing the ocular fundus and speaking of the retinal vessels, we are actually looking at the blood column circulating within the vessels, and not at the vessels themselves. Their walls, in normal cases, are transparent and, therefore, not visible by ophthalmoscopy. That means that any observable opacity in direct contact with the blood column is located in the wall of the vessel. The pathological phenomenon of the SRV goes through different degrees of severity. The first ophthalmoscopic appearance is a white streak along the retinal vein; its width is one or two tenths of that of the blood column, and can attain one half or more. At the same time, the density of the 'white' colour increases. Then, the white streak appears on both sides of the vein and, finally, the two streaks join to form a complete sheathing, hiding the red blood column. This last aspect was very infrequent.

In only one case have we observed the signs of a true periphlebitis, that means not only a complete sheathing, but haemorrhages and exudates around limited segments of the vein or at the periphery. The phenomenon appears along only one, or along all the first branches of the central vein of the retina. It rarely begins at less than one or two papillary diameters of the papilla and remains observable till the second or third division of the vein. It seems that the relative width of the white streak increases to the periphery. But along veins of little diameter, the SRV is difficult to observe with any accuracy.

The SRV was noted at its higher intensity in about ten cases only: streaks along all the veins, easily visible with the white light of the opthalmoscope, beginning from the papilla, in both eyes. Table 1 shows the occurrence of the SVR in the four groups of patients. One of us (H. A. De Laet)[2] in a group of 214 cases of MS observed 31.8% of SRV. Our present percentage of 24.7% has a good chance of approaching the reality, because of the number and the duration of our observations. This percentage lies at about the mean of the two extreme values found by other observers: 11% found by Wybar[3] in 81 cases and 42% found by Orban[4] in 50 cases.

Table 1 Distribution of venous sheathing in multiple sclerosis and other neurological diseases

	Patients	
Diagnosis	No.	%
Characteristic MS (1180 cases)	292	24.7
Presumed MS (270 cases)	47	17.4
Uncertain MS (53 cases)	9	17.0
Negative MS (225 cases)	7	3.10

In 45% of the cases of positive MS with SVR, optic atrophy was observed. The SRV rarely appears at the beginning of the disease, but is a feature of MS with a slow and long evolution, C. R. Bamford *et al* have made the same observation[5]. The phenomenon persists all through the duration of the disease, except in about 10% of the cases in which it slowly disappears.

The SRV is not absolutely pathognomonic of MS, we have found seven cases in 225 patients without MS. It is interesting to remember that Rucker[6], who observed SRV for the first time in 1944, in 33 patients found 21 cases of positive MS, seven of probable MS and six without any neurologic disorder (18%).

Among the seven patients without MS, there were two cases of Arnold–Chiari deformity, one of cerebral atrophy, one of Friedreich's hereditary ataxia, one of cervical medullopathic degeneration and two patients with no positive diagnosis.

SRV–uveitis–MS relation

We have found eight cases of active uveitis (six anterior and two posterior) in the group of positive MS, this is 0.7%. Of these eight cases, three showed SRV (37%). Porter[7] found 15% of SRV linked with uveitis in patients with MS. Two other cases of uveitis have been observed in two other groups: one in a patient without MS and one in a patient with questionable MS. The low occurrence of uveitis in our MS patients would indicate that it is not higher than in any other group. However, Petrochilos *et al*[8] found 3.5% cases of uveitis among 112 MS patients.

SRV and optic atrophy

We have noted the occurrence of optic atrophy among our patients with SRV within the four groups. We find, for our patients with positive, probable or questionable MS, 45, 38 and 66% cases of optic atrophy respectively. Only one of the seven patients with SRV but with negative MS had an optic atrophy.

We conclude that SRV and optic atrophy occur together much more often in MS than in any other neurological disease.

This relationship is shown in Table 2.

Table 2 Incidence of optic atrophy in neurological patients presenting venous sheathing

Diagnosis	Venous sheating No.	Optic atrophy No.	%
Characteristic MS	292	133	45.5
Presumed MS	47	18	38.2
Uncertain MS	9	6	66.6
Negative MS	7	1	14.2

OPTIC DISC ATROPHY

Table 3 shows the incidence of optic atrophy in our four groups of patients, indicating the number with one discoloured disc, those with two discoloured optic discs and the total.

Table 3 Frequency of optic atrophy in patients with multiple sclerosis or other neurological diseases

Neurological cases			Number of optic atrophies		
Diagnosis	No.	1 disc	2 discs	Total	%
Typical MS	1180	137	385	522	44
Presumed MS	270	29	62	91	34
Uncertain MS	53	5	16	21	40
Negative MS	225	15	27	42	19

The discolouration of the optic disc was estimated by ophthalmoscopy and, in doubtful cases, we have also made a compression/decompression test: pressure is applied for a few seconds to the eyeball in order to increase the intra-ocular pressure up to the level of the systolic blood pressure in the papilla. As soon as the pressure is relieved, a clearly visible hyperaemia appears on the normal papilla, due to the dilatation of the capillaries. In the case of local and/or doubtful optic atrophy, this simple procedure enhances the contrast in colour between the atrophied zone, which remains white, and the normal one which shows normal hyperaemia. 44% (Table 3) of the patients with positive MS show atrophy on one or both sides.

MOTOR DEFICIENCIES

Anterior internuclear ophthalmoplegia (AIO)

We have looked especially for the most significant motor syndrome of MS, i.e. anterior internuclear ophthalmoplegia. Following the criteria of Larmande[9], AIO shows the following particular signs:

(1) paresis of the adduction of one eye;
(2) dissociated (or ataxic) nystagmus of the other eye in abduction;
(3) conservation of convergence.

Table 4 summarizes the incidences of AIO in the four groups. They are, respectively, 7, 10 and 7% AIO in the first three groups, compared with 3.5% for patients without MS. In the first group there are 43 cases of unilateral AIO and 44 bilateral cases.

Table 4 Incidence of internuclear anterior ophthalmoplegia in patients with multiple sclerosis or other neurological diseases

Neurological cases		Anterior internuclear ophthalmoplegia	
Diagnosis	No.	No.	%
Typical MS	1180	87	7.37
Presumed MS	270	29	10.74
Uncertain MS	53	4	7.54
·Negative MS	225	8	3.55

Other oculo-motor paralysis

We also found the following:

(1) paralysis of the external rectus: 18 cases (1.43%) of which: 15 were unilateral and 3 bilateral.
(2) paralysis of the internal rectus, of which: 19 were unilateral and 3 bilateral.

These 3 cases of bilateral palsy of the internal recti with complete divergent nystagmus may be severe or extreme anterior internuclear ophthalmoplegia where it is not more possible to elicit a nystagmus because of the divergence.

Our results show a marked difference in the frequency of AIOs between MS and non-MS patients, and thus AIO is, basically, a symptom of MS.

CONVERGENCE PARESIS OR PALSY

We have counted cases of loss of convergence, although one must be careful with this symptom. Indeed, convergence may be lost either through a true paralysis or paresis, or through asthenia or/and psychasthenia, not taking into account eventual congenital defects. Nevertheless, as shown in Table 5, loss of convergence occurs with the same frequency (8–10%) in all neurological diseases.

Table 5 Incidence of convergence abolition in patients with multiple sclerosis or other neurological diseases

Neurological cases		Convergence abolition	
Diagnosis	No.	No.	%
Typical MS	1180	98	8.30
Presumed MS	270	19	7.10
Uncertain MS	53	5	9.50
Negative MS	225	24	10.70

HORNER'S SYNDROME

Table 6 indicates that only 1% of the patients with MS and 4% of those with other neurologic disorders present with Horner's syndrome. This syndrome is an exception in MS.

Table 6 Incidence of Horner's syndrome in patients with multiple sclerosis or other neurological diseases

Neurological cases		Horner's syndrome	
Diagnosis	No.	No.	%
Typical MS	1180	13	1.1
Presumed MS	270	3	1.1
Uncertain MS	53	0	0
Negative MS	225	9	4.0

NYSTAGMUS

We have listed in Table 7 all forms of nystagmus identified in our four groups, the nystagmus associated with an ophthalmoplegia as well as those not linked with it. One patient in three with positive, probable or uncertain MS has a nystagmus.

Table 7 Incidence of nystagmus (all forms) in patients with multiple sclerosis or other neurological diseases

Neurological cases		Nystagmus	
Diagnosis	No.	No.	%
Typical MS	1180	392	33
Presumed MS	270	73	27
Uncertain MS	53	18	34
Negative MS	225	43	19

Table 8 gives details of the different types of nystagmus in 392 patients with confirmed MS. Dissociated (ataxic) nystagmus is the most common with 241 cases, followed by 81 jerky types, 44 pendular types and 30 nystagmus of the rotatory type. Several patients had several types simultaneously, for example ataxic, pendular and rotatory, or ataxic on one side and jerky on the other side combined, moreover, with a pendular type. All combinations have been found.

Table 8 Distribution of different types of nystagmus in the group of 392 patients presenting typical multiple sclerosis with nystagmus

Type of nystagmus		No.
Ataxic type		241
with anterior internuclear ophthalmoplegia	87	
without anterior internuclear ophthalmoplegia	154	
Pendular type		44
Jerky type		81
Rotatory type		30

PERIMETER DEFECTS – SCOTOMAS

The kinetic perimetry test (with the Goldmann Perimeter) was performed on all patients able to withstand it. The following indexes have been generally used: V/4, I/4, I/2 and even I/I.

Table 9 Incidence of perimetric scotomas in patients presenting multiple sclerosis with optic atrophy and visual acuity lower than 0.7

Cases with optic atrophy and acuity of 0.7 and lower No.	Cases with scotomas	
	No.	%
393	197	50.12

Results of concentric narrowing of the visual field without objective reasons were not taken into account (approximately 2% of cases).

50% of patients suffering from confirmed MS showed in the Goldmann perimeter a central or caeco-central scotoma. Hawkins[10] in 1975 had the same results. Ohoka *et al*, in 1974[11] also obtained the same results.

At first sight it seems surprising that about 50% of patients with a positive MS, with an optic atrophy and visual acuity less than 0.7 exhibit no central or caeco-central scotoma. One must again point out the difficulties of performing a thorough perimetric examination of asthenic patients, with a low power of concentration, and suffering from some sort of nystagmus.

We remained, nevertheless, convinced that in the great majority of observed cases there was really no scotoma. For a scotoma to be present, a retina zone, more or less central, must be surrounded by a zone of higher sensitivity. This is the case of the retrobulbar neuritis, in its acute and inflammatory period. In the optic atrophy phase, the macular zone displays a reduced sensitivity, which is, however, not inferior to that of the surrounding zone. In the normal individual, the visual acuity falls to 0.1 at 2 or 3 ° from the foveola. To take the wellknown image of Traquair who compares the visual field to an island, with its level curves corresponding to the isopters of the visual field, a scotoma corresponds to a well or a crater in the island; whereas a levelling of the sharp central peak corresponds to a lowering of the visual acuity but does not result in a scotoma.

We have met, among our 1180 MS patients, five cases of homonymous hemianopsia. This frequency is very low compared with that of 1.3% found by Hawkins[10].

CONCLUSION

This work is intended to give good statistical evidence on the frequency of occurrence of ocular symptoms in a significantly large group of patients with severe multiple sclerosis. Only 239 (or 20%) of the 1180 patients of our sample with confirmed multiple sclerosis showed no ocular defects.

References

1. Schumacher, G. A., Beebe, G., Kibler, R. F., Kurland, L. T., Kurtze, J. F., McDowell, F., Nagler, B., Sibley, W. A., Tourtelotte, W. W. and Willmon, T. L. (1965). Problems of experimental trials of therapy in Multiple Sclerosis: report by the panel on the evaluation of experimental trials of therapy in Multiple Sclerosis. *Ann. N.Y. Acad. Sci.*, **122**, 552
2. De Laet, H. A. (1963). Engainement des veines rétiniennes et sclérose en plaques. *Bull. Soc. Ophtal. Fr.*, **76**, 611–622
3. Wybar, K. (1952). The ocular manifestations of disseminated sclerosis. *Proc. R. Soc. Med.*, **45**, 315
4. Orban, T. (1955). Beitrage zu den Augenhintergrundsveränderungen bei Sclerosis Multiplex. *Ophthalmologica*, **130**, 387
5. Bamford, C. R., Ganley, J. P., Sibley, W. A. and Laguna, J. E. (1978). Uveitis, perivenous sheating and multiple sclerosis. *Neurology*, **28**, 119
6. Rucker, W. C. (1944). Sheating of retinal veins in Multiple Sclerosis. *Staff Meet, Mayo Clinic*, **19**, 176

7. Porter, R. (1972). Uveitis in association with Multiple Sclerosis. *Br. J. Ophthal.,* **56,** 478
8. Petrochilos, M., Tricoulis, D. and Zitis, H. (1975). *Arch. Soc. Ophthal. Grèce Nord,* **22,** 484
9. Goddi-Jolly and Larmande, A. (1973). *Le Nystagmus,* pp. 994-1024. (Paris: Masson Edit)
10. Hawkins, K. and Behrens, M. M. (1975). Homonymous Hemianopia in Multiple Sclerosis. *Br. J. Ophthal.,* **59,** 334
11. Ohoka, R., Komoto, M., Tanahashi, Y. and Kawana, H. (1974). Ocular manifestations of Multiple Sclerosis: a retrospective statistical survey. *Rinsho Ganka,* **28,** 527

57
Flight of colours-test in MS and NRB patients

J. M. MINDERHOUD, M. Y. SMITS, J. KUKS and G. ter STEEGE

The study on after-images or the flight of colours (FOC) started with Aristoteles, Ptolemaeus and other ancient philosophers, but Goethe and many after him reported these phenomena. Depending on the intensity of stimulation, the level of dark-adaptation and other variations illumination of the retina evokes after-images of a complex nature. They start with what is called positive after-images having the same colour as the stimulating light. After that the real flight of colours starts. The use of the FOC in diseases of the optic systems was described by Feldman et al [1]. They examined the FOC, judging the duration of the total period of after-images and the number of changes of colours during the first minute. We studied, using the FOC, healthy people, patients with multiple sclerosis and patients who had had a retrobulbar neuritis in the past 10 years. After explanation of the procedure the patient was adapted to a semi-dark room for 5 minutes with eyes closed. Then one eye was illuminated for 10 seconds. The patient was then asked to focus on the light, which is held in front of the cornea, at a fixed distance of 1 cm. After closing the eyes the patient is blindfolded. Each 10 seconds thereafter he is asked to report the after-images, describing colour, brightness and changes of the colours. The colours are scored being in the red, blue, green or purple range. The test ends after less than 5 minutes if no after-images are reported for more than 40 seconds or if only grey colours are left. Sometimes, especially in the case of poor results the test is repeated after 10 minutes and the best results are used for further calculation. Ten minutes later the other eye is examined. Results are expressed in the duration of the after-images and the kind and number of colours reported. Visual stimulation was performed with a stable source of 30 lux.

Regarding the duration of the after-images, the results in 37 healthy people (21 males and 16 females, aged 31–55 y) showed a sex-difference. The mean duration in females was 228 seconds and in males 209 seconds. So it was decided to use different values for normal results over 190 seconds in females and over 160 seconds in males (Figure 1). We also examined 61 definite MS patients and 25 patients who had a retrobulbar neuritis (RN) in the past 10 years.

Figure 1 FOC normal values

females	228 sec	s.d.	24.0 sec.
males	209 sec.	s.d.	24.0 sec.

abnormal in females < 190 sec.
in males < 160 sec.

Figure 2 FOC abnormal length

NORMALS	5.4%
MS *without* visual defect	46.6%
MS *with* visual defect	68.8%
RBN *without* visual defect	35.7%
RBN *with* visual defect	53.1%

So we can present the results of 122 MS-eyes and 50 RN-eyes. They were divided into four groups according to sex and visual defect. In healthy people a small percentage of the eyes scored abnormal results, but in MS patients as well as in RN patients the percentages of abnormal results were remarkably higher (Figure 2). The results in MS patients were not related to a history of acute visual defect, age, sex or handicap. Eyes with a history of an acute visual defect showed often after-images as abnormal as eyes in which a gradual visual defect had occurred. In eyes with a history of a retrobulbar neuritis the time period after the acute accident was found to be of no importance (Figure 3).

Figure 3

Visual defect	FOC abn.
acute	67.5%
slowly progr.	70.8%

Time relapse RN and FOC	FOC abn.	n
0–2 y	58.8%	17
3–5 y	72.7%	12
> 5 y	67.7%	36

Figure 4 Abnormalities in MS

palette only	4.7%
duration only	34.0%
combined	67.9%

In 37 healthy people and 53 MS patients the flight of colours was performed more comprehensively. The first positive after-image, which has the same colour as the stimulus, was found to be of the same duration in patients as in healthy people. In MS patients however, as compared to healthy people, the duration of individual colours was clearly shorter, especially the duration of red, purple and blue and to a lesser extent that of green. In 31% of the MS patients the after-images were restricted to one colour or were even totally absent. Regarding this palette, a flight of colours could only be called normal if at least two of the colours blue, red, green and purple were seen and of which at least one should be blue or red. It proved, however, that the scoring of the duration of the flight was more sensitive than the palette (Figure 4).

The results of the FOC could be compared with the results of the visual evoked potential (VEP) in these people and patients. These visual evoked potentials were obtained using flash-stimulation, and the latency of the P-100 was used for measurements. In our material the FOC gave more frequent abnormal results than was obtained using the VEP.

To summarize: The FOC proved to be rather easy to obtain at a low price, being more sensitive than the VEP. The VEP, however, can be proposed to be a more objective method.

Reference

1. Feldman, M., Todman, L. and Bender, M. B. (1974). 'FOC' in lesions of the visual system. *J. Neurol. Neurosurg. Psychiat.*, **37**, 1265

58
The early diagnostic yield of multimodality evoked potentials: a 4.8 year prospective study on 171 patients

P. DELTENRE, C. VAN NECHEL, S. STRUL, A. CAPON and P. KETELAER

SUMMARY

The diagnostic yield of the described EP battery has been clearly demonstrated through this prospective study. The use of EP combined with CSF analysis is strongly advised, in view of the 96.5% detection thus obtained in a Def sub-group and of the results of the Pending group where a lower EP hit rate could be due to a slower form of the disease.

It is stressed that we still badly need such studies investigating patients in the very early days of their clinical manifestations.

INTRODUCTION

As far as the acute and chronic forms of experimental allergic encephalo-myelitis are valid models for multiple sclerosis (MS), the reports of attenuation or even suppression of the experimental disease by early therapy[1-3] emphasize the need for precocious positive diagnostic criteria in MS.

Evoked potentials (EP)[4,5] and CSF analysis[6,7] are the most widely used diagnostic aids. However, most of the studies demonstrating the interest of these two procedures have been performed on patients at various stages of the disease, so that one may still wonder about their value at the onset of the disease. This led to the design of this prospective study involving patients at the earliest possible stage of differential diagnosis.

MATERIAL AND METHODS

The study was started in 1977. 273 patients suffering from a neurological condition were examined, on an out-patient basis, by neurologists who considered MS as part of the differential diagnosis using combined multi-modality EP.

Normal data were gathered for each modality from at least 30 normal subjects chosen from the hospital staff, and whose ages ranged from 17 to 50 years. Abnormality was defined as an elevation of more than 3 SD from the mean for the considered parameter.

Pattern reversal visual evoked potentials (PRVEP) were elicited by the rotating mirror technique, with the whole screen subtending a visual angle of 17.9° horizontally and 16.7° vertically, individual squares covering 37 minutes. Luminance levels were 490 candela/m² for the white squares and 10 candela/m² for the black ones. Absolute latencies and inter eye latency differences of $P\overline{100}$ were measured.

Somatosensory evoked potentials (SEP) were recorded after electrical stimulation of the median nerve at the wrist and the peroneal nerve at the fibula head. Brachial plexus activity, spinal and cortical potentials were simultaneously recorded, and latency differences between $N\overline{9}$, $N\overline{13}$ and $N\overline{20}$ were computed. An anomaly of the spinal SEP was also recorded if its amplitude was less than $0.8\,\mu V$. After leg stimulation the cortical potential only was recorded.

Brainstem auditory evoked potentials (BAEP) were elicited by unipolar monaural $100\,\mu s$ wide clicks of 65 dB HL. Interpeak latencies were computed on ipsilateral vertex to mastoid tracings.

The blink reflex (BR) was recorded as the surface EMG activity of both orbicularis oculi muscles after stimulation of the supra-orbital nerves. Abnormal latencies of R_1 were considered to reflect intrapontine disease, provided a pattern of Vth or VIIth nerve involvement was excluded[8].

EP results were analysed in terms of the 'Hit rate', defined as the proportion of patients in which at least one subclinical lesion was demonstrated, thus proving the multifocal nature of the disease.

At the time of EP recording, patients were attributed to one of the four lower categories of McDonald's and Halliday's classification[9].

The time elapsed since the appearance of the first neurological symptoms reasonably attributable to the actual disease was deduced from the patient's interview and recorded as the pre-EP delay, if reliably established.

After a follow-up period of up to 4.9 years (mean 80 months, SD 38 months), the fate of the patients was reassessed by consulting current medical files, or, if necessary (for disability scaling only) by phone calls or writing to patients and/or their neurologist or general practitioner. At this stage patients were attributed to one of the three following classifications:

(1) clinically definite MS (Def)
(2) still pending diagnosis (Pending)
(3) other neurological disease (Ond)

The patients were also attributed an initial index (Ki) according to Kurtzke's functional disability scale[10] as estimated during the remission closest to EP testing, and a final one (Kf) at the time of reassessment.

An index of evolution was computed whenever possible as $I_{ev} = \dfrac{Kf - Ki}{dt}$

dt being defined as the time elapsed between EP testing and reassessment.

CSF data were collected during the follow-up from patient's files: results from samples obtained within 5 months of EP testing were retained for analysis. As different laboratories and techniques were involved in producing CSF data, these were reduced to 'positive' for elevation and/or oligoclonal fractionation of the γ-globulins compatible with the diagnosis of MS and 'negative' for normal or abnormal but not suggestive of MS. The IgG index was unfortunately only exceptionally used.

RESULTS

After the elimination of patients with incomplete clinical data, and of those lost for follow-up, 171 cases remained for analysis.

Clinically eventual definite patients (Def)

Among these 56 patients who evolved to a clinically definite MS during the follow-up period, the hit rate of the EP battery attained 48/56 or 85.7% (see Table 1 for details).

Table 1 Eventual clinically definite MS ($n = 56$)

Initial classification		EP Results		
EPOL	46/56	[+]	=	40/46 (86.9%) (hit rate)
		+	=	6/46 (13.4%)
		n	=	0/46 (0%)
Suspected	10/56	[+]	=	8/10 (80%) (hit rate)
		+	=	1/10 (10%)
		n	=	1/10 (10%)

Global hit rate : 85.7%; difference in hit rate between EPOL and suspected not significant at the 0.05 level
[+] Symbolizes the hit rate
  + Symbolizes the proportion of patients for which EP abnormalities merely reflect already known localizations
  n Symbolizes the proportion of patients for which the entire EP battery was normal

The respective yield of each EP modality was defined as the hit rate that would have been achieved should this modality have been applied alone: (Table 2). In accordance with other multimodal studies, it was found that PRVEP is the best test, since its hit rate would have been of 37/56 or 66%. The next best modality was the somatosensory one with a hit rate of 13/56 or 23.2%, followed by BAEP: 10/56 or 17.8% and BR with 12.5%.

Conversely, it can be shown that BR is the only test that could have been omitted without reducing the battery hit rate of 85.7%. Omission of any of the other three modalities would have reduced the hit rate as computed in the right part of Table 2.

Table 2

	Isolated modality hit rate	Hit rate after omission of one modality
VEP	37/56 (66%)	26/56 (45.6%)
SEP	13/56 (23.2%)	42/56 (75%)
BAEP	10/56 (17.8%)	44/56 (78.5%)
BR	7/56 (12.5%)	48/56 (85.7%)

Comparison with CSF data

Reliable CSF data were obtained from 29 of the eventual 56 Def patients. Among this subgroup the CSF analysis was considered suggestive of MS in 26 cases (89.6%), while the EP hit rate attained 24/29 or 82.7%. Two patients were detected by the EP battery and not by CSF analysis, and three others were detected by CSF analysis only, so that the proportion of patients that have been picked up by one or the other test is as high as 28/29 or 96.5%. Only one (3.4%) patient developed a definite MS despite escaping detection by the two tests.

PENDING DIAGNOSIS GROUP

The hit rate of the EP battery was considerably lower for these 69 patients: 18/69 or 26%; a highly significant ($p < 0.001$) difference from the Def group. The general pattern of differential sensitivity of each modality as observed in the Def group was again encountered as shown in Table 3.

Table 3   Pending diagnosis group ($n = 69$)

	Isolated modality hit rate
VEP	14/69 (20.2%)
SEP	5/69 (7.2%)
BAEP	2/69 (2.8%)
BR	1/69 (1.4%)

Global hit rate of the EP battery: 18/69 (26%)

Comparison with CSF analysis

39 cases were suitable for CSF data analysis, which showed, in 17/39 or 43.6% of the patients, a CSF profile positive for MS. Among the 39 patients with reliable CSF data, the EP battery had a hit rate of 15/39 or 38.5%.

Combining the two tests 24/39 or 61.5% of the patients would have been detected by one or another.

In this subgroup of clinical pending diagnosis with suggestive CSF, the proportion of entirely normal EP results was 4/17 or 23.5%.

Other neurological diseases group

47 patients could be ascribed a diagnosis other than MS. The EP battery has,

nevertheless, diagnosed a multifocal disease in eight of them (17%). The final diagnoses and the tests that revealed a subclinical lesion are listed in Table 4.

Table 4 Demonstration of a multi-focal disease by the EP battery in the OND group

[+] Test	Final diagnosis
VEP	Subacute combined degeneration of the spinal cord
VEP – SEP	Friedreich's disease with lactic acidosis and myoclonic epilepsy
VEP	Hereditary cerebellar degeneration
BAEP	Cervical herniated disc
VEP	Familial spastic paraparesia
VEP	Isolated sporadic cerebellar atrophy
VEP – SEP	Frontal hygroma

DISCUSSION

A high (85.7%) diagnostic yield of the EP battery has thus been demonstrated. The probable advantage of coupling EP and CSF analysis is suggested by the elevation of the detection rate to 96.5% in a Def subgroup and from 43.6% to 61.5% in a Pending subgroup.

The striking difference in hit rate between the Def and Pending groups deserves some comments. This difference can hypothetically be linked to several factors:

(1) The Pending group probably contains a substantial proportion of non-MS patients without multifocal CNS disease

(2) A shorter pre EP delay could lower the EP hit rate, not having allowed a sufficient number of plaques to develop. The mean pre EP delay was indeed significantly shorter ($\bar{x} = 29.3$ months, SD $+49.7$) for the pending group vs. ($\bar{x} = 86$ months, SD 96.5) $p < 0.001$ for the Def group.

(3) The difference between the two subgroups could be partly linked to a qualitative difference, as a slower evolutive form of the disease delaying the establishment of a definite clinical diagnosis and offering fewer lesions to be detected by the EP.

To try to discriminate between these factors a comparison was made between hit rates, pre EP delays and I_{ev} (evolution indexes) of the Def patients, and those in the Pending group whose CSF was positive for MS (subgroup Pending CSF +). This would lower the influence of factor A but could cause a bias in selecting a peculiar subgroup of patients in the Pending group. Nevertheless, this analysis showed that if the mean pre EP delay remained very significantly different between these two subgroups (pre EP delay Def = 86 months SD 96.6; pre EP delay Pending CSF + = 13.3 months, SD 22.6, $p < 0.0005$), the difference in hit rate (85.7% for Def and 60% for Pending CSF +) was less significant ($0.025 < p < 0.05$).

That the pre EP delay is not the major factor contributing to the EP hit rate was further suggested by the finding that the hit rate among the eight definite patients with a pre EP delay below 100 days was 100%; and that among the

Pending CSF + patients, the pre EP delays were not statistically different between four patients with a hit rate of zero, and the six patients where it was 100%, being even slightly longer (14.1 months vs 12.8) for the null hit rate subgroup. One had, therefore, to study the I_{ev} parameter to find support for factor C hypothesis, after the correction for factor A effect. This parameter was found rather difficult to use with confidence, partly because of the method of reassessment and partly because of the crudeness of Kurtzke's scale. The mean I_{ev} of the Def group (0.0142; SD 0.02794) was found to be significantly higher than that of the Pending CSF + subgroup (-0.00031; SD 0.000654) with $0.025 < p < 0.05$.

Comparison of I_{ev} between other subgroups was hampered by too few reliable data. It thus remains possible that the Def and Pending CSF + groups of this study contain an uneven proportion of patients with different forms of the disease.

A striking result of this study has been the finding of rather long pre EP delays as assessed by retrospective anamnestic data. Typically, the first episode did not bring the patient to a neurologist, so that only eight patients of the Def group were examined less than 100 days after clinical onset.

It is thus felt that studies like this one must continue to be applied, especially to patients in the very early days of the clinical manifestations of the disease in order to help to unravel the hypothesis of an early critical period in human MS, and the potential value of EP results in predicting the type of functional disability course.

The present results indeed suggest that escaping detection by the EP battery may be due to a slower form of the disease rather than to a short pre EP delay.

ACKNOWLEDGEMENTS

This work has been made possible thanks to the collaboration of the following physicians: Andriane, Baonville, Beauherz, Capon, Coërs, Dajez, Dumoulin, Duret, Gerard, Hildebrand, Joffroy, Ketelaer, Khoubesserian, Moerman, Monseu, Rétif, Seeldrayers, Soeur, Tugendhaft, Teleman-Toppet, Visée, who referred the patients and contributed to the follow-up.

References

1. Bolton, C., Borel, J. F., Cuzner, M. L., Davidson, A. N. and Turner, A. M. (1982). Immunosuppression by cyclosporin of experimental allergic encephalomyelitis. *J. Neurolog. Sci.*, **56**, 147
2. Hashim, G. A. (1978). Myelin basic protein: structure, function and antigenic determinants. *Immunol. Rev.*, **39**, 60
3. Teitelbaum, D., Webb, C., Bree, W. *et al* (1974). Suppression of experimental allergic encephalomyelitis in rhesus monkeys by a synthetic basic copolymer. *Clin. Immunol. Immunopathol.*, **3**, 256
4. Kjaer, M. (1982). The value of a multimodal evoked potential approach in the diagnosis of Multiple Sclerosis. In Courjon, J., Mauguière, F. and Revol, M. (eds.). *Clinical Applications of Evoked Potentials in Neurology*, pp. 507–512. (New York: Raven Press)
5. Purves, S. J., Low, M. D., Galloway, J. *et al* (1981). A comparison of visual, brainstem

auditory and somatosensory evoked potentials in Multiple Sclerosis. *Can. J. Neurol. Sci.,* **8,** 15

6. Delmotte, P. and Gonsette, R. (1977). Biochemical findings in Multiple Sclerosis. IV Iso-electric focusing of the CSF gamma globulins in M.S. (262 cases) and other neurological diseases (272 cases). *J. Neurol.,* **215,** 27

7. Hershey, L. A. and Trotter, J. L. (1980). The use and abuse of the cerebrospinal fluid IgG profile in the adult: A practical evaluation. *Ann. Neurol.,* **8,** 426

8. Kimura, J. (1973). The Blink Reflex as a test for brainstem and higher central nervous system function. In Desmedt, J. E. (ed.). *New Developments in Electromyography and Clinical Neurophysiology.* Vol. 3, pp. 682–691 (Basel: Karger)

9. McDonald, W. I. and Halliday, A. M. (1978). Diagnosis and classification of Multiple Sclerosis. *Br. Med. Bull.,* **33,** 4

10. Kurtzke, J. F. (1970). Clinical manifestations of Multiple Sclerosis. In Vinken, P. J. and Bruyn, G. W. (eds.). *Handbook of Clinical Neurology. Multiple Sclerosis and Other Demyelinating Diseases.* Vol. 9, pp. 161–216. (Amsterdam: Elsevier)

11. Halliday, A. M. (1981). Visual Evoked Potentials in Demyelinating Disease. In Waxman, S. G. and Ritchie, J. M. (eds.). *Demyelinating Diseases: Basic and Clinical Electrophysiology.* pp. 201–215 (New York: Raven Press)

59
Effect of heating on VER of multiple sclerosis patients apparently free of optic neuritis

M. P. DELPLACE and J. GUILLAUMAT

INTRODUCTION

By warming up the temperature of the room, the symptoms of the multiple sclerosis patient can be modified. Since Uhthoff many authors have taken an interest in its ophthalmological application.

We have studied the influence of warming-up on the latency of the visual evoked potentials of nineteen MS patients compared with fifteen healthy people.

MATERIALS

We have studied 15 people: 13 females and 2 males, apparently in good health. Of 19 patients with MS, 12 females and 7 males, classified according to McAlpine characteristics, we noted seven certain (typical), three probable (suspected) and nine possible (uncertain). But all of them appear, during the investigative period, free of any apparently evolving optical neuritis.

The 38 eyes were examined by settling: visual acuity was measured at 10/10 in 37 eyes and 3/10 in a keratoconus. Pupillar diameters were equal in 37 eyes and unequal in a patient with a certain MS. Pupillar movements, assessed by the pupil induction test (according to Safran's technique) were normal in 32 eyes; slow, R.L.E., once (the patient had received anafranil); diminished on one side, twice; and was not tested in one patient.

Paradoxal pupillar dilatation (Kestenbaum technique) was encountered in three eyes (one of them already included among the modified pupil induction test). Looking at the fundus of the eye we noted 20 normal eyes, atrophic papilla in six, temporal atrophy in four and we encountered retinal fibres in 9 eyes.

METHODS

The visual evoked responses (VER) were established in a room where the temperature could be increased from 20 °C to 39 °C.

The first sequence took place at 20 °C, the second one at 39 °C.

Before starting VER registration the patient sat for 10 minutes in a special room looking at a screen 2 m away. The registration took place in another room without modification of temperature.

Two sorts of stimulation were used:

(1) Black and white chessboard pattern on a TV screen exhibiting the following features:
    (a) contrast, 100%
    (b) chessboard, 4
    (c) frequency, 1 Hz
    (d) number of reversals, 100.

(2) Red and black chessboard pattern realized with a telescope, with diodes at one end; the procedure of the stimulation is as follows:
    (a) 100 reversals
    (b) frequency, 1 Hz.

This technique of stimulation may be considered as an intermediate procedure between flash and pattern stimulation.

Reception and detection of VER are managed as usual with a medial setting, by placing an active electrode 2 cm above the inion, an electrode at the vertex, and an indifferent electrode between them. All of them are of the needle model.

The light stimulator is a Medelec and the occipito–cortical responses are registered on an on-line oscilloscope.

Binocular, right and left monocular responses were successively monitored.

RESULTS

In healthy controls

Without warming-up

As a reference for pattern stimulation we selected the latency of the P2 spike wave; in our check sample, it fluctuated from 95 to 118 ms, with an average value of 105 ms.

For the black-red chessboard, the latency of the first positive spike was considered (DR +) at 95–130 ms with an average value of 116 ms.

After warming-up impairment

The latency delay of P2 fluctuated from 93 to 116 ms, with an average value of 106 ms. The DR + fluctuated from 95 to 103 ms, with an average time of 116 ms.

Looking for fluctuations in augmentation or a decreasing of the latency delay, we noticed a Gaussian repartition of the P2 wave registration, with a spike at +2 ms (Figure 1). However, the average increasing time is only +0.05 ms on warming-up. The spike wave of DR + is located from 0 to 4 ms, with an average wave of +0.34 ms (Figure 2).

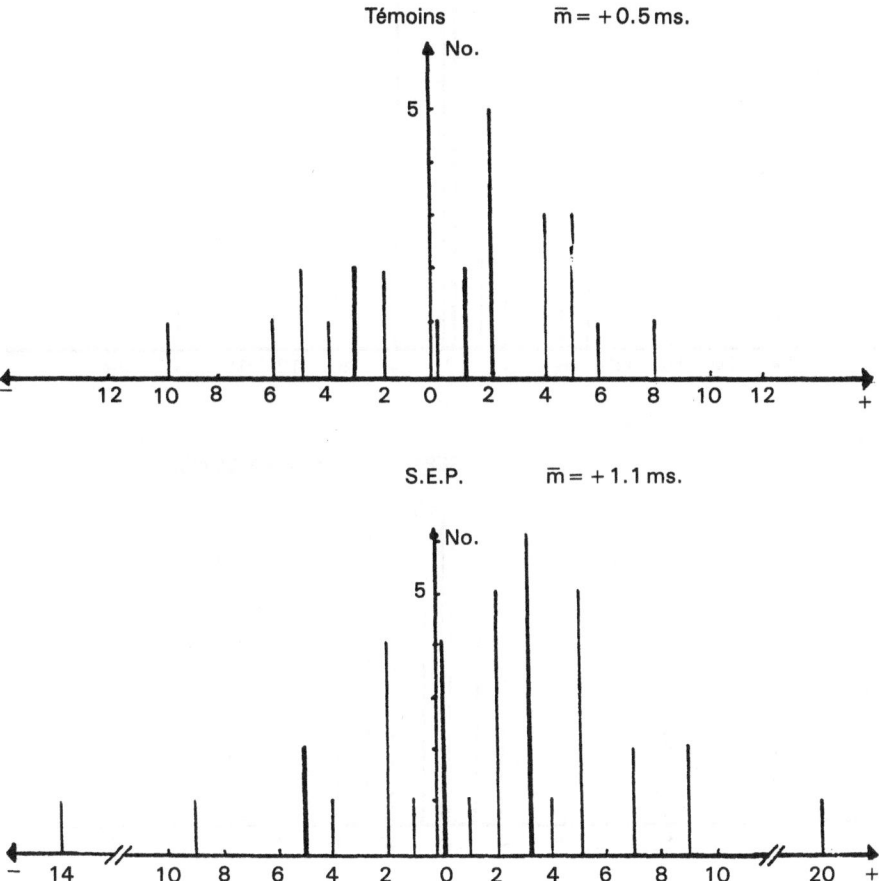

Figure 1   Changes in P2 latency as a function of temperature

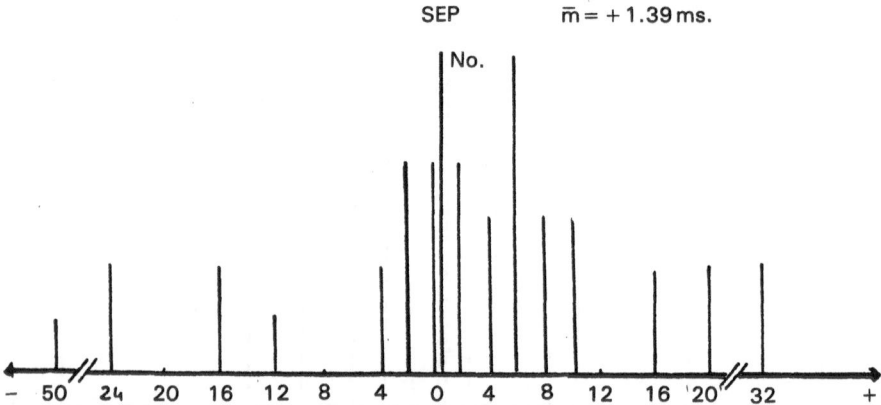

Figure 2   Changes in DR + latency as a function of temperature

In multiple sclerosis patients sequence

Without warming-up

The P2 spike wave is found from 95 to 156 ms with an average wave of 112 ms. We found that the DR + wave fluctuates from 105 to 165 ms (average value = 123.5 ms).

With warming-up

Here the P2 spike wave fluctuated from 99 to 152 ms (average value = 113 ms). DR + varied from 103 to 105 ms (average wave = 112 ms).

Looking for the more or less value of the latency delay time, we noticed for P2 wave, an increased latency time according to a Gaussian wave-curve response, maximum at $+3$ ms and average at $+1.1$ ms (Figure 1). The latency delay time for DR $+$ wave is increased by 1.39 ms (Figure 2). However, further investigation is needed to obtain a significant statistical ratio. Nevertheless, among our patient registrations, four conclusions dealing with the P2 response could be elicited.

Four plottings were modified:

(1) in one case a normal latency became abnormal,
(2) in one case a subnormal latency became abnormal,
(3) in one case a subnormal latency became normal,
(4) in one case an abnormal latency remained abnormal.

Dealing with DR $+$, we conclude from 38 records that 17 were modified in a significant way (Table 1).

Table 1

Final	Initial		
	Normal	Subnormal	Abnormal
Normal	0	3	1
Subnormal	3	0	0
Abnormal	2	1	7

So the two modes of stimulation don't lead to the same results.

According to McAlpine's assumption we compared the variation of the latency of P2 and DR $+$ in four certain MS and four healthy people (HP) of the same age, with normal latency following the two modes of stimulation.

	P2	DR $+$
MS	$+2.5$	$+7.75$
HP	$+2.75$	-0.35

In the same way, two probable MS and two HP of the same age were compared:

	P2	DR $+$
MS	$+6.5$	$+1.5$
HP	$+3.75$	-2.0

We also compared three possible MS and three HP with a normal and subnormal latency:

with normal latency

	P2	DR+
MS	0	+ 7.0
HP	+ 2.5	+ 0.3

with subnormal latency

	P2	DR+
MS	+ 1.0	− 5.3
HP	+ 2.5	+ 0.3

These results are not actually significant and need further investigation.

DISCUSSION

We disagree with the opinion of Galvin, Heron and Regan[1], Person and Sachs[2], and of Bajada, Mastaglia, Black and Collins[3], who did not notice any alteration in the latency by the VER with increasing temperature.

However, these authors observed a decreasing of the *amplitude* of the P2 wave of the VER. On the other hand, we noticed greater variations of P2 and DR+ *latency time* among MS patients free of evolving optic neuritis than among healthy people. And that is ratified both by individual modification and by average fluctuations.

The age distribution differs in our check sequence and among MS patients, but this fact does not interfere with the plottings according to Glaser. We could be blamed for not evaluating the effect of body temperature, but that technical procedure needs sophisticated instruments which we were deprived of. Besides, human homeothermical regulation is very powerful, and keeps the temperature of the body at the same level whatever the external temperature. In some healthy people this measure was performed and did not exhibit any alteration.

In our opinion, this test may yield a complementary sign of an alteration of optical pathways in borderline diagnostic cases of optic neuritis.

It could also lead from a prognostical point of view, to a new classification of patients.

But one must say that the Uhthoff sign is in no way specific of MS, and increasing the surrounding temperature may extend many other neurological syndromes.

References

1. Galvin, R. J., Regan, D. and Heron, J. R. (1976). A possible means of monitoring the progress of demyelination in multiple sclerosis: effect of body temperature on visual perception of double light flashes. *J. Neurol. Neurosurg. Psychiatry*, **39**, 861

2. Person, H..E. and Sachs, C. (1978). Provoked visual impairment in multiple sclerosis studied by visual evoked response. *Electroencephalogr. Clin. Neurophysiol.,* **44,** 664–668
3. Bajada, S., Mastaglia, F. L., Black, J. L. and Collins, D. W. K. (1980). Effects of induced hyperthermia on visual evoked potentials and saccade parameters in normal subjects and multiple sclerosis patients. *J. Neurol. Neurosurg. Psychiatry,* **43,** 849–852

Section VI
Free Communications

60
Multiple sclerosis: a case-control study. A preliminary report

D. CAPUTO, P. FERRANTE, G. DEL CORNO, M. ZAFFARONI
and C. L. CAZZULLO

INTRODUCTION

The aetiology of multiple sclerosis (MS) is yet unknown, despite the large numbers of research projects and the variety of approaches[1]. Several theories have been expressed about the putative causes of the disease, concerning virus involvement, metabolic abnormalities (particularly of certain unsaturated fatty acids), alterations of the immune response and a possible genetic predisposition. Such hypotheses, although all are likely and even though they have permitted some notable findings, contain many unproved and controversial facts. We believe that the epidemiological approach is very important because it could suggest the best trends of research.

Epidemiological investigations have formerly provided evidence of some peculiarities of MS. Namely: its close correlation with latitude[2] the higher risk among the relatives of a patient[3], the critical age of 15 years among migrating populations for acquiring the risk of developing the disease[4]. The latter datum suggests that MS is a symptomatologic expression of a process that begins before the age of 15. This is the reason why we focused our attention on the first 15 years of life of the patients, in order to find even a minimal sign of 'something' that, once it had primed the pathogenetic mechanism of MS, disappeared leaving few and poorly decipherable traces.

We are carrying out a case-control study in which a patient's sibling and a patient's childhood friend were chosen as controls. Such a choice was made in order to individualize that 'something' which might have started the development of the disease. Indeed these three subjects presumably lived in the same environment, and were exposed to the same viral agents responsible for childhood diseases, and to the same physical and social factors.

In conclusion, we are trying to understand why only one among the three persons developed MS.

Actually, there are remarkable immunological and genetic implications within the virus–host relation[5]: this is the reason why we chose the (patient's) sibling as one of the controls.

SUBJECTS AND METHODS

Until now 47 patients have been interviewed with clinically defined MS according to the criteria of McDonald and Halliday[6]. The questionnaire we utilized is reproduced in Figure 1. Each group of three subjects has been interviewed simultaneously by the same interviewer. As it concerns infectious diseases, we investigated whether mumps, measles, both or none were present and considered also whether measles was contracted before or after the age of 6 years, according to what is postulated for subacute sclerosing panen-cephalitis[7].

Furthermore, we took into account tonsillectomy, when done before the onset of MS, and the number of surgical operations as an index of stress and/or trauma[8,9] as follows: no operations; up to two operations; more than two operations. Contacts with animals before MS onset were analysed as follows: no contacts; presence of pets; presence of farm animals; presence of both. All items were also compared with respect to the age of onset (before or after 30 years).

The various items were analysed as follows: when the item had two alter-natives the χ^2 test for multiple matching was used[10]; when the item had 3 modalities, the χ^2 test for simple matching was applied according to Stuart–Maxwell[11,12].

RESULTS AND DISCUSSION

The results of this study are obviously incomplete, owing to the limited number of subjects interviewed until now.

We think that almost 100 patients and relative controls have to be investigated for a statistically correct data processing. Antibodies against measles, mumps, rubella, herpes simplex 1 and 2 will be titred next in each subject according to our previous studies[13,14].

Nevertheless, it seemed to us opportune to point out this epidemiological approach to a case-control study. Six items have been examined (Table 1). As can be observed, the preliminary results are not encouraging: the distributions of the above considered six factors do not differ statistically from the distribution in controls. Furthermore, the preliminary data concerning the degree of instruction (index of the social status)[8] and the exposure to toxic chemicals[15] did not reveal any difference between the considered groups (Table 2). Thus patient group and controls can be assimilated, for the items considered until now.

Nevertheless, before conclusions are assumed, we have to interview the whole series and examine all the items we programmed, paying special attention to the age when exanthematous diseases were contracted and to relative antibody titres and, possibly, to HLA typing.

Patient n.
Sibling of the patient n.
Control of the patient n.

Surname..................
Date of birth...............

Name.................
Place of birth..............

Infectious diseases: yes   no   age
  measles
  rubella
  mumps
  streptococcal
  hepatitis
  chickenpox
  others

Vaccinations: yes   no   age
  measles
  rubella
  diptheria–tetanus
  smallpox
  pertussis
  BCG.
  polio

Allergies
  to drugs
  to foods
  urticaria
  asthma
  hay fever

Father's birth place............birth rate........profession.......
Mother's birth place............birth rate........profession.......
Parent's neurological diseases........

Sibs:
  date of birth   sex   diseases   CNS diseases
1 ....
2 ....
3 ....
4 ....
5 ....
6 ....

Place of residence of birth..Province.......................

Place of residence at MS beginning...............................Province.......................

Present-day place of residence......................................Province.......................

House location (city, hinterland, village, country):

at birth...

possible variations................................

at onset of disease................................

at present..

bathroom: (absent, outside, inside)

at birth...

possible variations................................

at onset of disease................................

at present..

years of transfer:

year and place...................... from .... to

  ,, ,, ,, ...

  ,, ,, ,, ...

  ,, ,, ,, ... place

School state: yes no

Nursery school

Primary school

Secondary school

High school

University

Sports activity: agonistic not agonistic

Hobbies: yes no

Use of chemicals yes no

mastic

dyestuffs

solvents

others

Travels and/or stays (in other countries, in Italy only if lasting more then 6 months)

Year	length	place
....	....	....
....	....	....
....	....	....

Notes about jobs (kind of jobs, periods, tasks within the work place)

....

....

Use of chemicals

    yes   no

mastic

dyestuffs

solvents

others

Surgical operations before the disease (year and kind of operation):

....

Presence of animals:

    yes   no

farm animals..............................

pets...

ovines

swine

caprines

cattle

poultry

rabbits

others

dogs

cats

birds

at birth..

possible variations   –   until 4 years..................

  "   9   " ....

  "   14   " ....

at onset of disease..

at present..

Neurological diseases in subjects who lived in contact with the patient:

....

Clinical notes

onset year..

precipitating factors..

onset age..

modality of onset..

symptoms at onset..

period between 1st and 2nd episode..

Course of disease:

  remitting

  remitting and progressive

  progressive from onset

Kurtzke disability scale: P:.............   C:.............   T:.............   S:.............   SF:.............   V:.............

  M:.............   SP:.............   I:.............

Year: when MS was diagnosed:.............

Therapies during the last year:

  corticosteroids

  ACTH

  immunosuppressives

  others

Compilation date:..

kind   period

Figure 1

324

Table 1

		case-friend			*Matched pairs*	*case-sibling*		
Characteristics	No.	χ^2	d.of f.	p^a	No.	χ^2	d.of f.	p^a
Infectious diseases	47	3.1*	3	n.s.	47	2.1*	3	n.s.
Age of measles onset	32	3.9*	2	n.s.	31	0.7*	2	n.s.
Tonsillectomy	47	0.2**	1	n.s.	47	0.4**	1	n.s.
Surgical operation	47	0.8*	2	n.s.	47	0.4*	2	n.s.
Contact with animals	47	0.6*	3	n.s.	47	—	—	—
MS onset	47	0.3**	1	n.s.	47	2.1**	1	n.s.

[a] level of statistical significance $p = 0.05$
* according to McNemar's test[10]
** according to Stuart–Maxwell's test[11,12]
n.s. not significant

Table 2

Characteristics		
Degree of education	*Patient vs. sibling* No. 37 χ^2 2.5 (n.s.)	*Patient vs. friend* No. 37 χ^2 0.45 (n.s.)
Exposure to chemicals	*Patient vs. sibling and friend* No. 37 χ^2 0.67 (n.s.)	

n.s. = not significant

References

1. McFarlin, D. E. and McFarland, H. F. (1982). Multiple sclerosis. *N. Engl. J. Med.*, **307**, 1183
2. Kurtzke, J. F. (1975). A reassessment of the distribution of multiple sclerosis. Part one, Part two. *Acta Neurol. Scand.*, **51**, 110
3. Kurtzke, J. F. (1965). Familial incidence and geography in multiple sclerosis. *Acta Neurol. Scand.*, **41**, 127
4. Dean, G. and Kurtzke, J. F. (1971). On the risk of multiple sclerosis according to age at immigration to South Africa. *Br. Med. J.*, **3**, 725
5. Cazzullo, C. L. (1983). Opening remark. In *New trends in MS research*, (Milan: Masson Italia) (in press)
6. McDonald, W. I., Halliday, A. M. (1977). Diagnosis and classification of multiple sclerosis. *Br. Med. Bull.*, **33**, 4
7. Caputo, D. and Ferrante, P. (1981). Indagini virologiche nella sclerosi multipla. *Atti XXII Congresso Nazionale SIN*, p. 255 (Milano: Crippa and Berger)
8. Leibowitz, U. and Alter, M. (1973). *Multiple sclerosis. Clues to its cause.* (Amsterdam, North Holland: Elsevier)
9. Sharon, W., Greenhill, S. and Warren, K. G. (1982). Emotional stress and the development of multiple sclerosis: case control evidence of a relationship. *J. Chron. Dis.*, **35**, 821
10. McNemar, Q. (1947). Note on the sampling error of the difference between correlated proportions or percentages. *Psychometrika*, **12**, 153
11. Stuart, A. (1955). A test for homogeneity of the marginal distribution in a two-way classification. *Biometrika*, **42**, 412
12. Maxwell, A. E. (1970). Comparing the classification of subjects by two independent judges. *Br. J. Psychiat.*, **116**, 651
13. Caputo, D., Ferrante, P., Fasan, M. and Procaccia, S. (1981). Measles antibodies in multiple sclerosis patients. *Boll. Ist. Sieroter. Milan.*, **60**, 57

14. Ferrante, P., Caputo, D., Barbesti, S. and Fasan, M. (1982). Viral antibodies in multiple sclerosis. *Ital. J. Neurol. Sci.,* **2,** 115
15. Amaducci, L., Arfaioli, C., Inzitari, D. and Martinetti, M. G. (1977). Another possible precipitating factor in multiple sclerosis: the exposure to organic solvents. *Boll. Ist. Sieroter. Milan.,* **56,** 613

61
Numerical classification of multiple sclerosis

C. M. POSER

INTRODUCTION

The diagnosis of multiple sclerosis (MS) remains a clinical one based upon the interpretation of historical data, neurological signs and the results of ancillary laboratory procedures. The recent publication of new criteria for the diagnosis of MS, designed primarily for use in research protocols[1] has reduced somewhat the need for subjective interpretation which characterized some of the previous diagnostic schemes. Nevertheless, there appears to still be a need for an even more rigid system to isolate a core of cases, in particular in the definite category, about which there would be no questions whatsoever among investigators in different parts of the world.

In 1979, such a numerical score was proposed[2] based upon the examination of the entire detailed clinical course of 111 cases of autopsy-proved MS from England, Norway and the United States.

Upon re-examination of this scoring system, it seemed that too much weight had been given to the clinical signs and symptoms resulting from involvement of the corticospinal tracts, and to other relatively minor manifestations of the disease. A revised system is now being offered which is simpler to use and ascribes more realistic values to various sign–symptom combinations. The same criteria are used for the scoring system as previously described. The scoring system does not constitute a truly diagnostic tool, since it should be applied only in such patients with a very strong suspicion of the diagnosis of MS, in fact patients whose diagnosis would be classified as either probable or definite by the clinical classificatory schemes.

MATERIAL AND METHODS

The scoring system is based upon the same 111 proved cases of MS reported previously[3] (Table 1). For each clinical feature, a numerical value was assigned

Table 1 Clinical characteristics: autopsy series

Clinical feature	U.S. (n = 25) %	Norway (n = 31) %	England (n = 55) %	Total (n = 111) %
Remission	68.0	74.2	72.7	72.1
Pyramidal tract	100.0	100.0	98.2	99.1
Ocular	92.0	80.6	83.6	84.7
Urinary	52.0	87.1	92.7	82.0
Non-equilibratory	76.0	80.6	80.0	79.3
Vibration/position	64.0	64.5	78.2	71.2
Nystagmus	68.0	67.7	72.7	70.3
Paresthesiae	68.0	54.8	70.9	65.8
Dysarthria	52.0	61.3	52.7	55.0
Gait ataxia	60.0	67.7	45.5	55.0
Mental/cognitive	44.0	51.6	41.8	45.0

which corresponds to the percentage of occurrence of the particular item among the 111 patients.

The scoring system (Table 2) is cumulative, i.e. once a symptom has occurred or a sign has been elicited its value is retained even though it may no longer be present. Evidence of lesions obtained by means of ancillary clinical diagnostic procedures (paraclinical evidence of anatomic lesions) such as evoked response studies, hot bath tests, colour vision and neuropsychologic testing are awarded appropriate scoring values for the corresponding sign–symptom combinations. The presence of oligoclonal IgG bands or

Table 2 Scoring system

Clinical feature		Scoring value
Age of onset	20–29	1
	30–39	2
First symptom	weakness	4
	ocular	3
	paresthesiae	2
	cerebellar	1
Remission		7
Sign-symptom combination	pyramidal tract	10
	ocular/VER	8
	urinary	8
	non-equilibratory	8
	vibration/position/SSER	7
	nystagmus/BAER	7
	paresthesiae	7
	dysarthria	6
	gait ataxia	6
	mental/cognitive	5
	CSF OB/IgG	9
	CT Scan I+	5

Classification	Score
Definite	49 or above
Probable	36–48
Possible	35 or below

evidence of increased immunoglobulin G production in cerebrospinal fluid (CSF OB/IgG) is given the value of 9; in regard to tissue imaging, only contrast-enhancing lesions (I+) of white matter by CT scanning are acceptable and are given the value of 5.

It is not unusual for the onset of the disease to be characterized by more than one symptom. Scores are given only for first symptoms of weakness, ocular, paresthesiae and cerebellar (Table 2). In that event, the symptom scoring highest should be recorded: if a patient starts out with weakness and paresthesiae of the right arm, the first symptoms should be given a value of 4 for weakness. It must also be pointed out that the first symptom is scored *twice*: once as the first symptom and simultaneously given the appropriate value in the list of sign–symptom combinations: for example, for the individual whose first symptoms are that of weakness and paresthesiae of the right arm, the scoring is a value of 4 in the first symptom portion, plus a value of 10 for pyramidal tract involvement and a value of 7 for paresthesiae. The term weakness applies to specific paresis, not a general fatigue. It may be scored for facial weakness as well as limb weakness. The term ocular refers to any and all signs and symptoms involving the visual and ocular motor systems including loss or diminution of visual acuity, scotoma, blurring of vision, hemianopsia, diplopia, ptosis, loss of colour vision, pupillary abnormality, optic atrophy or definite disc pallor. Paresthesiae are what are often described by the patient as numbness, tingling, prickly or pins and needle sensation, formication, Lhermitte's symptom, etc. Certain types of pain may be included, specifically, trigeminal neuralgia or tabetic-like pains. Cerebellar symptoms must be divided into those that disturb equilibrium and the non-equilibratory ones which impair coordination. True vertigo may be considered to be a cerebellar symptom (scored under nystagmus) in this system once the physician is satisfied that it is not secondary to labyrinthine disease.

A remission is defined as the complete disappearance or significant decrease in severity for a period of at least 1 month of a symptom which lasted continuously for a period of at least 24 hours. Symptoms which last for less than 24 hours, however, may be scored: for example, an individual who has a well documented transient paraparesis or diplopia or dysarthria during exposure to extreme heat will be scored with the appropriate value for that sign–symptom combination, but *not* for a remission.

Involvement of pyramidal tracts should be scored when any of the following signs or symptoms have been recorded: hyperreflexia only if it is unilateral; spasticity regardless of the number of limbs involved; sustained clonus (transient clonus only if it is unilateral); Babinski signs; a plantar response which is equivocal on one side as compared to a definitely normal on the other one, should also be recorded and scored.

Ocular includes all symptoms described above as well as evidence of optic atrophy by funduscopic examination. Diplopia found only as a result of red glass testing must be scored positively, but dysconjugate gaze without a history of diplopia should be disregarded. Significant abnormalities of visual evoked response studies (VER) should also be scored under this rubric as should any disturbances of psychophysiologic tests of vision such as flicker-fusion, contrast sensitivity, flight of colour, etc.

Urinary disturbances refers to frequency, urgency and stress incontinence as well as urinary retention. Bowel incontinence (but not constipation) may be scored here as well as may the results of electromyographic examination of muscles of micturition. Significant sexual disturbances such as impotence, if clearly due to the illness, can also be scored under this rubric. Care must be taken to exclude such symptoms resulting from urinary tract infection.

Non-equilibratory signs and symptoms include incoordination secondary to cerebellar involvement such as head tremor, intention tremor, dysmetria, disorganization of movement, etc. Care must be taken to insure that such problems are not due to weakness or disturbance of position sense.

Diminutions in vibratory or position sensations must be scored only after specific examination of these modalities. In regard to testing of position sense, it must be pointed out that a positive Romberg test or significant widening of the base with eyes closed, or definite difficulty with tandem gait with eyes closed provides better evidence for loss of position sense in the feet than the inability to correctly indicate the position of the toes. Conversely, in the upper extremities, correct testing of position sense measures the extent of movement of the fingers rather than its direction: a displacement of just 2 or 3 degrees will be detectable by a normal individual, but impairment of position sense will increase this angle long before the patient is unable to describe the direction of motion. Abnormalities of peripherally induced somatosensory evoked response studies (SSER) indicative of central conduction delays are to be scored under this rubric.

Nystagmus must be scored only if it is sustained. Care must be taken to assure that it is not secondary to drugs or labyrinthine disease. Abnormalities of brainstem auditory evoked response studies (BAER) indicative of brainstem (but not of cochlea or auditory nerve) lesions are to be scored under this rubric.

Paresthesiae as described above, but pain problems which are non-specific such as headaches or backpain should not be included.

Dysarthria includes scanning speech or other articular disturbances, but not cortical aphasia problems; thus, the content of speech should be normal.

Gait ataxia is to be scored only when there is reasonable assurance that the disturbance represents equilibratory cerebellar ataxia as determined by history and examination. Titubation, drunken gait, leg incoordination are common descriptions, but may be quite difficult to separate from the gait disturbance due to loss of position sense, weakness or spasticity.

Mental changes are to be scored only if in the opinion of the physician these alterations exceed the commonly observed reactive depression seen with this illness. Only blatant euphoria should be scored, such as a definite 'belle indifference'. In addition, evidence of cognitive impairment detected clinically, or preferably by means of formal neuropsychological testing should be included. Obviously, signs of dementia, not uncommon late in the illness should also be scored under this rubric.

RESULTS

Clinical characteristics of autopsy-confirmed series (Table 1)

It is noted that the incidence of various sign–symptom combinations is remarkably uniform in the three series, with the exception of the relatively low occurrence of urinary tract disturbances in the American group.

Applying the scoring system to the 111 autopsy-confirmed cases, results in a mean value of 62 with a standard deviation of 13. On the basis of these data, the category of definite MS was chosen as encompassing those cases with scores above 48 (mean ± 1 SD). Cases listed as probable would be those with scores between 36 (mean ± 25 SD) and 48 while cases with scores with 35 or less would be listed as possible.

Using the scoring system, on the 111 autopsy-proved cases, results in the following classifications: definite 85.6%, probable 10.8% and possible 3.6%. The scoring system was also applied to a series of 60 clinically diagnosed cases of multiple sclerosis published by Thygesen[4] in Denmark and results in 80.0% definite, 15.0% probable and 5.0% possible cases.

DISCUSSION

It should be stressed that this scoring system is to be applied only in such instances where the clinical diagnosis of MS is suspected, and all other diseases of the nervous system have been reasonably excluded. It will not resolve the classic dilemma of differentiating MS from disseminated encephalomyelitis, unless there is evidence of peripheral nervous system involvement.

The system has a built-in rigidity which some clinicians and investigators may consider to be a drawback. No provisions are made for additions to the scoring system under the following circumstances: (1) appearance of a new sign or symptom involving the same system: thus, if paresthesiae of the right arm have been scored, the occurrence of paresthesiae of other body parts cannot be recorded; similarly, weakness of another limb or the appearance of a Babinski sign on the other side, or loss of vision in the other eye. (2) For aggravation of previously recorded signs and symptoms such as increased paresis to paralysis, loss as opposed to diminution of sensory modality.

On the other hand, its very value may be enhanced by the fact that it records *only* new sign–symptom combinations, thus avoiding the ever present dilemma of determining if an exacerbation represents a real extension of illness, the formation of new plaques or the extension of old ones, or simply a physiologically induced exacerbation.[5] Increasing awareness of the existence of asymptomatic lesions, demonstrable by paraclinical means, re-emphasizes the difficulties in evaluating the significance of symptomatic exacerbations in terms of evolution of the disease itself. Thus, the scoring system primarily reflects involvement of multiple systems within the CNS rather than the presence of multiple lesions. In view of Thygesen's[4] finding that clinical evidence of new lesions occurs in only 19% of exacerbations, the loss may be less important than the benefit accruing from keeping the scoring system uncomplicated and easy to use. This scoring system does not eliminate the need for subjective judgement in the interpretation on the part of the clinician. Its greatest value may well lie in providing an easily standardized means of evaluating the effect of therapeutic agents in arresting or stabilizing the course of the disease.

References

1. Poser, C. M., Paty, D., Scheinberg, L., McDonald, W. I., Davis, F., Ebers, G., Johnson, K., Sibley, W., Silberberg, D. and Tourtellotte, W. (1983). New diagnostic criteria for multiple sclerosis. *Ann. Neurol.,* **13,** 227
2. Poser, C. M. (1979). A numerical scoring system for the classification of multiple sclerosis. *Acta. Neurol. Scand.,* **60,** 100
3. Poser, C. M., Presthus, J. and Horsdal, O. (1966). Clinical characteristics of autopsy-proved multiple sclerosis. *Neurology,* **16,** 79
4. Thygesen, P. (1953). *The course of disseminated sclerosis: A close-up of 105 attacks.* (Copenhagen: Rosenkilde and Bagger)
5. Poser, C. M. (1965). Clinical diagnostic criteria in epidemiological studies of multiple sclerosis. *Ann. NY Acad. Sci.,* **122,** 506

62
HLA-determination in twins with multiple sclerosis

A. HELTBERG

Only a few studies of HLA-determination on MS-twins have appeared in the past. As part of a genetic study on twins with MS, HLA-typing, including DR, was performed.

MS-twins were ascertained by screening the files and by record linkage in two nationwide registers, the Danish twin-register, and the Danish multiple sclerosis register. 62 probands with clinically definite MS, according to the diagnostic criteria of Schumacher from 57 twin pairs were ascertained. All co-twins were followed up to death or to the age of at least 50 years, but no additional cases of MS were revealed. Different factors about the proband material is shown in Tables 1–3.

Table 1

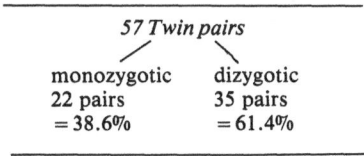

57 Twin pairs

monozygotic	dizygotic
22 pairs	35 pairs
= 38.6%	= 61.4%

Table 2

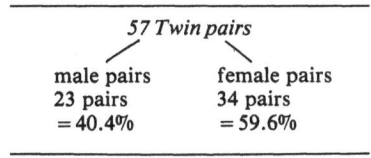

57 Twin pairs

male pairs	female pairs
23 pairs	34 pairs
= 40.4%	= 59.6%

Table 3

Both twins alive:	18 pairs
Only MS twin alive:	9 cases
Only mz. co-twin alive:	5 cases
Only dz. co-twin alive:	11 cases

Table 4 Included in the study:

30 probands from 28 MS twin pairs.

HLA determination on both twins:	14 pairs
HLA determination on MS twin alone:	10 cases
HLA determination on mz co-twin alone:	4 cases

Included in this study were 30 probands from 28 MS-twin pairs. As can be seen from Table 4, HLA determination was performed on 10 MS-twin patients, four monozygotic twin partners to deceased MS patients and 14 twin pairs, both alive. The ratio monozygotic/dizygotic for twins reported here is, therefore, different from the proband material, where this ratio corresponds to expectation.

Further details about the twins, included in this HLA-study, appear in Tables 5–8. Also the clinical condition and the course of the disease were

Table 5

Age at onset: 14–50 years
     mean: 32 years

Duration of disease at the time of the investigation:
          9–55 years
     mean: 19 years

Table 6

Monozygotic: 13 pairs

concordant:	2 pairs		discordant:	11 pairs	
DR2+	DR2−		DR2+	DR2−	
2	0		6	5	

Dizygotic: 15 pairs

concordant:	0 pairs		discordant:	15 pairs	
			DR2+	DR2−	
			9	6	}probands

334

evaluated, according to the functional system scale and the disability status scale. This can be seen from Tables 9 and 10. 63.3% of the probands were HLA-DR2 positive as compared to 28.7% in the normal Danish population.

No statistically significant difference in HLA-DR2 frequency was found between monozygotic concordant and discordant twin pairs.

No statistically significant difference in HLA-DR2 frequency was found between monozygotic and dizygotic twin probands. No statistically significant difference was found in HLA-DR2 frequency in dizygotic discordant twins, between proband and twin partner, but more probands were HLA-DR2 positive. No correlation between severity or course of disease and HLA-DR2 could be demonstrated.

Table 7

Monozygotic: 15 probands
DR2+   DR2−
  10   5

Dizygotic: 15 probands
DR2+   DR2−
   9   6

Table 8   Dizygotic pairs, all discordant for MS, both typed = 8 pairs

MS/not MS	DR2 +/+	DR2 +/−	DR2 −/+	DR2 −/−
	3 pairs	2 pairs	0 pairs	3 pairs

Table 9

FSS after 10 years: (27 probands)
   DR2+ (16 probands): mean 8.4
   DR2− (11 probands): mean 8.5

DSS after 10 years (27 probands)
   DR2+ (16 probands): mean 3.6
   DR2− (11 probands): mean 4.3

Table 10

FSS after 20 years (21 probands)
   DR2+ (13 probands): mean 9.2
   DR2− (8 probands): mean 10.1

DSS after 20 years (21 probands)
   DR2+ (13 probands): mean 4.2
   DR2− (8 probands): mean 6.1

CONCLUSION

(1) 63.3% of MS probands were HLA-DR2 positive as compared to 28.7% in the normal Danish population.

(2) No statistically significant difference between HLA-DR2 frequency in monozygotic concordant and monozygotic discordant twin pairs could be demonstrated.

(3) No statistically significant difference between HLA-DR2 frequency in monozygotic and dizygotic MS twin probands was found.

(4) No statistically significant difference in HLA-DR2 frequency in dizygotic discordant twins between proband and twin partner was demonstrated.

(5) No correlation was found between severity or course of disease and HLA-DR2.

63
Multiple sclerosis and myasthenia gravis

A. HERODE and S. BORENSTEIN

A number of earlier authors have suggested the possibility of a multiple sclerosis–myasthenia overlap syndrome. The following case suggests the true existence of this clinical association, but immunological studies gave puzzling results which are discussed.

CASE REPORT

V.B. was 12 years old when she noted the gradual onset of weakness and easy fatiguability. The symptoms worsened progressively with ptosis, diplopia, facial paresis, falling of the head and difficulty in climbing stairs and speaking. The diagnosis of myasthenia gravis was established in 1959, by testing the clinical response to prostigmine injection and by the electromyography decrements to repetitive stimulation with a favourable response to anticholinesterase drugs. She was initially managed medically, but because of an insufficient response, a thymectomy was done in 1971. Postoperatively, there was gradual but progressive improvement in her myasthenic status.

She had almost completely recovered from myasthenia when, on September 1, 1980, she complained of blurred vision in the left eye. Two days later, she consulted outside our institution, and she was admitted on September 5 to our hospital with suspicion of a left-sided optic neuritis. In fact on this date, visual acuities were 6/10 in the right eye, and reduced to counting fingers in the left eye. Kinetic visual field disclosed RE: a dense upper temporal quadrantic defect with a paracentral relative scotoma and LE: a large scotoma including the central area as well as the whole nasal field except a little area which seemed spared in the upper nasal quadrantic field.

On September 12, the visual impairment was worsening with total hemianopsy and visual acuity of 3/10 in the right eye. In the left eye visual field, only a little area in the upper nasal field was spared, and visual acuity deteriorated to light perception. Retrobulbar pain on rotation of eyes appeared, and at this date the corticotherapy was started in the form of prednisolone 60 mg 1 day/2.

She had a slight decreased left corneal reflex. The colour vision examination yielded disturbed results from the right eye, but was impossible to test in the left eye because of the magnitude of the visual impairment on this side. There was paresis of upward conjugate gaze with dissociated nystagmus of the abducting eye (more striking on the left eye). Pupil examination revealed a relative afferent defect in the left eye and pupil cycle time, when performed from the right eye it gave a normal level of 937 ms. The optic disc and retina appeared to be normal in both eyes. Visual evoked potentials recorded either with flashes or with checker-board pattern revealed a notable delayed response, especially from the left eye.

Electronystagmography revealed a spontaneous left nystagmus at the resting point with left nystagmus greater than right in vestibular trials (caloric irrigation and pendular test). An electroencephalogram obtained on September 9 showed diffuse poorly regulated waves, but gave a normal result 6 days later. Brainstem auditory evoked responses and blink reflex were normal.

At acute phase of optic neuritis, sedimentation rate was 48 mm/h with a fibrinogen level of 557 mg%. The following tests were normal: WBC/mm^3, RBC/mm^3, lymphocytes, sugar, urea, creatinine, ionogram, serum protein electrophoresis and immunoelectrophoresis, CRP, VDRL, latex, electrocardiogram, skull and chest radiography and brain scan. Lumbar puncture showed 2 RBC/mm^3, 15 WBC/mm^3 with 40% lymphocytes, sugar 54 mg% and protein 70 mg% with a γ-globulin level of 20% and which showed the existence of a paraprotein among this latter group.

The following clinical ophthalmologic evolution was noted: normal ocular motility 9 days after the onset of the disease. Progressive but complete recovery of visual acuity and visual field in the right eye, whereas remission was incomplete in the left eye with visual acuity still reduced to counting fingers at one metre and with the persistence of four scotomas in the visual field. Progressive left-sided disc pallor developed, and it was merely evident 7 months after the onset of retrobulbar neuritis.

The patient's condition remained unchanged until February 13, 1982, when a right-sided hemiparesis developed. She had right Babinski sign, absent abdominal reflexes and decreased appreciation for pin prick from C5 to C8 on the left. Computerized tomography and radiography of the spinal column gave normal results, and then corticotherapy was readministered in the form of prednisolone 200 mg/d, intravenously. The right-sided symptoms nearly completely remitted over 2 weeks but the hospital course was complicated by the development of a rapidly regressive paresis in the left arm. Laboratory studies of peripheral blood showed first some similar results to those collected in 1980, but an immunological study was made and gave the following results: presence of a paraprotein among the γ-globulins. The antinuclear antibody test was positive in a titre of 1/2560 with presence of antibodies to native DNA and LE cells. The research of antibodies anti-SM gave dubious results, and rheumatoid factor was absent. Lumbar puncture showed: 42 RBC/mm^3, 14 WBC/mm^3 with 12% lymphocytes, sugar 94 mg% and protein 86 mg% with α_2-globulin of 13.5% and γ-globulin of 23% with division into fractions.

On July 18, 1982, she experienced some haziness over the right eye just after a warm bath. She complained of some discomfort on moving this eye but visual acuity was 13/10 with normal ophthalmologic findings, except a perturbed reading of Boström and Kugelberg charts with the right eye and residual optic atrophy on the left side. Two weeks later, she denied any complaint but paradoxically ophthalmologic examination revealed a rotatory nystagmus in both eyes on lateral gaze.

COMMENT

At the age of 34, this woman had bilateral optic neuritis 22 years after the onset of a myasthenia gravis. In addition, she had oculomotor troubles with dissociated nystagmus which evoked brainstem lesions, but myasthenia may mimic this symptom[1]. However, according to the CSF abnormalities and the VEP delayed response, this patient was discharged with the diagnosis of possible multiple sclerosis.

This diagnosis seemed clinically confirmed when she developed regressive hemiparesis and later episodic blurred vision after a warm bath. So, we were in the presence of a particularly demonstrative case of multiple sclerosis associated with myasthenia gravis, but immunological studies gave puzzling findings which suggested a mixed collagen vascular disease.

DISCUSSION

Retrospectively, the diagnosis of systemic lupus erythematosus is evoked by the immunological findings but antineural antibodies (ANA) are also reported in myasthenia gravis[2]. In fact, if the optic neuritis and the myelopathy are imputed to systemic lupus erythematosus, we have to admit that they are uncommonly described in association, and completely isolated from other symptoms[3,4]. Indeed, there was no arthritis, no butterfly rash, no alopecia, no nephritis, no dermatologic sign, no particular fundi findings except the left optic atrophy. But otherwise examined, systemic lupus erythematosus is one of the diseases most often associated with myasthenia gravis while multiple sclerosis association is only suggested by some previous communications[5-9], where, to the best of our knowledge, a complete screening for hidden auto-immune disease was never performed.

We wonder if it is conceivable to associate multiple sclerosis with systemic lupus, or if such immunological results as we found should be introduced as exclusion criteria of multiple sclerosis diagnosis.

From another point of view, intensive corticosteroid therapy is required in systemic lupus[10], while spontaneous recovery without treatment is the rule in multiple sclerosis[11]. That is why such patients with clinical and laboratory features of multiple sclerosis should always be examined for systemic lupus erythematosus.

References

1. Glaser, J. S. (1966). Myasthenia pseudo-internuclear ophthalmoplegia. *Arch. Ophthalmol.,* **75,** 363
2. Kornguth, S. E., Hanson, J. C., Chun, R. W. M. (1970). Antineuronal antibodies in patients having myasthenia gravis. *Neurology* (Minneap.), **20,** 749
3. Vitale, C., Kahn, M. F., de Sèze, M., de Sèze, S. (1973). Névrite optique, myélite et maladie lupique. *Ann. Med. Intern.,* **124,** 211
4. Contamin, F., Singer, B., Mignot, B., Mougeot-Martin, M., Duhamel, G., Saraux, H., Nizak, J., Metzger, P. (1978). Sur un cas de lupus érythémateux disséminé avec atteinte de la moelle épinière et des deux nerfs optiques. *Ann. Med. Interne,* **129,** 463
5. Margolis, L. H., Graves, R. W. (1945). The occurrence of myasthenia gravis in a patient with multiple sclerosis. *N.C. Med. J.,* **6,** 243
6. Simpson, J. A. (1966). The biochemistry of myasthenia gravis. In Kuhn, E. (ed.). *Progressive muskeldystrophic, myotonic und myasthenie,* pp. 339–349 (Berlin: Springer-Verlag)
7. Keane, J. R., Hoyt, W. F. (1970). Myasthenic (vertical) nystagmus: verification by edrophenium tomography. *JAMA,* **212,** 1209
8. Patten, B. M., Hart, A., Lovelace, R. (1972). Multiple sclerosis associated with defects in neuromuscular transmission. *J. Neurol. Neurosurg. Psychiatry,* **35,** 385
9. Aita, J. F., Synder, D. H., Reichl, W. (1974). Myasthenia gravis and multiple sclerosis: an unusual combination of diseases. *Neurology,* **24,** 72
10. Dutton, J. J., Burde, R. M., Klingele, T. G. (1982). Autoimmune retrobulbar optic neuritis. *Am. J. Ophthalmol.,* **94,** 11
11. Glaser, J. S. (1978). Neuro–ophthalmology. In Duane, T. D. (ed.). *Clinical ophthalmology.* Vol. 2, p. 107 (Hagestown: Harper and Row)

Additional references

Andrianakos, A. A., Duffy, J., Suzuki, M., Sharp, J. T. (1975). Transverse myelopathy in systemic lupus erythematosus. Report of 3 cases and review of the literature. *Ann. Intern. Med.,* **83,** 616

April, R. S., Vansonnenberg, E. (1976). A case of neuromyelitis optica (Devic's syndrome) in systemic lupus erythematosus. Clinico–pathologic report and review of the literature. *Neurology,* **26,** 1066

Beutner, E. H., Chorzelski, T. P., Hale, W. L., Hausmanowa-Petrusewicz, I. (1968). Auto-immunity in concurrent myasthenia gravis and pemphigus erythematosus. *JAMA,* **203,** 845

Bloomer, L. C., Bray, P. F. (1981). Relative value of three laboratory methods in the diagnosis of multiple sclerosis. *Clin. Chem.,* **27,** 2011

Cendrowski, W., Stepien, M. (1974). Clinical variant of lupus erythematosus resembling multiple sclerosis. *Eur. Neurol.,* **11,** 373

Cinefro, R. J., Frenkel, M. (1978). Systemic lupus erythematosus presenting as optic neuritis. *Ann. Ophthalmol.,* **10,** 559

Connor, R. C. R. (1970). Causes of disseminated sclerosis. *Lancet,* **i,** 724

Duffy, J., Andrianakos, A., Lipsky, M. *et al* (1974). Low spinal fluid glucose in systemic lupus with spinal cord disease (abstract). *Clin. Res.,* **22,** 610

Flament-Durand, J., Coers, C., Van Bogaert, L. (1969). Remarques sur une observation de sclérose en plaques atypique à évolution subaiguë. *Acta Neurol. Psych. Belg.,* **59,** 788

Fulford, K. W. M., Catterall, R. D., Delhanty, J. J. (1972). A collagen disorder of the nervous system presenting as multiple sclerosis. *Brain,* **95,** 373

Gerson, B., Cohen, S. R., Gerson, I. M., Guest, C. H. (1981). Myelin basic protein, oligoclonal bands, and IgG in cerebrospinal fluid as indicators of multiple sclerosis. *Clin. Chem.,* **27,** 1974

Gold, D. H., Morris, D. A., Henkind, P. (1972). Ocular findings in systemic lupus erythematosus. *Br. J. Ophthalmol.,* **56,** 800

Hackett, E. R., Martinez, R. D., Larson, P. F., Paddison, R. M. (1974). Optic neuritis in systemic lupus erythematosus. *Arch. Neurol.,* **31,** 9

Hart, R. G., Sherman, D. G. (1982). The diagnosis of multiple sclerosis. *JAMA,* **247,** 498

Holmes, F. F., Stubbs, D. W., Larsen, W. E. (1967). Systemic lupus erythematosus and multiple sclerosis in identical twins. *Arch. Intern. Med.,* **119,** 302

Husain, M., Neff, J., Daily, E., Townsend, J., Lucas, F. (1974). Antinuclear antibodies. Clinical significance of titers and fluorescence patterns. *Am. J. Clin. Pathol.,* **61,** 59

Johnson, K., Nelson, B. (1977). Multiple sclerosis. Diagnostic usefulness of cerebrospinal fluid. *Ann. Neurol.,* **2,** 425

Kinney, E. L., Berdoff, R. L., Rao, N. S., Fox, L. M. (1979). Devic's syndrome and systemic lupus erythematosus. A case report with necropsy. *Arch. Neurol.,* **36,** 643

McAlpine, D. (1929). A form of myasthenia gravis with changes in the central nervous system. *Brain,* **52,** 6

Macrae, D., O'Rhilly, S. (1957). On some neuro-oto-ophthalmological manifestations of systemic lupus erythematosus and polyarteritis nodosa. *Eye, Ear, Nose, Throat, Mon.,* **36,** 721

Maumence, A. E. (1956). Ocular manifestations of collagen disease. *Arch. Ophthalmol.,* **56,** 559

Michels, R. G. (1974). Ocular manifestation in connective tissue disorders (CTD). In Ryan, S. J. (ed.). *The eye in systemic disease,* pp. 301–313 (New York: Grune & Stratton)

Mott, Sir F. W., Barrada, Y. A. (1923). Pathological findings in the central nervous system of a case of myasthenia gravis. *Brain,* **46,** 237

Perkin, G. D., Rose, F. C. (1979). *Optic neuritis and its differential diagnosis,* p. 144. (Oxford: Oxford Medical)

Petz, L. D., Sharp, G. C., Cooper, N. R., Irvin, W. S. (1971). Serum and cerebral spinal fluid complement and serum autoantibodies in SLE. *Medicine,* **50,** 259

Schneck, S. A., Claman, H. N. (1969). CSF immunoglobulins in multiple sclerosis and other neurologic diseases. Measurement of electroimmunodiffusion. *Arch. Neurol.,* **20,** 132

de Sèze, M., Kahn, M. F., Auvert, B., Solnica, J. (1964). Survenue d'une névrite optique au cours d'un lupus érythémateux disséminé méconnu. Intérêt de l'enquête familiale. *Bull. Soc. Méd. Hôp. Paris,* **15,** 1017

Shepherd, D. I., Downie, A. W., Best, P. V. (1974). Systemic lupus erythematosus and multiple sclerosis (abstract). *Arch. Neurol.,* **30,** 423

Simpson, J. A. (1966). Myasthenia gravis as an autoimmune disease: clinical aspects. *Ann. N. Y. Acad. Sci.,* **135,** 506

64
Intellectual impairment in multiple sclerosis

L. DE SMEDT, M. SWERTS, J. GEUTJENS and R. MEDAER

Intellectual impairment is hardly known or studied in multiple sclerosis (MS). For the last 3 years intellectual impairment in multiple sclerosis patients has been the subject of systematic research in the MS clinic of Overpelt. Psychometric testing in MS encounters many difficulties due to the patients' visual and motor deficits and also their psychological problems.

In this study we compared the premorbid intellectual functioning with the actual level to get a better insight into the existence and the extent of the intellectual impairment. In addition this intellectual impairment is correlated to other variables such as actual age, age at onset and progression rate.

POPULATION

46 patients with a definite diagnosis of multiple sclerosis were examined, 26 were women and 20 were men. These patients were selected from a large group on the basis of their ability to perform WAIS tasks, without any consequence for standardization of the test. At the same time as the psychometric research the patients had a neurological examination and were scored according to the 'Kurtzke disability status scale'. During the tests most of them were hospitalized in Overpelt. Others were out-patients following a rehabilitation programme. In this group the Kurtzke disability rate varied from 3 to 8 points, with an average of 6.0 and a SD of ± 1.1. The age at entry to the study ranged from 14 to 52 years, average 31.1 years and SD ± 9.5. Duration of illness varied

Table 1

Variable	Average	Limits	± SD
Age at examination	47.1	20–61	10.4
Age at onset	30.6	14–52	9.5
Duration of illness	15.7	2–41	10.0
Kurtzke disability rate	6.0	3–8	1.1
Progression rate	0.61	0.14–3	0.61

from 2 to 41 years, average 15.7 years and SD ± 10.0. Progression rate (Kurtzke disability rate divided by duration of illness) was calculated, and resulted in an average of 0.61 SD ± 0.61.

METHODS

The patients were tested on the WAIS 'Wechsler Adult Intelligence Scale' which is the most widely used intelligence test. It is composed of 11 different subtests. Wechsler classified six of them as 'verbal tests' the others as 'performential tests'.

For each of the examined patients a premorbid level of intellectual functioning was estimated according to three universally accepted methods:

(1) IQ based on attained educational level.
(2) IQ calculated on the highest WAIS subtest score.
(3) IQ calculated on the 'vocabulary' subtest of the WAIS.

Out of these three estimations an average was made and was considered as the best attempt at the premorbid level of the patient.

RESULTS

The mean promorbid IQ of the whole group was 102.9 with SD ± 10.9. *The total mean IQ at the time of testing* was 84.10.

In the Table 2 we have presented the results of the mean values of the subtests (verbal and performance scales) and the full scale IQ on the WAIS.

The mean results on subtests of the WAIS were divided into qualitative categories.

Multiple sclerosis patients seem to obtain low scores on subtests measuring

Table 2

	$\bar{x}$	± SD	Pc
Information	4.89	1.92	31/50
Comprehension	5.15	2.38	50/65
Arithmetic	4.50	3.76	16/31
Similarities	4.43	2.44	31/50
Digit span	3.95	2.55	15/31
Vocabulary	4.44	1.88	31/50
Digit symbols	2.56	2.76	7/16
Picture completion	3.04	1.94	16/31
Black design	3.04	1.95	16/31
Picture arrangement	3.84	1.80	16/31
Object assembly	2.09	2.19	7/16
Verbal IQ	90.73	19.72	25/30
Performance IQ	76.45	16.47	5/10
Full scale IQ	84.10	14.76	15/20

Pc = percentile points

Table 3

Qualitative interpretation	Subtest of the WAIS
Average	comprehension
Low average to average	information, similarities, vocabulary
Borderline to low average	arithmetic, digit span, picture completion, block design, picture arrangement
Borderline	object assembly, digit symbols

Table 4 Difference between actual IQ and premorbid IQ, points

	1	2	3
Deficit	0–14	15–29	30
Number of patients	16	26	4
%	34.7	56.5	8.5

visual-motor coordination and motor speed with, in addition, a loss of tempo in both verbal and performance subtests.

On subtests which among other things, measure attention, they get low scores; namely on substitution digit span and digit symbol.

The lower scores on arithmetic and digit span give evidence of immediate memory impairment.

Subtests that ask more of their verbal capacities, are performed much better than visuo-spatial tasks.

Then the patients were *divided according to the severity of the intellectual deterioration.*

A first group shows a deficit smaller than one standard deviation (SD ± 15) the second group lies between 1 and 2 SD, in the third this difference is greater than 2 SD.

A difference smaller than 1 SD which means less than 15 IQ points was

Table 5

	1	2	3
Mean actual IQ (full scale)	95.5	78.5	73.2
Mean premorbid IQ (estimated)	104.1	101.3	108.4
Mean deficit	8.63	22.69	35.17

Table 6

Disability	$p<0.05$	
Duration of illness	0.12	n.s.
Age	0.08	n.s.
Age at onset	0.01	n.s.
Verbal IQ	−0.03	n.s.
Performance IQ	−0.25	n.s.
Total IQ	−0.26	n.s.

n.s. = not significant

Table 7

Intellectual impairment		
Duration of illness	− 0.08	n.s.
Age	− 0.08	n.s.
Age at onset	− 0.05	n.s.
Progression rate	− 0.05	n.s.

n.s. = not significant

regarded as insufficient to prove mental deterioration. Out of each group we calculated the mean actual IQ and a mean premorbid IQ.

We looked for correlation between the intellectual deficit and duration of illness, age at onset, actual age, and progression rate. This nowhere revealed a significant correlation. Even correlation between disability and verbal performance or total IQ was not significant.

CONCLUSION

In this study on intellectual impairment in MS we examined 46 patients.

In 30 patients, or 65%, an intellectual deficit of more than 15 IQ points was found, compared to their estimated premorbid intellectual functioning. Out of this group a small to moderate deficit was apparent in 87%, in 13% the deficit was serious.

No significant correlation between intellectual impairment and duration of illness, age, age at onset or progression rate was found. Nor was there a significant relationship between disability and actual intellectual functioning.

We think that intellectual impairment can be considered as an isolated and frequent symptom in multiple sclerosis. It appears in young as well as in older multiple sclerosis patients and can start at an early or late stage of the disease. It is important that there is no correlation between intellectual impairment and a high progression rate of the illness, or with the severity of the disability.

Finally, we think that psychological testing of intellectual functioning should become a routine in the investigation of multiple sclerosis patients.

65
Multiple sclerosis: a conceptual reappraisal

E. J. FIELD

INTRODUCTION

Although an extended, detailed and accurate account of the clinical evolution of classical, recurrent multiple (disseminated) sclerosis is given in the diary of Sir Augustus d'Esté (1794–1848)[1] and a strikingly modern clinical and pathological account of the disease recorded by Charcot[2,3] no consensus exists, even today, as to the precise nature of the disease. Characteristically, it leads to widespread, patchy scarring within the neuraxis with, however, sites of predilection, e.g. at the lateral angles of the ventricles; and symmetry of lesions is often striking. In the majority of instances there are recurrent bouts or episodes of disability, though the picture is notoriously protean and experts agree that a high proportion of misdiagnosis occurs during life[4] and even more at ultimate uncovering at autopsy[5-8]. There is also, not uncommonly, little, if any, correlation between clinical symptoms and location of widespread multiple lesions in the nervous system. Opinion regarding aetiopathogenesis falls into three main categories.

(1) That the disease is an auto-immune response, gainsaying Ehrlich's *Horror autotoxicus*;[8a] more recently this has been subtly modified to suggest a basic disturbance of immunological reactivity in MS.

(2) That the disease is viral in origin, perhaps involving 'slow' infections, enthusiasm for which now rivals the popularity enjoyed by auto-immunity some two decades ago; and (inevitably)

(3) a combination of both viral and immunological factors – the former perhaps engendering products insufficiently different from normal to induce mistaken attack upon normal tissues.

The evolution of these ideas and the stimulus given by the elaboration of experimental allergic encephalomyelitis (EAE) have been discussed by Field[9]. Suffice it to say that the discovery of a specific virus or viroid has so far baffled

346

the most ingenious laboratory devices; the measles hypothesis is now to be seen in terms of an unusually hyperactive non-specific immunological response in MS[10], and sharing of antigenic determinants between brain material and viral components[11]. Sever[12], indeed, has written a refreshing article on 'Viruses which do not cause MS'.

Naturally, the neurologist's opinion will colour his management of the MS patient; immunosuppression – not uncommonly with far from innocuous drugs – follows from a belief that EAE is either fundamentally a model for the disease (a favourite opening gambit in applications for work-grants, largely destined to add still further to the morass of *post-hoc* phenomena painstakingly analysed and confusingly designated); or that an immunological process is carrying on recurrent episodes; dietary recommendations, from a belief that 'good foods' will allay or cure the disease; and so on.

CURRENT HYPOTHESIS

In this essay there is presented the hypothesis that MS is essentially of the nature of an Abiotrophy and the evidence discussed. In many aspects the hypothesis rests upon experimental results and offers testable derivatives. Clinically 'probable' MS is a syndrome in which most cases rest upon the congenital anomalies outlined below. A small proportion of patients with the syndrome are suffering recurrences of an acute disseminated encephalomyelitis (ADEM), and will not show laboratory tests given by the mass and outlined below. A still smaller number result from mimicry by neurosarcoidosis[13], sometimes limited to the CNS and without systemic signs[14]. Left atrial myxoma may, on rare occasions, give an embolic picture limited to the CNS (Carson and Gumpert – unpublished).

The great majority of cases of MS are based upon an inborn mishandling of unsaturated fatty acids of the linoleic (LA) (18:2 (n–6) 9.12 octadecaenoic) acid type and arachidonic (AA) (20:4 (n–6) 5.8.11.14 icosatetraenoic) acid and the elongated acids derived from them[15,16] leading to the formation of myelin of poor quality which does not last the normal life span. This major category of MS is, therefore, an example of 'Abiotrophy' in the sense of Gowers[17], i.e. results from poorly put together myelin, the lamellae being weakly welded by electrostatic forces so that there may be 'spontaneous' slippage along the intra-period line. From reasoning set out below three laboratory tests for this possibility of spontaneous slippage (MS diathesis) have been elaborated (Table 1). It is interesting that Gowers (*loc. cit*) seems to have been unaware of Charcot's penetrating reference to 'la famille neuropathologique[18]' or the antecedent ideas of Féré[19], and Revington[20] mentioned by Charcot (*loc. cit.*).

Those which are *not* based upon abnormal UFA (unsaturated fatty acid) handling give negative results in the above tests: indeed, very careful history taking of the first attack of ADEM will commonly alert the physician as to the nature of the illness he is dealing with[21].

Table 1 Laboratory tests for MS

MEM–LAD		Field et al[38]	1974
	confirmed by	Jenssen et al[70]	1976
E–UFA		Field et al[39]	1977
	confirmed by	Bisaccia et al[40]	1977
		Seaman et al[42]	1979
		Tamblyn et al[43]	1980
		Jones et al[71]	1981
PGE$_2$		Field and Joyce[72]	1977

Indicates workers who have confirmed the original MEM–LAD test and the E–UFA test in each case on double-blind specimens. Ref. 71 is of especial interest since Dr A. J. Forrester (a senior worker in the group) had previously dismissed the E–UFA test as utterly valueless[46] – though in 1981 he was working with Seaman et al's.[42] modification of it.

EVIDENCE FOR PRIMARY ABIOTROPHY

Histological study of MS

Examination of really early lesions shows disintegration of myelin *in situ*. Scharlach R staining globules are present within local glial cells or lying freely between the fibres. *No lymphocytes are present at this early stage,* whatever may be the case in EAE[22]. The macrophages, as we may call them, are clearly of local glial origin[23,24], and not haematogenous. Some are local microglia. They quickly migrate to adjacent small veins where cuffing with small round cells – lymphocytes, small fat containing macrophages and a few plasma cells – is present. It may be mentioned that none of the detailed descriptions of MS[25-34] give prominence to lymphocyte intervention at an early stage. Indeed, attention was drawn by Charcot[25], Müller[28], Anton and Wohlwill[29], Jakob[30], Field[31] and Lumsden[32] to early proliferation of astroglial cells.

Field[32], and more recently Allen[35,36] in beautiful morphological and histochemical studies, has drawn attention to changes in the seemingly normal white matter between lesions where both morphological and biochemical changes are regularly found, substantiating earlier and cruder gross biochemical estimates. Thus MS is *a disease of the whole white matter* with focalization around small blood vessels. This is in accordance with the Abiotrophy hypothesis outlined; astrocytes are known to work in close harmony with oligodendrocytes.

LABORATORY TESTS FOR MS

Three tests now exist (Table 1) but are hedged about with precautions (see below). The E–UFA test is the simplest to carry out, demanding no more than expertise in the accurate determination of erythrocyte electrophoretic mobility from MS suspected and normal subjects. All are based upon Thompson's hypothesis noted above. UFA are important constituents of phospholipids, and as such, constituents of all animal cell membranes. Membranes in classical MS should, therefore, be unusual in their constitution, and this might be reflected in their surface charge. (Such reasoning would not be valid for the MS picture derived from recurrent ADEM). MS thrombocytes have long been known to have unusual membrane properties[37]; the MEM-LAD (macrophage electrophoretic mobility–linoleic acid depression) test brings out an anomaly in the surface membrane of MS T-lymphocytes[38]; and the erythrocyte–unsaturated fatty acid (E-UFA) test[39] shows the different arrangement of surface electrical groupings on MS red blood cells from that on normal or OND (other neurological disease) erythrocytes.

RESULTS OF E-UFA TEST (Table 2)

Table 2 E-UFA test results

| | | Concentration of UFA | |
		0.08 mg/ml LA	0.02 mg/ml
MS	LA	S	F
	AA	S	F
Non-MS	LA	F	S
	AA	F	S
'Anomalous' e.g. mother of MS:	LA	S	S
eldest daughter, etc.	AA	F	S

Note: 'Anomalous' is 'half way' between MS and normal, but shows unexpected failure to reverse with 0.02 mg/ml LA.

LA = Linoleic Acid (C18 : 2 (n–6))
AA = Arachidonic Acid (C20 : 4 (n–6))
Note clear differences between MS and non-MS subjects
S = slow: decreased RBC mobility
F = fast: increased RBC mobility
($p \ll 0.001$).
Note intermediate or 'anomalous' results and failure to reverse with LA but not AA at 0.02 mg/ml concentration. The concentrations are the final ones in the RBC suspensions. Both MS and non-MS reverse fully at 0.02 mg/ml.

Those of the MEM-LAD test have been set out in detail and follow closely those of E-UFA[39–43]. The E-UFA test has been fully confirmed in double blind trials[40,41] at the 0.08 mg/ml and 0.02 mg/ml levels. More recently Seaman *et al*[42,43] wrote 'We have been able to confirm the test for multiple sclerosis described by Field *et al* . . .', whilst emphasizing their initial scepticism. They go on to give good reasons why other, much less experienced workers[44–46], had been unable to confirm the work. 'Unless the individual operating the electrophoretic apparatus is experienced and the equipment is functioning very reliably, the small changes can readily be lost in instrument or operator "noise" '. Seaman *et al*[47] attributed the MS phenomenon to an unstable plasma factor and this we have been able to confirm thus producing an 'Office Test' for immediate diagnosis or exclusion of MS at the patient's first visit[48].

MS

The test was intended initially for the diagnosis or exclusion of MS at the first encounter with a patient referred to a neurological clinic, thus eliminating the 4 year interval which commonly elapses before a definitive diagnosis is established. Such patients may (if the general practitioner is astute or if the case is one of retrobulbar neuritis (RBN)) present only a single symptom or sign for the first time. Our earliest diagnosis has been in a patient 11 days after onset of distracting pins and needles in one arm. Such fresh cases are unlikely to be dosed with drugs which can interfere gravely with the test, since they adsorb to the surface of RBC. Currently we are compiling a 'Black Pharmacopoeia' (see below). It is of the greatest importance to learn what medicaments, both medical and herbal, the patient has been taking before testing. We have now developed methods, outside the scope of the present work, for detecting false results induced by medicamentation (Tables 3-6).

Well washed red blood cells in Hanks medium 199 (with glutamine) - PBS of known ionic strength etc. cannot be used for technical reasons - travel more slowly in an electric field when 0.08 mg/ml LA or AA is added to the ambient medium than they do when alcohol alone (the vehicle for LA and AA) is present (as control). $p \ll 0.001^2$. All non-MS RBC (normals: other neurological diseases - OND) travel more rapidly under like conditions ($p \ll 0.001$).

The importance of medicaments on the measurements made in the E-UFA test cannot be exaggerated. ACTH and prednisolone are still favourite drugs (though it is interesting to see how easy their life-long devotees have found it to abandon them in favour of the unequally proven azathioprine!). In some countries steroids may be purchased by patients themselves. The effects of ACTH are shown in Table 5. It will be seen that both MS and non-MS results can be reversed by therapeutic dosage. These materials probably adsorb to the surface of RBC (accounting for rapid clearance from plasma), and are only very slowly released over the space of about 3-4 weeks[48a]. But even more alarming is the effect of ferrous sulphate often dispensed so uncritically for 'anaemia'. It must be emphasized that iron is a potentially dangerous medicament and the cirrhosis etc. which may follow the breaking down of the body's defence against excessive intake are detailed in standard pathological works[48b]. A deliberate experiment is shown in Table 3. Not unexpectedly antibiotics, which must first attach to bacterial cell walls, also show marked affinity for RBC membranes, and again the result of exhibition of amoxil (a typical common antibiotic) to a normal subject shows the erroneous results with the E-UFA test.

Inderal-LA (not uncommonly being taken by parents of MS subjects) will give perverted results. *Very heavy* smoking shows itself clearly in the E-UFA test. Of course, quantitation of smoking on information given by the subject is notoriously an underestimate, Table 6.

It has been found in some cases that when drugs are exerting effect, reversals with 0.02 mg/ml, LA and AA does not take place; or only occurs after the washed cells have stood at 4 °C for some weeks. These phenomena will be expanded elsewhere.

All of some 300 mothers of MS patients show an unexpected anomalous

MULTIPLE SCLEROSIS: A CONCEPTUAL REAPPRAISAL

Table 3 Normal subject. Female aged 51. E-UFA test and drugs

Day	Control with alcohol	0.08 mg/ml LA	0.08 mg/ml AA	0.02 mg/ml LA	0.02 mg/ml AA	31.25 pg/ml PGE_2
1 Before FeSO$_4$	0.98 ± 0.02	1.06 ± 0.03	1.06 ± 0.03	0.87 ± 0.02	0.87 ± 0.03	1.09 ± 0.04
1 5 hours after beginning	0.99 ± 0.03	0.93 ± 0.02	0.93 ± 0.02	1.08 ± 0.03	1.07 ± 0.04	0.81 ± 0.02
4 Finish after am dose	0.99 ± 0.03	0.87 ± 0.03	0.84 ± 0.03	1.05 ± 0.04	1.06 ± 0.03	0.87 ± 0.03
6	0.98 ± 0.03	0.88 ± 0.02	0.90 ± 0.03	1.06 ± 0.04	1.05 ± 0.03	0.90 ± 0.02
8	0.98 ± 0.03	*0.95 ± 0.02	1.07 ± 0.04	1.07 ± 0.04	*0.94 ± 0.04	1.08 ± 0.02
11	0.98 ± 0.03	1.06 ± 0.03	1.07 ± 0.04	0.86 ± 0.02	0.87 ± 0.03	1.07 ± 0.04

Erythrocyte mobilities in $\mu s^{-1} v^{-1} cm^{-1}$ ± SD
Effect of ingestion of FeSO$_4$ in therapeutic dosage for 3 full days
*All changes significant at $p < 0.001$ except this, i.e. not fully recovered from iron treatment

Table 4 Normal subject. Male aged 67. E-UFA test and drugs. Therapeutic course of amoxil

Day	Control with alcohol	0.08 mg/ml LA	0.08 mg/ml AA	0.02 mg/ml LA	0.02 mg/ml AA	31.25 pg/ml PGE_2
1 Before amoxil begun Begin	0.97 ± 0.03	1.02 ± 0.03	1.06 ± 0.03	0.88 ± 0.02	0.87 ± 0.03	1.06 ± 0.02
3	0.98 ± 0.03	0.90 ± 0.02	0.87 ± 0.03	1.07 ± 0.03	1.06 ± 0.03	1.08 ± 0.03
7 —Finish						
8	0.97 ± 0.02	0.86 ± 0.02	0.86 ± 0.02	1.06 ± 0.04	1.05 ± 0.03	1.04 ± 0.03
11	0.97 ± 0.03	0.88 ± 0.03	0.89 ± 0.03	1.06 ± 0.02	1.07 ± 0.03	1.08 ± 0.02
14	0.97 ± 0.03	1.07 ± 0.03	1.05 ± 0.02	0.88 ± 0.03	0.88 ± 0.02	1.07 ± 0.04

Erythrocyte mobilities in $\mu s^{-1} v^{-1} cm^{-1}$ ± SD
Amoxil oral, 7 days
All changes significant at $p < 0.001$

Table 5 Effect of ACTH treatment

Patient		Days of treatment	% change	
			LA	AA
MS				
M.Sh. (F) 24		Before	− 11.82	− 12.15
		12	+ 5.73	+ 5.43
		20	+ 6.33	+ 6.23
		Finish		
		20	− 14.06	− 14.06

ACTH begun 80 U/day for 5 days; 60 U for 5 days; 30 U for 8 days; 10 U for 5 days; 5 U for 5 days

OND				
A.G. (F) 46		6	+ 5.38	+ 5.68
		23	− 12.53	− 10.30
(mother not		30	− 7.54	− 9.55
anomalous)	Finish	37	− 10.67	− 10.37
A.G. not MS	Days	7	− 9.85	− 9.35
	After	14	− 11.57	− 11.67
		21	+ 5.34	+ 5.64

Treatment (15 days × 80 U) + (7 days × 60 U) + (7 days × 40 U) + (7 days × 20 U)

All results significant $p<0.001$. Student's t-test with 39 degrees of freedom: Control (alcohol) vs. either LA or AA (in alcohol). Mean mobility in both directions of current. Seven MS patients have been followed through an ACTH course, one OND (subacute combined degeneration of the cord).
Solid underline = normal type result
Broken underline = MS type result

G.O. M 28

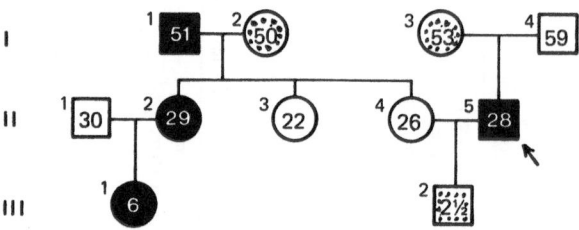

Figure 1 MS family in which II (5) is the male propositus (marked ✝). His mother, I (3), was the customary red circle; his wife, II (4), normal but the son, III (2) was a red square. This led to a further search and an eldest sister of the child's mother, II (2), was found to be detained in a hospital because of aggressive and antisocial behaviour. She gave a positive E–UFA test; her mother, as expected, I (2), was a red circle; her father, I (1), was a 'silent' MS; and her daughter, III (1), gave a positive E–UFA result. This illustrates (a) how proximity of two MS results leads to occurrence of a red square and the need for further search if a red square is found; (b) how MS may come in from both sides of a family. This is not really very surprising when (for example the North of England) about 1 in 800–1000 persons is suffering from MS.

Table 6 E-UFA test – Smokers

Name	Sex	Age	Smoking details given by subjects	Control with alcohol	0.08 mg/ml LA	0.08 mg/ml AA	0.02 mg/ml LA	0.02 mg/ml AA	31.25 pg/ml PGE_2
AS	M	43	20–25/day for 20 years	0.77 ± 0.02	0.85 ± 0.02	0.84 ± 0.03	0.86 ± 0.02	0.85 ± 0.02	1.08 ± 0.03
MH	F	51	40–75/day for 30 years	0.86 ± 0.02	0.78 ± 0.02	0.79 ± 0.02	0.81 ± 0.03	0.78 ± 0.02	1.07 ± 0.03
KG	F	79	40/day for 40 years	0.89 ± 0.03	0.82 ± 0.02	0.81 ± 0.03	0.82 ± 0.02	0.82 ± 0.03	1.08 ± 0.04
WJ	M	71	40/day for 50 years	0.92 ± 0.03	0.77 ± 0.03	0.78 ± 0.02	0.78 ± 0.02	0.77 ± 0.03	1.08 ± 0.04
EJ	F	33	20–30/day for 6 years	0.98 ± 0.04	0.91 ± 0.03	0.86 ± 0.02	0.87 ± 0.03	0.86 ± 0.03	1.08 ± 0.04
AM	F	60	20/day for 20 years	0.96 ± 0.03	1.03 ± 0.03	1.02 ± 0.03	0.86 ± 0.03	0.87 ± 0.04	1.07 ± 0.03

It will be seen that the really heavy smokers produce a change in the control electrophoretic mobility; and that, in general, reactivity with LA and AA is abnormal except in case AS. Curiously all tested showed normal PGE_2 reaction (see text) reaction. Their RBCs travel more slowly with LA, and more rapidly than control with AA ($p \ll 0.001$). A similar anomalous finding occurs with the great majority of elder daughters. Such females are called 'red circles': they can never develop MS themselves but can become the mothers of MS offspring.

'Red squares' (i.e. anomalous males) are relatively rare, but almost without exception ($\chi^2 < 0.01$) are found only when there are two MS subjects (overt or occasional covert) amongst the near relatives (Figure 1).

CLINICALLY 'PROBABLE' MS WITH NEGATIVE E–UFA RESULT

If very early cases are studied Fog's admission[4] (agreed by others with very extensive experience of the beguiling early presentation of MS) must be borne in mind. 'In my opinion the percentage of false diagnosis of MS is about 20% ... [and] is in both directions ... as long as the CSF is excluded.' Broman[49] has pointed out that if 'we wait 5–10 years the figures of false diagnosis will be much less than 20%'. Bauer[50] (*loc. cit.*) found 'a little over 5% (out of 1000 cases) remained questionable even after 12 years'.

There is a small but clear group of cases of neurosarcoidosis which may mimic MS closely and, indeed, be revealed only at autopsy[13]. Some are limited to the CNS and do not give a positive Kveim test[14], rendering diagnosis especially difficult even on CSF examination. The test described by Field and Caspary[51] can detect such cases, but a careful history is of paramount importance. Indeed, with increasing experience, the late Henry Miller's warning to beware of making a diagnosis of MS 'if the history is not right', gains added force. This is especially true of the group of E–UFA negative cases which *are recurrent ADEM*[52,53]. We have several of these and there is often a significantly different onset of the *first* attack from that in the true classical MS[54]. Introductory infections, especially respiratory, high temperature, periods of coma, or stupor, midbrain signs and so on must be carefully enquired for.

Hysteria (emphasized so forcibly by Charcot in his Leçons du Mardi), meralgia paraesthetica, carpal and other tunnel syndromes, migraine with marked somaesthetic manifestations have all been amongst the patients referred to us by their doctors as examples of MS together with cases in which psychiatric symptoms, especially depression, has been a presenting feature. Indeed, some 0.5–1.0% of MS cases appear first before the psychiatrist (personal communication by Dr H. L. Field).

Recurrent ADEM is distinguished from classical MS by testing of the mother (if available) or, less satisfactorily, the patient's children, especially an eldest daughter. In classical MS the mothers will always be a 'red circle' (except in the relatively few cases where she, herself, is MS). In recurrent ADEM the mother will be normal. The great majority of first daughters (and it is important to ask if there has been an antecedent miscarriage) are 'red circles'.

CLASSICAL MS

Here the patient shows slowing of RBC with 0.08 mg/ml LA and AA; increased speed with 0.02 mg/ml acids; and reduced RBC mobility in the presence of 31.25 pg/ml PGE_2. Non-MS RBC travel more rapidly under these circumstances. ($p \ll 0.001$).

In the histological section it was pointed out that MS thrombocytes, lymphocytes and RBCs have unusual membrane properties as brought out by their electrical charge in the presence of LA and AA, and that this difference from non-MS might be attributed to abnormal handling of unsaturated EFA. Our electrical measurements tell us only about the net negative charge on the membrane but nothing of the material rearrangement. However, from the point of view of electrostatic attractions between adjacent myelin lamellae (see Figure 1) these surface groupings must be of paramount importance. Indeed, there may be considerable internal variation in actual chemical make up in both MS and non-MS myelin within defined limits (ordinary biological variation) but when boundary conditions are overstepped the pathological state ensues. The important notion of variability has been emphasized by Bernsohn[55].

If now this anomaly is generalized to *all* cells of the body to include oligo-dendrocytes then central myelin, being largely made from the surface extensions of these cells around axons (with addition of certain materials, notably cholesterol), we would expect unusual myelin to be formed in MS. It is possible that the new surface molecular configurations on the oligodendrocyte

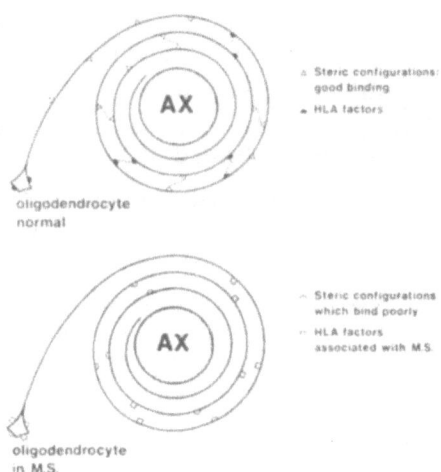

Figure 2 Hypothetical scheme which bases the origin of MS (a scattered localized disintegration of myelin sheaths within the CNS) in a poor stabilization of adjacent lamellae dependent upon reduced electrostatic binding charges between surface groupings following from altered oliogodendrocyte surfaces. The possible contribution of certain HLA haplotypes may also be involved (if present in the lamellae).

surface are unable to offer good electrostatic attractive forces between adjacent lamellae upon which the integrity of normal, tightly wound myelin depends (Figure 2). Under these conditions the myelin might persist for years – indeed, for a lifetime; but it is relatively unstable as compared with normal myelin and may, in response to some identifiable external stimulus (e.g. trauma, nearby antigen–antibody interaction, temporary platelet accumulation[56], puerperium, etc.) or even 'spontaneously' begin to unwind, i.e. disintegrate to produce the local destruction we call 'plaques'. The stimulus to such disintegration would appear to emanate from, or be associated with, small blood vessels – so that perivascular initial lesions are encountered. When such 'unwinding' or slippage of myelin lamellae occurs it will do so along the intraperiod line – the original oligodendrocyte surface.

A further interesting speculation is that certain HLA groupings contribute to the electrostatic forces holding adjacent lamellae whilst certain others (those associated with MS) may not do so (see Figure 2). In this way it is possible to offer an explanation for the association of certain 'non-binding' haplotypes more frequently than randomly expected with MS.

SUMMARY OF NEW CONCEPT OF MS

(1) MS is a syndrome rather than a single disease entity of uniform aetiopathogenesis. (Table 7)

(2) A few MS pictures may be mimicked by sarcoidosis; meralgia paraesthetica; somaesthetic migraine, etc.

(3) A small proportion are the result of recurrences of ADEM as discussed in detail by van Bogaert[52], Miller and Evans[53] and others.

(4) The vast majority of true MS pictures is due to 'Abiotrophy' of white matter. MS is a generalized disease of the central nervous system with focal perivascular myelin breakdown.

(5) Once breakdown has occurred 'spontaneously' it may be continued intermittently by an EAE-like process, though fresh lesions may occur from primary breakdown in new areas.

(6) Breakdown products of brain tissue are clearly not enough *per se* to induce an ongoing intermittent immunological process of focal degeneration in the brain; otherwise MS would follow with much greater frequency on injury or surgical intervention in the CNS. Some homeostatic mechanism must ordinarily be at work and possibly defective in MS.

(7) Children who are born disadvantaged with respect to UFA handling require more EFA. Human milk contains seven times as much linolenic acid as does cow's milk[57]. It may well be that the industrialized 40–60° latitude MS belt coincides with the region where breast feeding is least. Since the critical age for myelination is up to about 5 years, operation of the uncorrected biochemical defect in handling UFA during this

Table 7 Multiple sclerosis as a syndrome

Mimicry	Hysteria; somaesthetic migraine; meralgia paraesthetica; neurosarcoidosis. E–UFA − ve: mother not a red circle.
Recurrent ADEM (vs. Bogaert; McAlpine; Miller and Evans etc.)	E–UFA − ve: mother not a red circle
Neuromyelitis Optica (Devic)	E–UFA − ve: mother not a red circle
Behçet's disease	E–UFA − ve
Classical MS (Great majority) History (!)	E–UFA + ve: mother a red circle.

NB   Beware drugs and health store products; heavy smoking; $FeSO_4$; ACTH and steroids; SSO γ -linolenate; Inderal-LA β -blockers; etc.
Enquire carefully and note for a 'Black Pharmacopoeia'

period will be crucial. This 5 year period is precisely that which epidemiologists find to be significant in migration studies from high to low risk areas (e.g. Germany to Israel)[58].

IMPLICATIONS FOR THERAPY AND PREVENTION OF MS

Classical MS

All children born into an MS family should be tested for inheritance of pathological handling of UFA as early as feasible so that it may be corrected[59] and the γ-linolenate therapy should certainly be continued until the age of twenty, and in the absence of precise knowledge of turnover of myelin constituents in the adult human, it should be continued throughout life. Fortunately, other beneficial effects are accredited to this food supplement (e.g. upon cholesterol levels in blood) and, indeed, many people subject to stress take it as a routine. Whether therapy begun once the disease has manifested itself is of benefit is unknown. Anecdotally we have many highly successful cases but they are not controlled, and a (lesser) number can be matched by those who have done badly. A note of warning should be added in dealing with students and other young people who 'enlarge their experience' (as they put it) by using hallucinogenic drugs. These drugs have a direct damaging effect upon myelin[60] and such patients do badly.

'Almost insuperable difficulties surround any trial of therapy in MS'[61]. The present writer would omit the word 'almost'. A meaningful trial is, however, relatively easily established with young children who are candidates for MS as picked out in family studies; for there, the development or non-development of MS is a criterion. It is hoped that such a trial (already begun by us) will be continued and enlarged.

Tallis[61] gives a useful discussion of modern attempts at MS treatment and maintains that 'the therapeutic career of PUFAs in MS is by no means at an end'. We agree.

Recurrent ADEM

Foci of infection which might give adjuvants[62-64] should be eradicated, and attempts made to limit respiratory infections perhaps by large Vitamin C dosage (Pauling). Here immunosuppression therapy may be of value. There have, of course, been many attempts to determine an optimum regimen, combined or unitary, of immunosuppressive drugs. It is, however, remarkable that associated with γ-macroglobulin fraction of serum is a *physiological* suppressor able to prevent lymphocytes from interacting with an antigen first described by Cooperband et al[65] and since receiving inadequate attention. Much of this material is a by-product in IgG preparation, and in the writer's opinion deserves immediate attention. The suggestion by Field and Shenton[66] that attempts should be made to harness it for therapeutic purposes does not yet seem to have been acted upon, though analytical work has proceeded[67].

Another remarkable feature of T-lymphocyte suppression is the effect of total thymectomy. This procedure leads to very rapid disappearance of thymosin from the blood[68,69] which persists for considerable periods. Whilst thymectomy is not an operation to be contemplated lightly, and is not always total, the production of a monoclonal antibody to thymosin might be a way forward. In short, there should be more attempt made to co-operate with natural suppressor mechanisms rather than reliance placed upon essentially toxic drugs.

ACKNOWLEDGEMENTS

The author would like to express his deep gratitude to Miss Greta Joyce AILMS, upon whose very extensive electrophoretic mobility measurements the ideas brought forward in this work are based. The Naomi Bramson Trust supported this work throughout and a contribution from ARMS (Multiple Sclerosis Research) Ltd is acknowledged.

References

1. Firth, D. (1948). *The Case of Augustus d'Esté*. (Cambridge: Cambridge University Press)
2. Charcot, J-M. (1868). Histologie de la sclérose en plaques. *Gaz. Hôp. (Paris)*, **41**, 554
3. Charcot, J-M. (1872–1873). *Leçons sur les Maladies du Système Nerveux faites à Salpêtrière*. (Paris: Delahaye)
4. Fog, T. (1974). The International Symposium of Multiple Sclerosis: Göteborg, September 1972. *Acta Neurol. Scand.*, **50**, 63
5. Georgi, W. (1961). Multiple Sklerose: Pathologischanatomische Befunde multipler Sklerose bei klinisch nicht diagnostizierten Krankheiten. *Schweiz. Med. Wochenschr.*, **91**, 605
6. Ghatak, N.R., Hirano, A., Littmaer, H. and Zimmerman, H. (1974). Asymptomatic demyelinated plaque. *Arch. Neurol.*, **30**, 484
7. Castaigne, P., L'Hermitte, F., Escourelle, R., Hauw, J.J., Gray, F. and Lyon-Caen, O. (1981). Les scléroses en plaques asymptomatiques. *Rev. Neurol. (Paris)*, **137**, 729
8a. Ehrlich, P. and Morgenroth, J. (1901). Ueber Hämolysine V. *Berl. Klin. Wschr.*, **38**, 251–254
8b. Kurland, L.T. (1952). Epidemiologic Characteristics of Multiple Sclerosis. *Am. J. Med.*, **12**, 561

9. Field, E. J. (1975). The Brain and Nervous System in Allergic Disease. In Gell, P. G. H., Coombs, R. R. A. and Lachmann, P. J. (eds.). *Clinical Aspects of Immunology*, pp. 1545–1586. (Oxford, London, Edinburgh, Melbourne: Blackwell Scientific Publication)

10. Daniel, P. (1972). Profil virologique de la sclérose en plaques. *Nouv. Pr. Med.*, **1**, 1939

11. Field, E. J., Caspary, E. A., Shenton, B. K. and Madgwick, H. (1973). Lymphocyte sensitization after exposure to measles and influenza. Possible relevance to pathogenesis of Multiple Sclerosis. *J. Neurol. Sci.*, **19**, 179

12. Sever, J. L. and Madden, D. L. (1979). Viruses that do not cause Multiple Sclerosis. In Boese, A. (ed.). *Search for the Cause of Multiple Sclerosis and other Chronic diseases of the central nervous system*, pp. 414–424. First International Symposium of Hertie Foundation. Frankfurt/Main. Verlag Chemie Weinheim. Deerfield Beach, Florida. Basel

13. Zollinger, H. U. (1941). Groszellig-granulomatöse Lymphangitis cerebri (Morbus Boeck) unter dem Bilde einer multiplen Sklerose verlaufend. *Virch. Arch.*, **307**, 597

14. Matthews, W. B. (1979). Neurosarcoidosis. In Vinken, P. J. and Bruyn, G. W. (eds.). *Handbook of Clinical Neurology; Neurological Manifestations of Systemic Diseases; Part I* pp. 521–542. (Amsterdam, New York, Oxford: North Holland)

15. Thompson, R. H. S. (1966). A biochemical approach to the problem of Multiple Sclerosis. *Proc. R. Soc. Med.*, **59**, 269

16. Thompson, R. H. S. (1973). Fatty acid metabolism in Multiple Sclerosis. *Biochem. Soc. Symp.*, **35**, 103

17. Gowers, W. R. (1902). A Lecture on Abiotrophy. *Lancet*, **i**, 1003

18. Charcot, J-M. (1872–1873). *Lecons sur les Maladies du Systeme Nerveux faites à la Salpétrière.* pp. 1887–1888 (Paris: Delahaye)

19. Féré, C. H. (1884). La famille névropathique. In Publiée sous la direction de J-M. Charcot. *Archives de Neurologie*. Vol. 7, pp. 1–43 (Paris: Bureaux du Progrès Médical)

20. Revington, G. T. (1889). The Neuropathic Diathesis, or the Diathesis of the Degenerate. *J. Mental Sci.*, **34**, 33

21. McAlpine, D. (1932). Acute disseminated encephalomyelitis. *Lancet*, **i**, 846

22. Waksman, B. H. (1959). Experimental Allergic Encephalomyelitis and the 'Auto-Allergic' Diseases. *Int. Arch. Allerg. Appl. Immunol.*, **14**, (Suppl.), 1

23. Ferraro, A. and Davidoff, L. M. (1928). The Reaction of the Oligodendroglia to injury of the brain. *Arch. Path.*, **6**, 1030

24. Field, E. J. (1957). Histogenesis of compound granular corpuscles in the mouse brain after trauma and a note on the influence of cortisone. *J. Neuropath. Exp. Neurol.*, **8**, 48

25. Charcot, J-M. (1872–1873). *Lecons sur les Maladies du Système Nerveux faites à la Salpétrière.* pp. 196–219. (Paris: Delahaye)

26. Borst, M. (1903). Die multiple Sklerose des Zentralnerven systems. *Ergeb. Allgemein. Path.*, **9**, 67

27. Bielschowsky, M. (1903). Zur Histologie der multiplen Sklerose. *Neurol. Zbl.*, **22**, 770

28. Müller, E. (1904). *Die Multiple Sklerose des Gehirns und Ruckenmarks.* (Jena: Fischer)

29. Anton, G. and Wohlwill, F. (1912). Multiple nicht eitrige Encephalomyelitis und Multiple Sklerose. *Z. Ges Neurol. Psychiat.*, **12**, 31

30. Dawson, J. W. (1916). The histology of disseminated sclerosis. *Trans. R. Soc. Edinburgh.*, **50**, 517

31. Adams, R. D. and Kublik, C. S. (1952). The morbid anatomy of the demyelinating disease. *Am. J. Med.*, **12**, 510

32. Jacob, H. (1969). Tissue process in Multiple Sclerosis and para-infections and post vaccinal encephalomyelitis. Int. Arch. Allergy., **36**, (Suppl.) 22

33. Field, E. J. (1967). The significance of astrologial hypertrophy in scrapie, kuru, multiple sclerosis and old age, together with a note on the possible nature of the scrapie agent. *Dtsch. Z. Nervenhelk.*, **192**, 265

34. Lumsden, C. E. (1970). The neuropathology of multiple sclerosis. In Vinken, P. J. and Bruyn, G. W. (eds.). *Handbook of Clinical Neurology*. Vol. 9, pp. 217–309 (Amsterdam, New York, Oxford: North Holland)

35. Allen, I. V. and McKeown, S. R. (1979). A histological biochemical study of the macroscopically normal white matter in Multiple Sclerosis. *J. Neurol. Sci.*, **41**, 81

36. Allen, I. V., Glover, G. and Anderson, R. (1981). Abnormalities in the macroscopically normal white matter in cases of mild or spinal Multiple Sclerosis (MS). *Acta Neuropath.*, **VII**, (Suppl.), 176

37. Bolton, C. H., Hampton, J. R. and Phillipson, O. T. (1968). Platelet behaviour and plasma phospholipids in Multiple Sclerosis. *Lancet,* i, 99
38. Field, E. J., Shenton, B. K. and Joyce, G. (1974). Specific laboratory test for diagnosis of Multiple Sclerosis. *Brit. Med. J.,* 1, 412
39. Field, E. J., Joyce, G. and Smith, B. M. (1977). Erythrocyte–UFA (E–UFA) Mobility Test for Multiple Sclerosis: Implications for Pathogenesis and Handling of the Disease. *J. Neurol.,* 214, 113
40. Bisaccia, G., Caputo, D. and Zibetti, A. (1977). E–UFA test in Multiple Sclerosis. *Boll. 1st. Sieroter. Milan.* 56, 583
41. Caputo, D., Zibetti, A., Ghezzi, A., Cazzullo, C. L., Frosio, C. and Bertoni, G. (1979). Erythrocyte unsaturated fatty acid test (E–UFA): A biological test to detect optic neuritis as initial feature of multiple sclerosis. *J. Neurol.,* 221, 53
42. Seaman, G. V. F., Swank, R. L., Tamblyn, C. H. and Zukoski, C. F. (1979). Simplified red cell electrophoretic mobility test for Multiple Sclerosis. *Lancet,* i, 1138
43. Tamblyn, C. H., Swank, R. L., Seaman, G. V. P. and Zukoski, C. F. (1980). Red cell electrophoretic mobility test for early diagnosis of Multiple Sclerosis. *Neurol. Res.,* 2, 69
44. Stoof, J. C., Vrijmoed-de Vries, M. C., Koetsier, J. C. and Langevoort, H. L. (1977). Evaluation of the red cell cytopherometric test for the diagnosis of MS. *Acta. Neurol. Scand.,* 56, 170
45. Hawkins, S. A. and Millar, J. H. F. (1979). Erythrocyte electrophoretic mobility test for Multiple Sclerosis. *Lancet,* i, 165
46. Forrester, J. A. and Smith, W. J. (1977). Screening of children at risk of Multiple Sclerosis. *Lancet,* ii, 453
47. Seaman, G. V. F., Swank, R. L. and Zukoski, C. F. (1979). Red-cell membrane differences in Multiple Sclerosis are acquired from plasma. *Lancet,* i, 1139
48. Field, E. J. and Joyce, G. (1982). An office test for Multiple Sclerosis. *IRCS Med. Sci.,* 10, 560
48a. Field, E. J. and Joyce, G. (1981). Simplified E–UFA Test for Multiple Sclerosis (MS): Some Sources of 'False' Results. *J. Neurol.,* 226, 149–155
48b. Robbins, S. L. and Cotran, R. S. (1979). Systemic diseases – Iron Storage Disorders. In *Pathologic Basis of Disease.* p. 345 (Philadelphia, London, Toronto: W. B. Saunders)
49. Broman, T. L. (1974). The International Symposium of Multiple Sclerosis: Göteborg September 1972. *Acta Neurol. Scand.,* 50, 64
50. Bauer, H. (1974). The International Symposium of Multiple Sclerosis: Göteborg September 1972. *Acta Neurol. Scand.,* 50, 64
51. Field, E. J. and Caspary, E. A. (1971). Lymphocyte sensitization in sarcoidosis. *Br. Med. J.,* 2, 143
52. van Bogaert, L. (1950). Post-infectious encephalomyelitis and Multiple Sclerosis. *J. Neuropath. Exp. Neurol.,* 9, 219
53. Miller, H. G. and Evans, M. J. (1954). Prognosis in Acute Disseminated Encephalomyelitis with a note on Neuromyelitis Optica. *Q. J. Med.,* 22, 347
54. McAlpine, D. (1946). The problem of disseminated sclerosis. *Brain,* 69, 233
55. Bernsohn, J. and Stephanides, L. M. (1967). Aetiology of Multiple Sclerosis. *Nature,* 215, 821
56. Putnam, T. J. and Adler, A. (1937). Vascular architecture of the lesions of Multiple Sclerosis. *Arch. Neurol.* (Chicago), 38, 1
57. Field, E. J. (1979). Multiple Sclerosis: treatment and prophylaxis. *J. R. Soc. Med.,* 72, 487
58. Leibowitz, U. and Alter, M. (1973). Epidemiologic characteristics of Multiple Sclerosis. In *Multiple Sclerosis – clue to its cause.* (Amsterdam, London: North Holland)
59. Field, E. J. and Joyce, G. (1978). Effect of prolonged ingestion of γ–linolenate by MS patients. *Eur. Neurol.,* 17, 67
60. Carnegie, P. R., Smythies, J. R., Caspary, E. A. and Field, E. J. (1972). Interaction of Hallucinogenic drugs with encephalitogenic protein of myelin. *Nature,* 240, 561
61. Tallis, R. C. (1980). Some recent advances in the clinical aspects of Multiple Sclerosis. *Neuropath. Appl. Neurobiol.,* 6, 325
62. Burky, E. L. (1933). Production of lens sensitivity in rabbits by the action of staphylococcus toxin. *Proc. Soc. Exp. Biol.,* NY, 31, 445

63. Burky, E. L. (1934). The production in the rabbit of hypersensitive reactions to lens, rabbit muscle and low ragweed extracts by the action of staphylococcus toxin. *Allergy,* **5,** 466

64. Cavelti, P. A. and Cavelti, E. S. (1945). Studies on the pathogenesis of Glomerulonephritis. I. Production of autoantibodies to kidney in experimental animals. *Arch. Path.,* **39,** 148

65. Cooperband, S. R., Bondevik, H., Schmid, K. and Mannick, J. A. (1968). Transformation of human lymphocytes: Inhibition by homologous alpha globulin. *Science,* **159,** 1243

66. Field, E. J. and Shenton, B. K. (1973). Effect of fatty acids on lymphocyte activity. *Br. Med. J.,* **4,** 738

67. Ford, W. H., Caspary, E. A. and Shenton, B. K. (1973). Purification and properties of a lymphocyte inhibition factor from human serum. *Clin. Exp. Immunol.,* **15,** 169

68. Field, E. J., Bates, D., Shaw, D. A., Griffin, S. G., Shenton, B. K. and Smith, J. K. (1973). Lymphocyte sensitization in myasthenia gravis: function of the adult thymus gland. *Lancet,* **ii,** 675

69. Meyer-Rienecker, H. J., Ernst, K., Gundlach, J., Shenton, B. K. and Field, E. J. (1975). Prognosis after thymectomy for Myasthenia Gravis: A laboratory test? *IRCS Med. Sci.,* **3,** 105

70. Jenssen, H. L., Meyer-Rienecker, H. J., Köhler, H. and Gunther, J. (1976). The linoleic acid depression (LAD) test for multiple sclerosis using the macrophage electrophoretic mobility (MEM) test. *Acta Neurol. Scand.,* **53,** 51

71. Jones, R., Capildeo, R., Rose, C. F., Forrester, J. A., Luckman, N. P. and Preece, A. W. (1981). A diagnostic test for multiple sclerosis using glutaraldehyde fixed erythrocytes and laser cytopherometry. In Preece, A. W. and Light, P. A. (eds.). *Cell Electrophoresis in Cancer and other Clinical Research.* pp. 189–195. (Elsevier, Amsterdam: North Holland)

72. Field, E. J. and Joyce, G. (1977). Prostaglandin (PGE_2) and human erythrocyte mobility: a specific test for Multiple Sclerosis? *IRCS Med. Sci.,* **5,** 158

66
A rarely reported multifocal demyelinating disease: pancreatic encephalopathy

J. M. BRUCHER, Y. DE SMET and R. E. GONSETTE

The literature[1] contains very few pathological reports on pancreatic encephal-opathy (PE). The histological pattern seems to be specific and presents some resemblance to that of multiple sclerosis (MS), i.e. disseminated, patchy, often perivenular loss of myelin, occasional perivascular haemorrhages, moderate gliosis and no axonal destruction.

Reporting two cases of PE the authors emphasize the ability of enzymes to destroy myelin either directly, a hypothesis already suggested by Joseph Baló as far back as 1940 in a case of diffuse sclerosis of the Schilder type[2], or indirectly through released fatty acids, a recent hypothesis sustained by the evidence for subacute fat embolism as the cause of MS[3].

On the other hand, the undoubted occurrence of myelinotoxic factors cir-culating in the blood in MS and EAE[4] in the presence of a lowered blood–brain barrier might well be of significance in the development or extension of demyelinating lesions. Thus the old concept that the demyelination in MS is due to vascular features should not be rejected.

References

1. Sharf, B. and Levy, N. (1976). In Vinken, P. J. and Bruyn, G. W. (eds.). *Handbook of Clinical Neurology*. Vol. 27, i, pp. 449–458. (Amsterdam: North-Holland)
2. Baló, J. (1940). *J. Belge Neurol. Psych.*, **40**, 160–168
3. James, P. B. (1982). *Lancet*, **i**, 380–386
4. Grundke-Iqbal, I. and Bornstein, M. B. (1979). *Brain Res.*, **160**, 489–503

67
Plaques, necrotic myelopathy and Rosenthal fibre reaction: glial pathology in MS

P. C. BLUMBERGS and J. F. HALLPIKE

A 49 year-old white male came to necropsy after a closely studied 5 year course that seemed typical of a severe disseminated type of MS, progressive from outset. The neuropathological findings included: (1) MS plaques of varying chronicity in optic nerves, cerebrum, brainstem, cerebellum and spinal cord, (2) necrotic myelopathy, (3) numerous foci of intense Rosenthal fibre formation related to plaques and myelopathy and (4) paucity of perivenular and leptomeningeal cellularity. A subacute, progressive, pattern of MS in this case appears to be linked with degenerative/reactionary changes in astrocytic glial cells.

68
Comments on MS-compensation in West Germany

H. J. BAUER

Compensation for MS patients remains a dilemma if legislation requires any form of proof that there is a causal relationship between the manifestation or exacerbation of the demyelinating process and a noxious exogenic influence. This is a worldwide problem, especially in the case of war veterans and members of armed forces.

The MS-compensation situation that presents itself in West Germany, I think, is typical of the attempt to invoke at least a certain degree of logic in arriving at a conclusion, and to provide a legal basis for the moral obligation to help people who have had the misfortune of acquiring MS during military service, imprisonment, the particular hardships of war or – rarely – in the wake of injuries and noxious occupational influences.

I was not able to obtain from the responsible ministry official figures on the number of persons receiving compensation for MS acquired in connection with military service, but Professor Firnhaber and I collected 800 cases from the compensation files of World War II back in 1960. On the other hand, the German occupational insurance central agency (*Hauptverband der Berufsgenossenschaften*) could not name a single case of compensation granted for MS in connection with an occupational hazard. The problem of compensation for MS in West Germany is largely limited to military personnel, war veterans and the victims of political and racial persecution. The reason for this becomes evident in view of the accepted prerequisites for compensation.

Under West German legislation, the probability of a causal relationship is required between the acute manifestation or exacerbation of MS in close time relationship with severe hardships, injury or strain. For this statement to be meaningful, the two terms 'close time relationship' and 'severe strain or injury' require definition. A purely arbitrary period of 8 months is considered as the largest acceptable interval between the occurrence of severe strain or injury and the manifestation or exacerbation of MS. Admittedly, this is a criterion without any scientific basis whatsoever; I think it must be interpreted as a compromise between divergent medical opinions and administrative discretion. Severe injury or strain may implicate numerous things: serious

364

battle wounds, injuries due to accidents and resulting complications, severe exposure to cold, wet, heat, solar radiation or other physical duress, extreme exhaustion and fatigue, severe malnutrition, acute illness during critical situations, hardships of imprisonment and under certain conditions extreme psychomental strain and abuse.

A person is entitled to compensation if compatible with current knowledge concerning the disease, the probability of a causal relationship is greater than the lack of any connection with noxious exogenic influences. Taking into account the uncertainty concerning the aetiology and many aspects of the pathogenesis of MS, the law does not require proof, but the possibility of a causal connection is not adequate for compensation. However, as we all know, in most cases it is impossible to establish probability on a scientifically sound basis, and that is why so many protracted law suits result.

In view of this, West German legislation has introduced the *Kann-Versorgung*, the possibility to grant compensation if a sufficiently close time relationship can be established, even if there is doubt concerning the pathogenetic significance of the alleged noxious influence. This in a certain sense implies an *in dubio pro aegroti* decision; the lack of scientific knowledge concerning the disease is not to be the reason for denying compensation.

In West Germany this is in fact what most medical opinions concerning MS and compensation boil down to: the establishment of an acceptable time relationship. But here also it is often difficult to obtain reliable information in one or the other direction. Unquestionably, many initial manifestations have not been noticed, so that a close time relationship which actually existed cannot be adequately documented. On the other hand, the doubtful character of statements given under oath many years after the alleged noxious influence often poses a dilemma which is difficult to resolve.

Despite these difficulties, the *Kann-Versorgung* has provided a fairly useful instrument for handling the compensation problems in MS in a more liberal way. However, this modality is restricted to military personnel, conscientious objectors during conscript service in some civilian area, prisoners and persecuted individuals and persons with a communicable disease subject to compulsory supervision, such as tuberculosis. It is not applicable in the area of social insurance and especially in dealing with occupational hazards. This is one of the reasons why there are virtually no cases of MS-compensation in industrial medicine.

A special problem is posed by the manifestation of MS, occurrence of bouts or exacerbations following vaccinations. The problem has lost some of its major importance since smallpox vaccination is no longer obligatory; the two principal types of vaccination, in which the question of compensation arises, are rabies and poliomyelitis.

Rabies, the classical example of postvaccinal encephalomyelitis, usually poses no problems concerning the initial relationships, but recurrent encephalomyelitis – although not accepted as a sequel of vaccination according to accepted knowledge – raises some puzzling and pathogenetically possibly important questions. Can rabies vaccination initiate a relapsing–remitting type of encephalomyelitis, or are cases of this type already existing MS, in which the vaccination has triggered the activity of the demyelinating process?

In the past 2 years I have seen two cases of relapsing–remitting encephalo-myelitis following rabies vaccination. When an acute episode of the encephalomyelitis, for which he was receiving compensation, recurred, one of these patients tried to commit suicide by shooting a rifle bullet into his mouth. He suffered a moderate brain concussion, peripheral facial palsy and sensory disturbances, but the bullet did not enter the skull and his brain escaped critical injury. He was rehabilitated fairly well by surgery and physiotherapy, had one or two moderate bouts subsequent to the shot injury, but has been stable for more than a year now.

Much more dubious than in rabies are the cases of an alleged causal con-nection to polio vaccination. I presume that there is a fairly good consensus to the effect, that only those cases deserve serious consideration in whom an exacerbation occurs within an incubation period of not more than 3–4 weeks, and in whom the demonstration of transient titre elevations has been achieved. These are general prerequisites with respect to other vaccinations as well.

The question of post-vaccinal and para-infectious encephalomyelitis, which at the turn of our century pointed the way to some of the basic concepts con-cerning immune phenomena in MS, has been largely neglected in the immediate past. It appears desirable to devote more attention to such cases, especially in view of the new tools available in the scientific analysis of immune phenomena in MS. This is a classical area of clinical research which may reveal facts providing new insight into pathogenetic features of MS.

69
Multiple sclerosis and CT: a correlative study – preliminary results (43 cases)

M. T. IBA-ZIZEN, O. LYON-CAEN, E. ROULLET, J. TAMRAZ,
R. MARTEAU, E. A. CABANIS and F. LHERMITTE

MATERIAL AND METHODS

Forty-three patients (25 females) aged between 22–55 years old, all of them attending the Neuropsychological department (Professor F. Lhermitte), present a 'definite' MS disease: these patients have a CT examination (ND 8000 CGR, X-ray department, Dr E. A. Cabanis). The NOP (neuro-ocular-plane) orientation is the constant cephalic plane adopted. CT are performed after iodine i.v. injection (2 ml/kg).

RESULTS

Nine of the patients presented CT visible plaques; 21 of them had a cortical atrophy (three cerebellar); two large demyelination CT signs and ten showed atheromatous vascular curlings.

Optic nerves (in NOP, physiological study, coronal examination) presented densitometric alterations in seven cases (one 'railway' picture); 13 patients had a retrobulbar hyperdensity (CRA ?). Average diameter equalled 3 mm (± 1 mm).

DISCUSSION

One fact must be pointed out: the double-blind study without a clinical report in the preliminary series. We know how reduced the plaques may be, and how poor are the anatomical and clinical correlations. A second point is the low frequency of isolated plaques in comparison with the severity of the disease and the absence of optic nerve CT-lesion in the case of VEP disturbances. In all these cases, we hope the NMR approach will help.

70
Multiple sclerosis and CT: a correlative study – preliminary results (39 cases)

M. T. IBA-ZIZEN, E. ROULLET, M. H. RIGOLET, J. TAMRAZ,
O. LYON-CAEN, R. MARTEAU, E. A. CABANIS and F. LHERMITTE

INTRODUCTION

Computerized tomography (CT) visualization of the optic nerve is not an easy task, and this structure has not been routinely assessed in multiple sclerosis (MS) patients, making clinicoradiological correlations difficult. The 'neuro-ocular plane'[1] allowed us a prospective study of the optic nerves in MS and tentative correlations with the clinical course of the disease and the opthalmological examination (including visual evoked potentials – VEP). Now we report our preliminary results in 39 patients.

PATIENTS AND METHODS

This study was started in June 1982 and most of all suspected or newly diagnosed MS patients in the clinic of La Salpetriere are enrolled in it. Clinical evaluation VEP and CT scan are done on the same day in every patient. The examiners for the clinical examination, ophthalmological examination and VEP and CT scan are blind to each other.

Ophthalmological examination includes visual acuity, colour vision, fundus and, if necessary, visual field. Optic neuritis is considered if there is defective colour vision, central or caeco-central scotoma, or optic disc palor, or a combination of these three. Visual evoked potentials are studied with the pattern reversal technique; the size of the check is 8 and 20 minutes, the whole visual field, each hemi-visual field and each eye are studied. VEP are considered as abnormal if P_{100} latency exceeds 125 ms or if, under this range there is a marked asymmetry between both eyes.

CT scan is performed with ND 8000 CGR brain CT (thickness = 3–6 or 9 mm, 256×256 or 512×512 matrix, 40 or 80 s duration mode). The iodine i.v. perfusion is done before the beginning of the examination, with 2 ml/kg of Radioselectan 76%. In previous works, the usefulness of pre- and after enhancement CT has been established (scanning duration); furthermore, delayed CT (1.4 and 24 hours) after perfusion had been left. These data depend on the machine generation and the well known nuclear magnetic resonance (NMR) results. The most important technical point is the cephalic plane of examination: the neuro-ocular plane (NOLP) with lens-optic nerve heads – and optic canals (in primary gaze) is adopted. In the case of optic nerve involvement, coronal cuts and sagittal reformations are done. 'Dynamic' study of the orbit (NOP in right and left orientated gaze) allows a better approach of the optic nerves. Numerous metric functions are used (density profiles) on the diagnosis console.

The results reported here concern 39 patients (22 females) from 20 to 55 years (average = 39 y) with two spikes (30–35 and 50–55). All of them present probable or definite MS according to McAlpine's criteria.

RESULTS

30/39 patients had CT abnormalities. There were plaques in eight, cortico-sub-cortical atrophy in 16, pseudo-atheromatous vascular curlings in eight, abnormal optic nerves in eight and diffuse white matter density attenuation in two.

One to four plaques (10 and 14 in two cases) were found in eight patients, either unique (four cases) or multiple (four cases), with the usual CT features (2–15 mm large, + 30 UH enhanced hyperdensity). Most of them were dissemi-

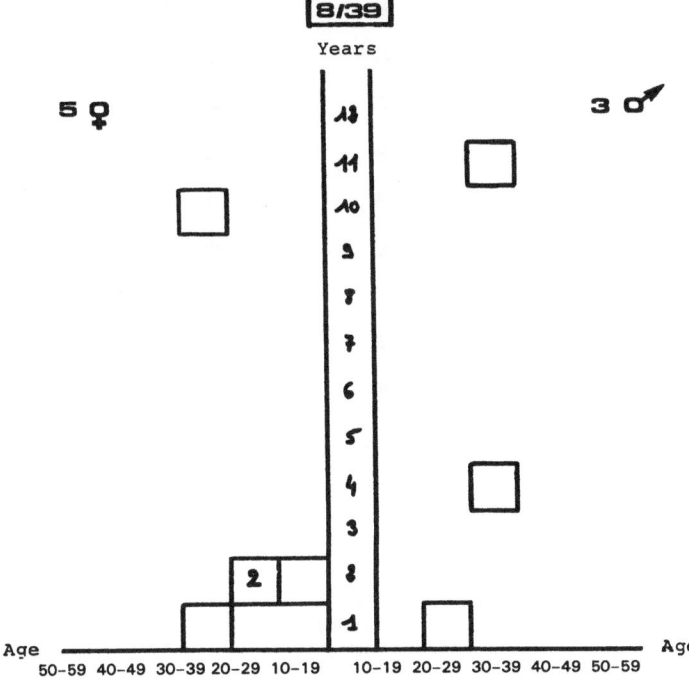

Figure 1 Alterations are more frequent when CT is completed at the beginning of the illness

nated in supra-tentorial white matter; in one case, two infra-tentorial plaques were visible (cerebellum and pons). Less frequent are hypodense (-15 UH relative) and 'ring enhanced' plaques (two cases). As has already been shown[2], plaques were more frequent early in the course of the disease, or in the acute phase.

This is in keeping with our previous experience: plaques were more frequent (14/26) in patients with isolated, 'pure', optic neuritis[3], in whom CT scan was made weeks to months after clinical onset (Figure 1), than in this series of 'neurological' patients (8/39), in whom CT scan was usually done years after onset.

There was no correlation on the other hand, between age, duration of disease and presence or absence of atrophy, neither could it be linked to corticosteroid therapy.

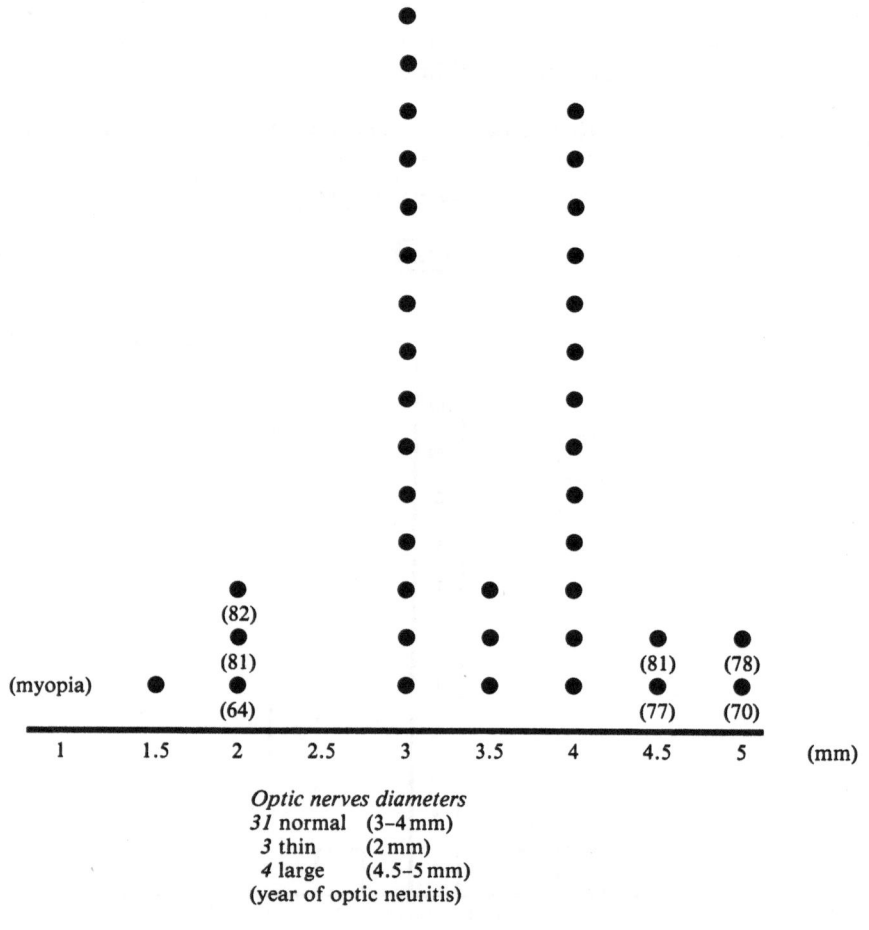

Optic nerves diameters
31 normal   (3–4 mm)
 3 thin   (2 mm)
 4 large   (4.5–5 mm)
(year of optic neuritis)

Figure 2 Correlation between optic nerve diameter and optic neuritin

Vascular 'curlings', i.e. abnormal visualization of intracranial arteries (mostly the anterior and middle cerebral arteries) such as those seen in old, 'atheromatous' patients, were seen in 8/39; we could find no satisfactory explanation for this fact, occurring in young patients (20–45 years).

Optic nerve abnormalities were found in eight patients. The size of the optic nerve was normal (2–4 mm) in 31, decreased (1.5–2 mm) in four, increased (4.5–5 mm) in four, with no correlation between diameter and the evolution (Figure 2) of the disease.

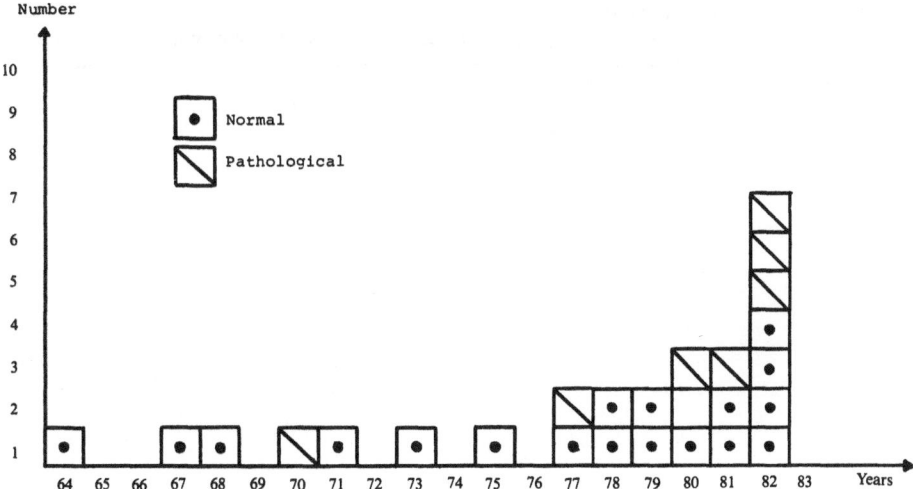

Figure 3 Correlation between optic nerves shape and optic neuritis

Two aspects were considered as signs of optic neuritis: a 'railway' feature in one case (linear high density aspect of the edges of the optic nerve, which means abnormal enhancement of the meningeal sheaths of the optic nerve), and 'hazy' limits of the optic nerve in seven cases. Other findings were localized high density lesions most frequently in the anterior third of the optic nerve, or a non-homogeneous aspect of the optic nerve, considered as non-specific. Optic nerve abnormalities are more frequent when CT scan is done not far from the onset of optic neuritis (Figure 3). As nearly all VEP were abnormal (31 out of 39), we could make no clear correlation between optic nerve abnormalities and VEP. All abnormal CT optic nerves had abnormal VEP however. We observed no plaques in this series, contrary to our previous one[4].

In conclusion, these preliminary results are in keeping with those of other workers regarding alterations to the brain parenchyma. We cannot, at this time, show any clear correlation between CT aspect of the optic nerve and the results of ophthalmological examination and VEP.

References

1. Cabanis, E. A., Pineau, H., Iba-Zizen, M. T., Coin, J. L., Newmann, N. and Salvolini, U. (1981). CT scanning in the 'neuro-ocular plane': the optic pathways as a 'new cephalic plane'. *Neuro-ophthalmology*, **1**, 237
2. Louizou, L. A., Rolfe, E. B. and Hewazy, H. (1982). Cranial computed tomography in the diagnosis of multiple sclerosis. *J. Neurol. Neurosurg. Psychiat.*, **45**, 905
3. Cabanis, E. A., Guillaumat, J., Baleriaux, D., Iba-Zizen, M. T., Benrabah, R., Lopez, A. and Salvolini, U. (1982). Aspects tomodensitométriques dans les atteintes ophtalmologiques de la Sclérose en placques. *Comm. Symposium 'Troubles visuels et oculomoteurs au cours de la Sclérose en Plaques'*, Bruxelles, 28 Feb. 1982. (Published in *Journal de la Société Belge d'Ophtalmologie*).
4. Brant-Zawadski, M., Davis, P. L., Crooks, L. E., Mills, C. M., Norman, D., Newton, T. H., Sheldon, P. and Kaufman, L. (1983). N. M. R. demonstration of cerebral abnormalities: comparison with C.T. *A.J.R.*, **140**, 847

71
Multiple sclerosis: some preliminary findings of a neurological and medical–sociological prospective research project

M. SAMPSON, S. POSER, P. EIBEN and H. FRIEDRICH

Since October 1981 our interdisciplinary research group from the Departments of Neurology and Medical Sociology at the University of Göttingen have been conducting a prospective research project with a group of newly-diagnosed MS-patients. The project will last 3 years. Our main objective is to analyse neurological and socio–medical aspects dealing with the onset and course of MS commencing at the time of initial diagnosis. For the purpose of our study every patient will be examined and interviewed at regular intervals, three times during the first year and once annually thereafter.

For our presentation we would like to focus on – in addition to the basic social data – a brief comparison of five categories in which it has been possible to observe some change during the past 6–12 months. These categories are:

(1) Degree of disability
(2) Changes in relationship
(3) Occupation
(4) Income and, finally,
(5) The attainment of handicapped status.

It must be noted that the findings presented here are preliminary in nature, they allow at most only a glimpse of trends now beginning to take shape.

SOCIAL DATA

The 61 patients now in our sample – 46 women and 15 men – represent nearly all of the MS-patients diagnosed in Göttingen during the past 2 years. Patients were selected only if they had learned their diagnosis within the last 2 years. The average age at onset of illness was 29.5; the diagnosis was made, on the average, 3 years after onset. Our interviews were normally conducted only shortly after the diagnosis.

43% of our patients are single, 56% are married, and one person is divorced. The average age of our patients is 36.

The list of occupations extends from assembly line workers through academic professions. The only striking feature in this category appears to be the relatively low percentage of housewives compared to the normal MS-population. This can possibly be explained by the fact that younger women today are more interested in careers.

Diagnosis

We were especially interested in the question of whether the fact of learning about a diagnosis of an incurable disease would affect the psychosocial situation of the patients during the first year after diagnosis. To provide a basis for this inquiry, we analysed the neurological changes (Figure 1). Here we see the percentage of patients and level of disability at each of three neurological examinations separated by 6 months each. It appears that the level of disability at the time of the initial examination is on the average higher than at the

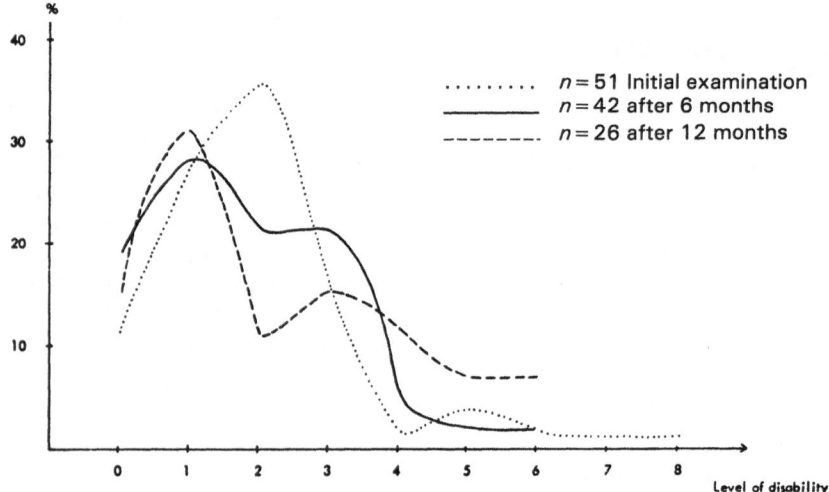

Figure 1 Percent in correlation to level of disability at initial examination. After 6 months and 12 months

following examinations. A closer look reveals that this is not the case, since the second examination shows two peaks which correspond to the trend that one would expect.

Social relationships

Figure 2 illustrates, in complicated sociological fashion, changes that have – or have not – taken place in patient–partner-relationships in the first 6–12 months after our initial interview.

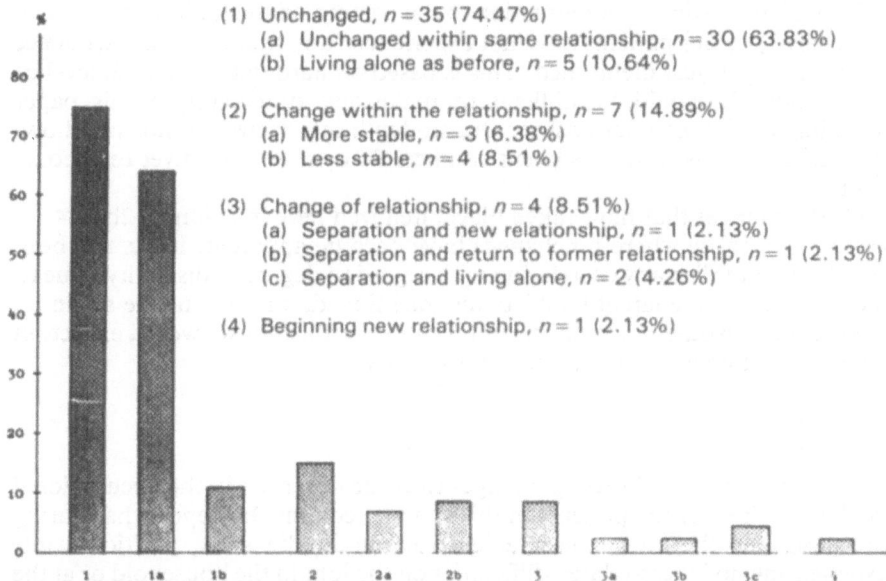

(1) Unchanged, $n = 35$ (74.47%)
    (a) Unchanged within same relationship, $n = 30$ (63.83%)
    (b) Living alone as before, $n = 5$ (10.64%)

(2) Change within the relationship, $n = 7$ (14.89%)
    (a) More stable, $n = 3$ (6.38%)
    (b) Less stable, $n = 4$ (8.51%)

(3) Change of relationship, $n = 4$ (8.51%)
    (a) Separation and new relationship, $n = 1$ (2.13%)
    (b) Separation and return to former relationship, $n = 1$ (2.13%)
    (c) Separation and living alone, $n = 2$ (4.26%)

(4) Beginning new relationship, $n = 1$ (2.13%)

Figure 2 Relationship $n = 47$

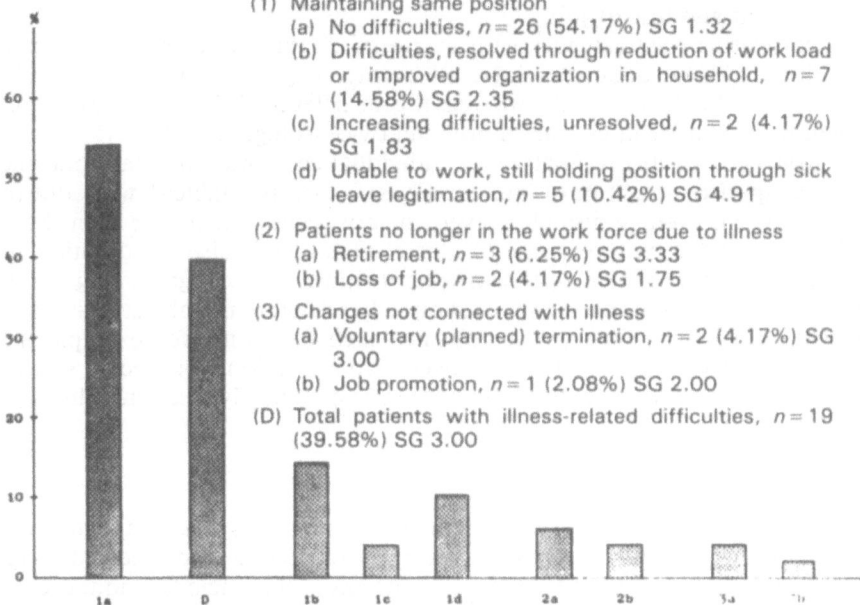

(1) Maintaining same position
    (a) No difficulties, $n = 26$ (54.17%) SG 1.32
    (b) Difficulties, resolved through reduction of work load or improved organization in household, $n = 7$ (14.58%) SG 2.35
    (c) Increasing difficulties, unresolved, $n = 2$ (4.17%) SG 1.83
    (d) Unable to work, still holding position through sick leave legitimation, $n = 5$ (10.42%) SG 4.91

(2) Patients no longer in the work force due to illness
    (a) Retirement, $n = 3$ (6.25%) SG 3.33
    (b) Loss of job, $n = 2$ (4.17%) SG 1.75

(3) Changes not connected with illness
    (a) Voluntary (planned) termination, $n = 2$ (4.17%) SG 3.00
    (b) Job promotion, $n = 1$ (2.08%) SG 2.00

(D) Total patients with illness-related difficulties, $n = 19$ (39.58%) SG 3.00

Figure 3 Changes in occupation/household/studies $n = 48$
(SG = Disability score)

I would like to draw your attention to the column on the far left. As you can see, nearly ¾ of our patients have not experienced any changes of consequence in the time span just mentioned. This is based on hard data on a high level of aggregation. It would be difficult to make any statements in this paper regarding quality of relationship. Our in-depth interviews do indicate, however, that in many instances latent conflicts do exist and have yet to become manifest.

Of the changes that have taken place, itemized here in columns 2b to 4, as well as with those where no changes have become apparent, it has not been possible to establish any correlation with regard to degree of disability. Due to the existence of the latent conflicts just mentioned, and due to the strain an MS-diagnosis would normally mean for any relationship, we would expect, in time, to see a considerable change in this area.

Occupation

Figure 3 attempts to illustrate changes thus far observed in the occupational field. Over 50% of the patients in this sample (column 1a) report that during the past year they have been able to maintain the same position while experiencing no illness-related difficulties on the job, in the household or at the university. On the other hand, nearly 40% have reported to us illness-related problems in this area. As we can see in columns 1(b)–2(b), which together comprise column D, these problems range from relatively minor difficulties that have in the meantime been resolved through a reduction in the work load to retirement and loss of job.

In correlating each category with degree of disability, our results indicate that those with no difficulties have an average degree of disability of 1.32 measured on the Kurtzke scale, whereas the mean level of disability for column D – those with difficulties – lies more than twice as high at 3.00.

It won't be possible to analyse the individual categories in detail, but one other comparison might be of interest: Those presently unable to work due to illness have an average disability level which is somewhat higher than those retired during the past year due to illness. One could raise the question of whether the degree of disability is an accurate indicator for legitimating retirement, or whether there are factors not directly related to the objective impairment caused by the illness that influence such decisions, for example the patient's motivation, family, employer, labour unions or social service agencies, some of which tend to view MS as a completely disabling illness.

Income

We felt it would be of interest to examine possible changes in regard to income, a matter which always reflects the nature of the respective economic and social system in which the patient lives. For instance, the socio–economic consequences of a chronic illness like MS in America and Western Europe can be very different indeed.

The details shown in Figure 4, in regard to income changes, will probably

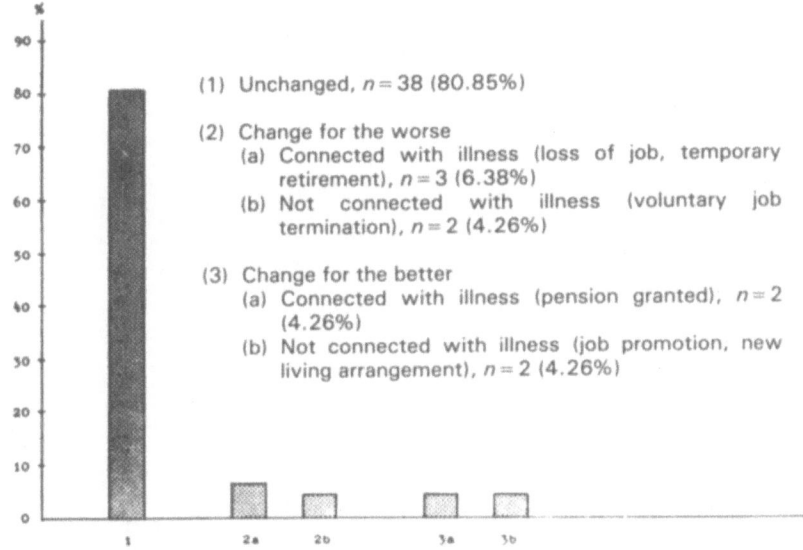

Figure 4 Income $n = 47$

not surprise anyone who lives in a country with a high level of social and particularly job security. Despite the changes we just observed in the field of employment, slightly over 80% of our patients have reported no change in their total household income. It will be very interesting to see whether in time there will be considerable change in this area, or whether other factors will serve to counteract possible reductions in income.

ID-cards

Our final Figure, 5, deals with a very puzzling problem. A person confronted with the fact of a chronic illness is also faced with the possibility of an alteration in his psycho–social identity. One question this raises is whether this individual will define himself as a handicapped person or as one who is stricken with an illness but still capable of functioning in his daily social activities. This involves coping strategies designed to protect himself against insecurity or loss of social influence.

In West Germany the social security system offers a special kind of social protection, in the form of an official identification card for handicapped persons. This ID-card offers its holder special privileges and rights, such as tax exemptions, free public transportation, and protection by law to a certain degree from being dismissed from their jobs.

This figure is divided into two parts. On the left we see the percentages of patients with and those without severely handicapped status. Just under half the patients have applied for and received this status, a little more than half have not.

The six columns on the right represent the average degree of disability –

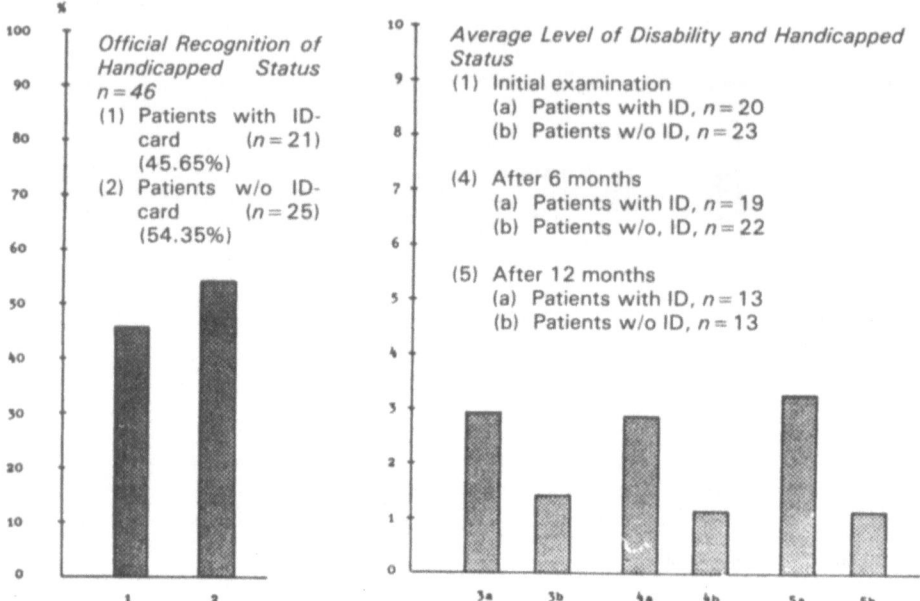

Figure 5 Disability

according to the Kurtzke scale – for those patients with and those without severely handicapped status, divided up into the first, second and third neurological examinations of the patients. At present it is uncertain what one should view as a significant difference between these figures. This question aside, the total average of these two groups very much resembles column 3(a) and 3(b), which means a total of 1.78 degrees separate the two (3.00 for those with and 1.22 for those without). We still can't determine if this is a real correlation or an artifact.

A closer look at the conditions leading to the acquisition of handicapped status reveals there are two sets of factors to be held responsible. First, the activities of the patients and their families to attain this status and second, and this was very surprising to us, the active role of social services professionals and some of the medical staff in various institutions, which to a certain degree counsel the patients to apply for handicapped status, thereby legitimizing their professional role.

This raises the question of whether in the early phases of the illness we should take into consideration which psycho–social factors influence the strategies of coping with MS and whether the different forms of coping do have an effect on the course of the illness.

Section VII
Posters

Poster 1
Measles antibodies, anti-proteinase and plasminogen distribution in serum and plasma from patients affected with multiple sclerosis and patients affected with non-neurological diseases

F. BOLLENGIER, A. MAHLER, G. CLINET and P. DELMOTTE

Neurochemical studies have shown that there is an increase of acid proteinase in MS-plaque and that the activity of neutral proteinases can be increased in the acute phase of plaque formation[1]. In serum neutral proteinases are normally inactivated by α_2-macroglobulin and α_1-antitrypsin[2]. For example serum levels of α_2-macroglobulin are raised in rheumatoid arthritis when proteolytic enzyme levels are high; serum levels of α_1-antitrypsin rise as a result of increased production in the liver in inflammation and other forms of physiological stress. It has been proposed that on the one hand demyelination may be initiated by plasminogen activator, released from activated macrophages and on the other hand that plasmin itself causes demyelination[3].

In order to establish whether multiple sclerosis (MS) patients present or not a particular profile in regard to these parameters, total protein, α_1-antitrypsin, α_2-macroglobulin, plasminogen contents and measles antibody titres were determined in serum and plasma from, on the one hand, patients affected with MS, and on the other hand patients affected with non-neurological diseases (NNP).

Comparison with 2 control groups was established; control group I consisted of healthy adult donors and control group II of medical students.

Total protein was measured with the biuret reaction; α_1-antitrypsin and α_2-macroglobulin were determined using NOR-Partigen plates and plasminogen (plg) using M-Partigen plates from Behringwerke. Haemagglutination inhibition and complement fixation tests were carried out as previously described[4,5].

Finally, the non-parametric Wilcoxon test was used to investigate the different populations (Table 1).

Table 1

	n	Total protein g/100ml median	α₁ Antrypsin mg/100ml median	α₂ Macroglobulin mg/100ml median	Plasminogen mg/100ml median	CF median	HI median
Controls I	20	7.4	332	236	13.9	1/16	1/16
Controls II	11	7.7	298	223	18.6†	1/128†	1/256†
Multiple sclerosis	29	6.6*	310	223	17.8*	1/64*	1.128*
No. of Patients	25	6.8‡	366	223	20.0‡	1/16	1/64§

* Multiple sclerosis values differ from Controls I for 0.05⩽2α<0.01
† controls II differ from Controls I for 0.05⩽2α<0.01
‡ No. of Patients differ from Controls I for 0.05⩽2α⩽0.01
§ No. of Patients differ from Controls I for 0.05⩽2α⩽0.02

RESULTS

(1) α_1-Antitrypsin and α_2-macroglobulin present similar profiles for the four groups under investigation, except four particularly high α_1-antitrypsin values for NNP.

(2) Plasminogen content is increased as well in NNP as in MS; this increase is most probably due to an equilibrating feedback system, to compensate for a higher turnover of plasminogen into plasmin, since it is an acknowledged fact that plasmin and plg-activators are implicated in a variety of biological processes such as fibrinolysis, cell transformation and inflammatory responses.

(3) For both CF and HI titres, the highest activity is systematically recorded not only for the MS patients, but also for controls II, and occasionally for NNP. In our opinion these facts add more evidence in favour of the hypothesis that increase of viral antibody titers may be the result of non-specific mitogenic stimulation[6], related in some unknown way with the disease process in the CNS, as far as MS is concerned.

(4) For the MS-cases there is no apparent correlation between the duration of the disease, the evolution type and the investigated parameters: the same random distribution is observed as for the NNP.

(5) For the parameters assayed, and significantly different from control group I, there is not a single one which is specific for MS.

CONCLUSIONS

If one looks for specificity in MS, it becomes more and more clear that it must be looked for in the mechanism leading to disturbed biochemical or immunological parameters, and especially the mechanism by which the central nervous system becomes the principal area of the disease.

References

1. Kipelainen, H. O., Halonen, T., Kekoni, G. K. *et al.* (1980). Acid proteinase, neutral proteinase and β-glucuronidase activity of cerebrospinal fluid in multiple sclerosis. *Acta Neurolog. Scand.*, **62**, 39
2. Starkey, P. M., Barret, A. J. (1977). *Proteinases in Mammalian Cells and Tissues.* (Amsterdam: North-Holland Publishing)
3. Norton, W. T., Cammer, W., Brosnan, C. F. *et al.* (1981). The role of macrophage secretion products in inflammatory demyelination. *Abstracts of the 8th Meeting of the International Society for Neurochemistry*, p. 265
4. Thiry, L., Dachy, A. and Lowenthal, A. (1969). Measles antibodies in patients with various types of measles infection. *Arch. Ges. Virusforsch.*, **28**, 278
5. Zissis, G. and Clinet, G. (1974). Viral antibody detection by a more sensitive complement fixation reaction. *Lancet*, **II**, 754
6. Poskitt, D. C., Frost, H., Cahill, R. N. P. *et al.* (1977). The appearance of non-specific antibody-forming cells in the efferent lymph draining antigen-stimulated single lymph nodes. *Immunology*, **33**, 81

Poster 2
The benign form of multiple sclerosis

**S. MARFORIO, A. GHEZZI, M. ZAFFARONI, D. CAPUTO and
C. L. CAZZULLO**

The large series of patients affected by multiple sclerosis (MS), in the MS Centre of Gallarate (Milan), shows many cases with a benign course. We define a benign course as a self-sufficient patient able to walk, even with a stick, and to stay on his feet for 12 hours a day (ranging from the first to the fourth degree of Kurtzke's invalidity scale[1]).

If this condition is sustained for several years after the onset of MS (we considered patients with at least 12 years of disease) there is a good chance of a favourable prognosis.

Table 1

		Benign MS	Controls	χ^2	
Age at onset (years)	<20	22	11		
	–40	38	40	12	$p<0.01$
	> 40	0	9		
Sex	M	19	41		
	F	27	33	2.26	$p>0.10$
Mode of onset	monosymptomatic	46	43		
	polysymptomatic	14	17	0.39	$p>0.10$
Symptoms at onset	visual	30	16		
	motor	20	21		
	sensory	15	21	4.5	$p>0.10$
	diplopia	7	9		
	cerebellar	5	5		
Interval between I and II attack	<6m	8	10		
	6m–5y	30	34	9.5	$p<0.01$
	> 5y	17	5		
	no interval	5	11		
Course	with relapses without sequelae	33	39		
	with relapses with sequelae	22	10	7.2	$p<0.05$
	progressive	5	10		

A comparative study of cases with a benign course and cases with the usual progression allowed us to outline some clinical parameters concerning the modality of onset and the degree of invalidity of the disease (Table 1).

We studied 60 cases (3.7%) of benign course of MS out of 1613 patients with MS hospitalized in our Centre. We assumed the diagnostic criteria of Schumaker, and considered only patients with clinically proven MS: 41 females (68.3%) and 19 males (31.6%). The control group consisted of 60 patients randomly collected from the whole series in our Centre. A prevalence of females was found (females/males ratio, 2.12), a finding not significantly different if compared with the total MS population. This was supported by similar findings reported by Bonduelle et al[2] (F/M ratio, 2.2).

The mean age of onset in our benign form series is 24.2 years (23.6 y in females and 25.6 y in males). These figures do not significantly differ from the mean age of onset in the control group (26.3 y). Nevertheless, if we subdivide the patients into three groups according to the age of onset (early: less than 20 y; typical: between 21 and 40 y; late: more than 40 y) we observe an earlier onset in patients with a benign course. Bonduelle et al[2] observed a mean onset age of 26 y, and a relatively larger number of cases with earlier onset. No familiarity was reported in our series. We observed a prevalence of mono-symptomatic onset (46 cases, 76.66%) with respect to multisymptomatic patients (14 cases, 23.3%). These figures do not significantly differ from the control group.

Among various onset symptoms, the most frequent in patients with a benign course was visual impairment (usually a unilateral amblyopia): it was present in half the cases. Among them, only 7 cases showed a visual failure associated with other symptoms. The incidence of this symptom is high if compared with the control group. Thus visual impairment is very frequent as monosympto-matic onset in benign course MS, as confirmed by McAlpine et al[3] who stated that an acute onset with optic neuropathy is very significant to formulate a benign prognosis of MS. The onset with motor disturbances, a frequent occurrence in MS, is in our series clearly less frequent as compared to visual impairment (20 cases, 33%). However, a comparison of this observation with the randomly collected control group does not show a significant difference. McAlpine found a less frequent incidence of motor disturbances in benign course MS. Similarly, Bonduelle found half of his series having a pyramidal onset (alone or associated with other symptoms) and half with an onset involving cranial nerves, particularly the optic nerve.

Sensitivity disturbances are relatively conspicuous (15 cases, 25%) at onset in our cases, always appearing together with other symptoms, except for two cases. This finding differs significantly from the control group. Similarly Bonduelle observed a small incidence of this symptom at disease onset (20% of his cases). Less significant are gaze derangement and ataxia at onset, showing percentages not differing from the controls. McAlpine too reports that ataxia at onset is a symptom as frequent in benign course MS as in typical MS.

The number of patients in our series, who presented a first clinical episode followed by a complete remission was 55 (92%); thus few cases (8%) had, since onset, a slow and progressive worsening of the initial symptoms. Also Bonduelle found few cases of benign course MS with a progressive evolution.

In fact significant differences were found in comparing our patients with the control group.

We observe that relapse/remitting progression of the disease is peculiar to a benign course MS, though this kind of clinical course is found to a large extent among typical MS.

As far as the duration of the first clinical episode is concerned we noticed that it was shorter in patients with benign MS than in the control group. This finding is undoubtedly linked to the eye symptom (amblyopia) which rapidly recovers, as compared with motor and sensory symptoms which have a more lasting duration.

The interval between the first episode and the stage of clinical progression is longer in patients with benign course than in controls. In assessing the evolution of the disease, MS with a benign course has a lower relapse rate and longer exacerbation-remission intervals of the initial symptoms, without new clinical manifestations, suggesting a less widespread involvement of the central nervous system. Comparing neurological signs after 12 years from onset, we found a reduced incidence of motor symptoms and signs of urinary system involvement. On the other hand, we observed a great number of cases with cerebellar involvement. Furthermore, we found a reduced deficit of cranial nerves, no cases of IX and X nerve involvement and only two cases with nystagmus, suggesting a rare involvement of the brainstem.

References

1. Kurtzke, J. F. (1965). Further notes on disability evaluation in multiple sclerosis with scale modifications. *Neurology*, **15**, 654
2. Bonduelle, M., Bouygues, P., Degos, C. F. and Gauthier, C. (1979). Les formes benignes de la sclérose en plaques. *Rev. Neurol.*, **135**, 593
3. McAlpine, D. (1961). The benign form of multiple sclerosis. A study based on 241 cases seen within three years of onset and followed up until the tenth years or more of the disease. *Brain*, **84**, 186

Poster 3
Optic neuritis: laboratory tests for diagnosis and prognosis for the development of multiple sclerosis

A. GHEZZI, M. ZAFFARONI, D. CAPUTO, S. MARFORIO and
D. GIUSSANI

INTRODUCTION

The probability of developing multiple sclerosis (MS) following uncomplicated retrobulbar optic neuritis (RBN) when toxic, degenerative, vascular,
compressive causes are excluded, varies in different reports[1-3], ranging from
13% (Kurland[4]) to 85% (McAlpine[5]). The risk seems to be related to the histocompatibility antigens[3,6] which seem to greatly influence the possibility of
developing MS in the years following RBN (70% for BT 101 carriers instead of
the 20% for non-carriers)[7,8]. Our report extends a previous observation[9] and
deals with:

(1) the comparison of electrophysiological and ophthalmological tests in
the assessment of damage to the optic pathways;
(2) the application of electrophysiological tests for MS and CSF examination in patients with RBN, to detect the possible role of an underlying
demyelinating pathogenesis.

MATERIAL AND METHODS

Twenty-one patients, from ophthalmological departments of our and other
hospitals, who had previously suffered from one or more attacks of RBN, were
observed. In 14 cases RBN was unilateral, in seven cases bilateral at different
times. Compressive and toxic causes were excluded by the appropriate investigations. The age at observation ranged from 14 to 40 years, the last attack
preceding the observation time from 1 month to 6 years. Cases were submitted
to visual evoked potential (VEP) recording in response to a LED pattern
reversal (total field 5.5 °, single check 55 ′) according to Epstein *et al*[10].

In normal subjects P_2 latency was 96.9 ms (SD 5.5), the amplitude 7.2 μV (SD 3), the interocular difference was 2.8 ms (SD 1.9)[11]. Flicker-fusion threshold was determined as the frequency at which an intermittent LED was seen as continuous; the fusion in normal subjects[12] appears at 35.8 Hz ± 1.8.

Somatosensory evoked potentials were recorded in response to medial nerve stimulation at the wrist, according to the techniques of Namerow[13] and Trojaborg and Peterson[14]. Latency of cerebral somatosensory evoked potentials was in normal subjects: N_1, 17.4 (SD 1.5); P_1, 22.9 (SD 3.6); N_2, 30.1 (SD 4.3), P_2, 37.6 (SD 4.5). Brainstem auditory evoked potentials were recorded in only a few cases and were omitted.

CSF examination was performed by isoelectrofocusing (IEF) on poly-acrylamide gel to detect the IgG oligoclonal pattern[15,16]. IgG Index[17] and *de novo* synthesis[18] were also determined. Visual field, acuity, fundus oculi were assessed in all the cases. Electrophysiological responses were considered abnormal if > 2.5 SD the normal values.

Ten cases were clinically surveyed at regular intervals, for a mean period of 3.8 years.

RESULTS

Results are reported in Table 1 and in Figure 1. Ophthalmological findings were abnormal in the affected eyes in 13 cases. The threshold of the flicker-fusion test (FFT) was reduced in nine cases. VEPs were abnormal in 20 out of 21 cases: also in four patients in the clinically and anamnestically unaffected eyes.

A CSF abnormal pattern was observed in 10 out of 21 cases. Ten patients (five with CSF oligoclonal bands) were surveyed for a mean time of 3.8 years: only one patient developed neurological dysfunction outside the optic nerve (a spastic paraplegia with bilateral Babinski's sign), belonging to the group of cases with a normal CSF (Table 2).

Table 1 Ophthalmological and electrophysiological results in 21 ON patients

	Visual field acuity fundus	Flicker fusion test	VEPs
Abnormal findings	13/21	9/21	20/21

Table 2 Clinical course after 3.8 years (m.v.) of follow-up with regard to CSF examination and the evolution toward multiple sclerosis

		MS
CSF oligoclonal bands +	no. 5	0
CSF oligoclonal bands −	no. 5	1

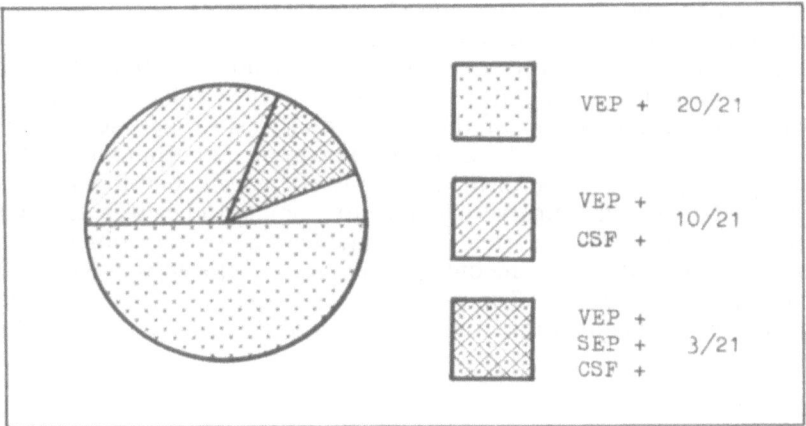

VEP + 20/21

VEP +
CSF + 10/21

VEP +
SEP + 3/21
CSF +

Figure 1   Results testing by VEP, SEP and CSF examination

DISCUSSION

The results from our series concern two questions:[1] the comparison of optic electrophysiological investigations with clinical findings and (2) the relationship between the tests, namely SEPs and CSF, and the possible demyelinating pathogenesis of RBN.

Concerning the first aspect, VEPs were found abnormal in 20 out of 21 cases, revealing the most sensitive test for the assessment of optic pathways lesions following RBN. Ophthalmological findings and FFT were abnormal in a lower number of cases. One case presented a normal VEP in spite of four attacks of RBN. Halliday[19] describing a similar case, interprets this fact as a consequence of the fact that only oedema took place in the acute phase, with no demyelination, or that remyelination of damaged fibres occurred. It is interesting to stress that four cases presented a delayed VEP in the unaffected eye: it could suggest a second subclinical involvement in another, though contiguous, site of CNS and, according to Halliday[20], it should increase the probability of developing MS.

The second aspect of our work concerns the possibility of detecting the underlying demyelinating process in RBN patients when applying tests for MS. It is well known that the clinical diagnosis of MS lies in the demonstration of two different lesions within the white matter and on the relapsing course[5]. When clinical data are lacking, neurophysiological tests can demonstrate a multifocal subclinical involvement of CNS[21]. CSF examination by IEF, in definite and suspected cases, can support the diagnosis, showing an intrathecal synthesis of oligoclonal IgG, which can often be demonstrated by an increased IgG index or *de novo* synthesis.

Applying SEP to medial nerve stimulation abnormal responses were found in three out of 21 patients.

The opportunity of testing several sensitive pathways by means of cerebral evoked potentials is emphasized by Tackmann *et al*[22], who found additional lesions in CNS outside optic nerve in 11 out of 32 RBN cases.

The interpretation of a CSF abnormal pattern in patients with RBN should take into account its non-specificity: Klingele[23] paid attention to the possibility of RBN caused by autoimmune vasculitis. But when collagen diseases are excluded, we believe that a CSF oligoclonal pattern is strongly suggestive for MS. A follow-up should clarify and add value to the importance of CSF and electrophysiological results for the prognosis of clinically developing MS.

Our preliminary data suggest that great attention must be given when interpreting the results. Ten cases (five CSF + and five CSF −) were observed for a mean period of 3.8 years. The only patient who developed signs of involvement of another site of CNS outside the optic nerve (spastic paraplegia at lower limbs with bilateral Babinski's sign) had a normal cerebrospinal fluid.

Acknowledgements

This investigation was supported by a CNR grant for 'Progetto Finalizzato Medicina Preventiva e Riabilitativa – Malattie S.N.C. – OB.26'.

References

1. Bradley, W. G. and Whitty, C. W. M. (1968). Acute optic neuritis: prognosis for development of multiple sclerosis. *J. Neurol. Neurosurg. Psychiat.*, **31**, 10
2. Hutchinson, W. M. (1976). Acute optic neuritis and the prognosis for multiple sclerosis *J. Neurol. Neurosurg. Psychiat.*, **39**, 283
3. Compston, D. A. S., Batchelor, J. F., Earl, C. J. and McDonald, W. I. (1978). Factors influencing the risk of multiple sclerosis developing in patients with optic neuritis. *Brain*, **101**, 495
4. Kurland, L. T., Beebe, G. W., Kurtzke, J. F., Nagler, B., Auth, T. L., Lessel, S. and Nefzger, M. D. (1966). Studies on the natural history of multiple sclerosis. *Acta Neurol. Scand.*, (Suppl.) **19**, 157
5. McAlpine, D., Lumsden, G. F. and Acteson, E. D. (1972). *Multiple sclerosis: a Reappraisal.* 2nd Edn. (London: Churchill Livingstone)
6. Sandberg-Wollheim, M., Platz, P., Ryder, L. P., Nielsen, L. S. and Thomsen, M. (1975). HLA histocompatibility antigens in optic neuritis. *Acta Neurol. Scand.* **52**, 161
7. Anonymous. (1979). Multiple sclerosis and optic neuritis. *Lancet*, **13**, 85
8. Innis, M. D. and Landy, P. J. (1979). Optic neuritis and multiple sclerosis. *Lancet*,
9. Ghezzi, A., Zaffaroni, M. and Caputo, D. (1983). Evoked potentials and CSF findings in optic neuritis and progressive spastic paraparesis. New trends in MS research. Masson Italia Ed. (in press).
10. Epstein, G. M. (1979). True checkerboard pattern reversal with light emitting diodes. *Electroenceph. Clin. Neurophysiol.*, **47**, 611
11. Ghezzi, A. and Orsini, O. (1981). Potenziali evocati visivi nella sclerosi multipla: confronto tra stimoli patterned e unpatterned. *Riv. It. EEG Neurofis. Clin.* **1**, (Suppl. 1), 157
12. Ghezzi, A. and Giussani, D. (1981). Il flicker fusion test nella sclerosi multipla: un semplice esame per lo studio funzionale delle vie ottiche. *Riv. It. EEG Neurofis. Clin.* **1**, (Suppl. 1) 155
13. Namerow, N. S. (1968). Somatosensory evoked responses in patients with varying sensory loss. *Neurology*, **18**, 1197
14. Trojaborg, W. and Petersen, E. (1979). Visual and somatosensory evoked cortical potentials in multiple sclerosis. *J. Neurol. Neurosurg. Psychiat.*, **42**, 322
15. Delmotte, P. and Gonsette, E. (1977). Biochemical findings in MS. IV: IEF of the gamma-globulins in MS and other neurological diseases. *J. Neurol.*, **215**, 27

16. Procaccia, S. and Caputo, D. (1980). Oligoclonal bands in cerebrospinal fluid. In Bauer, Poser and Ritter, (eds.). *Progress in MS Research*. (Berling, Heidelberg, New York: Springer-Verlag)
17. Link, H. (1976). The value of CSF immunoglobulin analysis in clinical neurology. *Riv. Pat. Nerv. Ment.*, **97**, 323
18. Tourtellotte, W. *et al.* (1980). MS *de novo* CNS IgG synthesis, measurement, antibody profile, significance, eradication, and problems. In Bauer, Poser, Ritter, (eds.). *Progress in M.S. research*. (Berlin, Heidelberg, New York: Springer-Verlag)
19. Halliday, A. M. and McDonald, W. I. (1977): Pathophysiology of demyelinating disease. *Br. Med. Bull.*, **33**, 21
20. Halliday, A. M. and McDonald, W. I. (1981). Visual evoked potentials. In Stalberg, E. and Young, R. (eds.). *Clinical Neurophysiology* (Butterworths)
21. Ghezzi, A., Caputo, D., Montanini, R., Procaccia, S., Zibetti, A. and Cazzullo, C. L. (1981). Multiple diagnostic tests in diagnosis of multiple sclerosis. *It. J. Neurol. Sci.*, **3**, 297
22. Tackmann, W., Ettlin, T. H. and Strenge, H. (1982). Multimodality evoked potentials and electrically elicited blink reflex in optic neuritis. *J. Neurol.*, **227**, 157
23. Klingele, T. G. and Burbe, R. M. (1982). Oligoclonal banding in autoimmune optic neuritis. *JAMA*, **248**, 1974

Poster 4
Detection of S-100 protein in the cerebrospinal fluid of animals with acute experimental allergic encephalomyelitis

J. A. CERF, E. CERF, G. CARELS and A.-M. MALFROID

INTRODUCTION

Experimental allergic encephalomyelitis (EAE) is a useful animal model for the study of immune-mediated demyelination. It has been clearly established that the induction of EAE is dependent on cell-mediated immune reactions requiring T-cell sensitization to myelin basic protein, although the possibility that an antibody (B-cell) response may have an important pathogenic role cannot be ruled out[1-3]. The histopathology of the ordinary, acute form of the disease is characterized by perivascular infiltrates of haematogenous mononuclear cells[4]. Demyelination is observed in the vicinity of the invading mononuclear cells, but its precise mechanism is still the subject of much speculation. Recent studies support the view that macrophages, activated within the central nervous system (CNS) by mediators released by sensitized T lymphocytes interacting with the appropriate antigen, secrete myelinolytic products including proteinases[5-7].

Another interesting hypothesis is that much of the myelin breakdown in EAE could be secondary to the death of oligodendrocytes, the myelin forming and supporting cells in the CNS. Besides, both myelin and its parent cell could be the target of the same immunopathological reaction, demyelination and oligodendroglial cell loss occurring simultaneously. Direct evidence for either mechanism is lacking. Actually, electron microscopic studies of the lesions of acute EAE have revealed degenerating cells, possibly oligodendrocytes, phagocytosed by macrophages[8,9]. A depletion of oligodendroglia was also noted. Whether these alterations result from a specific attack on the cells, or are secondary to myelinolysis, is still unclear.

At any rate, it is to be expected that damaged oligodendrocytes release soluble cellular constituents in the interstitial fluid of the nervous parenchyma. Some of these could diffuse into the cerebrospinal fluid (CSF). Michetti et al[10] recently reported the presence of S-100, a brain protein considered to be primarily located in glial cells[11], in the CSF of patients with multiple sclerosis (MS). Since oligodendroglial damage has been claimed to be an initial event in the pathogenesis of the MS plaque[12] (see however [13]), oligodendrogliolysis could conceivably account for the appearance of S-100 in CSF. Here we show that S-100 protein may also be found in the CSF of animals with acute EAE. As will be discussed, however, the origin of the S-100 occurring in CSF, both in EAE and MS, is probably not oligodendroglial in view of recent immunocyto-chemical data on the cellular localization of this protein in the CNS[14-16].

MATERIALS AND METHODS

Twenty outbred albino rabbits, weighing 2.5–3.5 kg, were used in this study. EAE was produced in 12 animals by a single intradermal injection into the footpads of 0.12 ml of an emulsion containing ox brain white matter in an equal volume of complete Freund's adjuvant. CSF (0.5–1.0 ml) was drawn by puncture of the cisterna magna under anaesthesia provided by a mixture of fluanisone and fentanyl (Hypnorm, Janssen, 0.6 ml/kg i.m.), and stored at −45 °C until assay. A CSF sample was taken from each EAE rabbit on the day of onset of clinical signs or the day after. In several animals, up to five additional samples were obtained during the disease. For control assays, CSF was removed from eight healthy rabbits, and in four of these animals a second sample was taken 10–12 days later.

S-100 protein from ox brain was isolated and purified according to Gombos et al[17]. An antiserum to S-100 was raised in rabbits[18], and its specificity tested by double diffusion in agar and complement fixation analysis using extracts of a variety of tissues as antigens. Cross-reactivity of the anti-ox-S-100 antiserum with rabbit brain extracts was verified. The amount of S-100 in rabbit CSF was measured by quantitative microcomplement fixation essentially as described by Moore and Perez[19], all reagent volumes being scaled up 10-fold. The anti-serum was used at a dilution of 1 : 6000, and purified bovine S-100 protein was the standard against which the amount of S-100 in CSF was measured in each test. The level of S-100 protein considered as the effective limit of detection in the assay was 6 ng/ml. Anticomplementarity, occurring in a number of CSF samples, was removed for the most part by a 90 min incubation at 60 °C in presence of 2 mmol/l 2-mercaptoethanol, and calculations of S-100 levels were corrected for any residual anticomplementary activity.

RESULTS AND DISCUSSION

S-100 antigen was not found in any of the 12 CSF samples drawn from healthy rabbits. In contrast, S-100 was detected in the CSF of 10 of the 12 rabbits experiencing EAE. As shown in Table 1, S-100 antigen did not occur regularly in the CSF of these 10 rabbits, but it was detectable in at least one of the samples from each animal. The presence of S-100 in CSF showed no apparent relationship to the clinical state of the animals. It was noticed, however, that

Table 1 S-100 antigen in CSF of rabbits with EAE

Animal No.*	Day of onset	Level of S-100 in successive samples† (ng/ml)					
1	11	12.5	18.4	ND‡			
2	13	9.0	13.6				
3	13	7.0	ND	ND	ND	15.2	
4	14	35.6					
5	15	70.4					
6	15	10.6					
7	17	ND	10.0	ND	6.5	ND	
8	18	ND					
9	20	ND	ND	ND	6.0	ND	
10	22	ND	29.6	ND	9.6		
11	24	ND	ND	ND	ND		
12	52	ND	ND	ND	24.9	ND	ND

* Animals arranged in order of increasing latencies of onset of clinical signs
† First sample drawn at onset. In several animals, additional samples were taken at different times during a period of 8–15 days following onset; intervals between cisternal punctures were at least 2 days
‡ ND = not detectable

the samples taken at the time of onset of the disease were positive for S-100 in animals presenting the shortest latent periods (11–15 days). Because of the small number of cases, the possible significance of this observation has yet to be determined.

The finding of S-100 antigen in some of the EAE-CSF samples cannot easily be related to a particular process in the pathogenesis of the disease. Yet it seems reasonable to suggest that S-100 protein is released in the extracellular fluid in damaged zones of the CNS, and subsequently diffuses into the CSF. In fact, S-100 could be suspected *a priori* to be a breakdown product of oligoden-drocytes, assuming that the degenerating cells seen in EAE lesions belong to this glial cell type[8,9]. A strong argument for considering the possibility of antibody-mediated destruction of oligodendrocytes comes from *in vitro* studies with sera from animals with EAE (induced by sensitization to white matter). In addition to their known demyelinating ability[1], such sera show an early, complement-dependent toxic effect on oligodendroglial cells in organotypic CNS tissue cultures[20] and on cultured neonatal glial cells[21]. In embryonic CNS cultures, the sera inhibit differentiation of oligodendrocytes and myelination[22]. Further analysis has shown that the gliotoxic activity of EAE serum resides in the immunoglobulin fraction[23,24], and that serum immunoglobulins bind *in vitro* to the plasmalemma of oligodendrocytes as well as to myelin[25,26], the neuro-antigen involved being possibly galactocere-broside[26]. Likewise, the notion that lymph node cells[27] and white blood cells[28] from animals sensitized with whole CNS tissue are able to destroy neuroglia in tissue culture is also of interest in this context.

However, recent immunocytochemical data apparently exclude oligoden-droglia as the source of the S-100 protein occurring in pathological CSF. Although S-100 has generally been thought to be present in various glial cell types (including oligodendrocytes, see [11]), several authors have recently reported that, in rat brain and cerebellum, the protein is exclusively localized in the astrocytes[14-16]. Therefore, the possibility has to be considered that astrocytes, in some way yet to be determined, release cytoplasmic constituents in the interstitial fluid in relation to lesion formation in EAE. Alternatively, it might be suggested that the S-100 protein appearing in CSF derives somehow from the haematogenous inflammatory cells infiltrating the perivascular spaces and adjoining parenchyma in EAE lesions. In fact, S-100 has of late been detected in several non-nervous tissues. Interestingly, its presence has been reported in human white blood cells, especially T lymphocytes, and in mouse macrophages[29].

SUMMARY

CSF was drawn by cisternal puncture from eight healthy rabbits and 12 rabbits with acute EAE produced with whole white matter and complete Freund's adjuvant. Some of these animals were sampled several times during the disease. A microcomplement fixation assay was used to test for the presence of S-100 protein in the CSF. In 10 of the rabbits experiencing EAE, S-100 antigen was detected in at least one of the CSF samples from each animal. S-100 antigen was not found in the CSF obtained from control rabbits. The possible origin of the S-100 appearing in the CSF of animals with EAE is discussed.

ACKNOWLEDGMENTS

The authors wish to thank E. Ponslet, F. Symons and J. Van Dale for technical assistance. This work was supported by a grant from the Belgian Research Group for Multiple Sclerosis.

NOTE ADDED IN PROOF

A recent study (Smith, M. E., Somera, F. P. and Eng, L. F. (1983). *Brain Res.,* **264,** 241) showed increased metabolic activity in astrocytes during the acute stage of EAE lends some support to the idea that an astroglial reaction may be involved in the release of S-100 protein appearing in the CSF.

References

1. Bornstein, M. B. (1978). Immunobiology of demyelination. In Waxman, S. G. (ed.). *Physiology and Pathobiology of Axons*, pp. 313–336. (New York: Raven Press)
2. Paterson, P. Y. (1978). The demyelinating diseases: Clinical and experimental studies in animals and man. In Samter, M., Talmage, D. W., Rose, B., Austen, K. F. and Vaughan, J. H. (eds.). *Immunological Diseases,* 3rd Edn., pp. 1400–1435. (Boston: Little, Brown and Co.)
3. Weigle, W. O. (1980). Analysis of autoimmunity through experimental models of thyroiditis and allergic encephalomyelitis. *Adv. Immunol.,* **30,** 159
4. Raine, C. S. (1976). Experimental allergic encephalomyelitis and related conditions. In

Zimmerman, H. M. (ed.). *Progress in Neuropathology, Vol. 3*, pp. 225–251. (New York: Grune & Stratton)

5. Cammer, W., Bloom, B. R., Norton, W. T. and Gordon, S. (1978). Degradation of basic protein in myelin by neutral proteases secreted by stimulated macrophages. A possible mechanism of inflammatory demyelination. *Proc. Natl. Acad. Sci. USA*, **75**, 1554

6. Smith, M. E. (1980). Proteinase inhibitors and the suppression of EAE. In Davison, A. N. and Cuzner, M. L. (eds.). *The Suppression of Experimental Allergic Encephalomyelitis and Multiple Sclerosis*, pp. 211–226. (London: Academic Press)

7. Brosnan, C. F., Bornstein, M. B. and Bloom, B. R. (1981). The effects of macrophage depletion on the clinical and pathologic expression of experimental allergic encephalomyelitis. *J. Immunol.*, **126**, 614

8. Lampert, P. (1967). Electron microscopic studies on ordinary and hyperacute experimental allergic encephalomyelitis. *Acta Neuropathol.*, **9**, 99

9. Dal Canto, M. C., Wisniewski, H. M., Johnson, A. B., Brostoff, S. W. and Raine, C. S. (1975). Vesicular disruption of myelin in autoimmune demyelination. *J. Neurol. Sci.*, **24**, 313

10. Michetti, F., Massaro, A. and Murazio, M. (1979). The nervous system-specific S-100 antigen in cerebrospinal fluid of multiple sclerosis patients. *Neurosci. Lett.*, **11**, 171

11. Zomzely-Neurath, C. and Walker, W. (1980). Nervous system-specific proteins: 14-3-2 protein, neuron-specific enolase and S-100 protein. In Bradshaw, R. A. and Schneider, D. M. (eds.). *Proteins of the Nervous System*, 2nd edn., pp. 1–57. (New York: Raven Press)

12. Lumsden, C. E. (1970). The neuropathology of multiple sclerosis. In Vinken, P. J. and Bruyn, G. W. (eds.). *Handbook of Clinical Neurology, Vol. 9: Multiple Sclerosis and Other Demyelinating Diseases*, pp. 217–309. (Amsterdam: North-Holland)

13. Raine, C. S., Scheinberg, L. and Waltz, J. M. (1981). Multiple sclerosis. Oligodendrocyte survival and proliferation in an active established lesion. *Lab. Invest.*, **45**, 534

14. Cocchia, D. (1981). Immunocytochemical localization of S-100 protein in the brain of adult rat. An ultrastructural study. *Cell Tissue Res.*, **214**, 529

15. Legrand, Ch., Clos, J., Legrand, J., Langley, O. K., Ghandour, M. S., Labourdette, G., Gombos, G. and Vincendon, G. (1981). Localization of S100 protein in the rat cerebellum: An immunoelectron microscope study. *Neuropathol. Appl. Neurobiol.*, **7**, 299

16. Haan, E. A., Boss, B. D. and Cowan, W. M. (1982). Production and characterization of monoclonal antibodies against the 'brain-specific' proteins 14-3-2 and S-100. *Proc. Natl. Acad. Sci. USA*, **79**, 7585

17. Gombos, G., Zanetta, J.-P., Mandel, P. and Vincendon, G. (1971). Etude de la fraction protéique neurospécifique S 100: II – Hétérogénéité moléculaire de la fraction protéique S 100. *Biochimie*, **53**, 645

18. Zuckerman, J. E., Herschman, H. R. and Levine, L. (1970). Appearance of a brain specific antigen (the S-100 protein) during human foetal development. *J. Neurochem.*, **17**, 247

19. Moore, B. W. and Perez, V. J. (1966). Complement fixation for antigens on a picogram level. *J. Immunol.*, **96**, 1000

20. Raine, C. S. and Bornstein, M. B. (1970). Experimental allergic encephalomyelitis: An ultrastructural study of experimental demyelination *in vitro*. *J. Neuropathol. Exp. Neurol.*, **29**, 177

21. Berg, O. and Källén, B. (1962). An *in vitro* gliotoxic effect of serum from animals with experimental allergic encephalomyelitis. *Acta Pathol. Microbiol. Scand.*, **54**, 425

22. Bornstein, M. B. and Raine, C. S. (1970). Experimental allergic encephalomyelitis. Antiserum inhibition of myelination *in vitro*. *Lab. Invest.*, **23**, 536

23. Berg, O. and Bergstrand, H. (1968). Different types of antibodies with a gliotoxic effect in serum from animals with experimental allergic encephalomyelitis. *Acta Pathol. Microbiol. Scand.*, **73**, 195

24. Grundke-Iqbal, I., Raine, C. S., Johnson, A. B., Brosnan, C. F. and Bornstein, M. B. (1981). Experimental allergic encephalomyelitis. Characterization of serum factors causing demyelination and swelling of myelin. *J. Neurol. Sci.*, **50**, 63

25. Johnson, A. B., Raine, C. S. and Bornstein, M. B. (1979). Experimental allergic encephalomyelitis: Serum immunoglobulin binds to myelin and oligodendrocytes in

cultured tissue. Ultrastructural-immunoperoxidase observations. *Lab. Invest.*, **40**, 568
26. Lisak, R. P., Saida, T., Kennedy, P. G. E., Saida, K., Silberberg, D. H. and Leibowitz, S. (1980). EAE, EAN and galactocerebroside sera bind to oligodendrocytes and Schwann cells. *J. Neurol. Sci.*, **48**, 287
27. Koprowski, H. and Fernandes, M. V. (1962). Autosensitization reaction *in vitro*. Contactual agglutination of sensitized lymph node cells in brain tissue culture accompanied by destruction of glial elements. *J. Exp. Med.*, **116**, 467
28. Berg, O. and Källén, B. (1963). White blood cells from animals with experimental allergic encephalomyelitis tested on glia cells in tissue culture. *Acta Pathol. Microbiol. Scand.*, **58**, 33
29. Kanamori, M., Endo, T., Shirikawa, S., Sakurai, M. and Hidaka, H. (1982). S-100 antigen in human T lymphocytes. *Biochem. Biophys. Res. Commun.*, **108**, 1447

Poster 5
Estimation of levels of IgG to multiple sclerosis specific brain antigens in the cerebrospinal fluid of MS patients

S. C. RASTOGI, J. CLAUSEN, H. J. HANSEN, E. PEDERSEN and W. W. TOURTELOTTE

The binding of partially purified multiple sclerosis (MS) specific brain antigens (MSG2) and of the corresponding antigens of non-MS brains (KG2) to the IgG in cerebrospinal fluid (CSF) of patients with MS and other neurological diseases were assayed employing sandwich enzyme linked immunosorbent assay (ELISA) technique. The brain antigens were bound to the wells in micro-ELISA plates, followed by the binding of CSF-IgG to the antigens, and finally peroxidase labelled rabbit antihuman IgG was bound to the CSF-IgG. The activity of peroxidase expressed as optical density (OD) of the enzyme released chromophore was considered as a measure of antigen-antibody binding. Initial studies revealed an antigen dose dependent increase in the binding of brain antigens with the IgG in undiluted CSF until an optimal (maximal) binding was achieved. Assay of antigen-antibody binding revealed that the concentration of MSG2 required for the optimal binding with the IgG in the undiluted MS CSF was significantly lower than that of KG2. The index for IgG binding capacity of an antigen (IgBC) was expressed as a ratio of the OD of the colour formed at the optimal antigen-antibody binding to the lowest concentration of the antigen required for the optimal binding. The IgBC of MSG2 was found to be linearly correlated with the IgG concentration in the CSF of MS patients. These results indicate that IgG with specificity to various antigens in the MSG2 may be present in the CSF of MS patients.

Poster 6
Increased T-helper cell levels in cerebrospinal fluid

J. DE SAEDELEER, R. DOM, J. RAUS, J. STRAGIER, H. CARTON and
A. A. VANDENBARK

ABSTRACT

Utilizing fluorescein-conjugated monoclonal antibodies and flow cytometry, lymphocyte subsets in cerebrospinal fluid (CSF) and blood from 25 active neurologic disease patients, and in blood from 21 healthy donors were evaluated. CSF showed increased percentages of the T-helper/inducer (T_H) and decreased percentages of the T suppressor/cytotoxic (T_{SC}) subsets, as well as increased ratios of T_H/T_{SC} compared with paired or normal blood values. CSFs with increased cell counts had significantly higher levels of T total and T_H subsets than those with baseline counts, but no differences were observed in levels of T_{SC} or HLA-DR ($+$) subsets. Of particular significance, both the CSF and blood of neurologic disease patients (but not blood of healthy donors) demonstrated increased T_H/T_{SC} ratios as the % of total T-cells increased. The increase in total T cells was due almost entirely to increases in the T_H subset, while the T_{SC} subset remained nearly constant. Taken together these data suggest that increased levels of the T_H subset in neurologic disease patients anticipates a selective migration of these cells into the CSF, resulting in altered T_H/T_{SC} ratios and escape from regulation by T-suppressor cells.

INTRODUCTION

The availability of monoclonal antibodies that detect functionally related lymphocyte subpopulations has helped to describe the nature of immuno-regulatory abnormalities in a number of diseases. In multiple sclerosis (MS), for example, there appears to be a relationship between clinical activity and decreases in T_S suppressor/cytotoxic (T_{SC}) cell populations[1-3]. These data suggest that lack of adequate suppressor activity may contribute to increased T helper/inducer (T_H) activity, which in turn may stimulate disease-associated cell mediated or humoral effector mechanisms. Although several reports have described T_H and T_{SC} levels and activity in the blood of MS and other neurologic disease patients[4-11] few reports have investigated these subsets in cerebrospinal fluid[1,12], especially in patients with low cell counts. In this study, T_H, T_{SC}, and T total subsets in the CSF and blood of 25 patients with a variety of acute neurologic diseases were compared with similar values obtained from clinically healthy individuals.

METHODS

CSF and blood specimens were obtained from 25 patients with acute neurologic disorders, including MS (5); possible MS (2); Guillian–Barré (2) herniated disc (2); and one each of transverse myelitis, syringomyelia, spinal cord compression, polyneuropathy, megadolichobasilaris, migraine, tumour, cardiovascular accident, cerebral hypoperfusion, dementia, thrombosis, arthrosis, epilepsy, and an hysterical disorder. CSF samples ranged 0.8–7.5 ml ($\bar{x} = 3.7$ ml) and contained from <1 to 78 cells/mm^3. Five ml heparinized blood were collected from neurologic disease patients and 21 healthy individuals. Cells from 50 μl blood or $\frac{1}{3}$ of the total CSF cells were stained with fluorescein-labelled-anti Leu 2 (T_{SC}), anti-Leu 3 (T_H) or anti-Leu 4 (T total), the red cells lysed with 1 ml NH$_4$Cl, and the fluorescent cells detected using a FACS IV flow cytometer. The entire sample of CSF cells (> 700 cells per monoclonal, average) and > 5000 cells from blood were evaluated.

RESULTS

Using the normal blood values as a reference, the neurologic disease patients as a group had increased levels of T_H cells (52% vs 43%) and decreased levels of T_{SC} (16% vs 22%) in their CSF, producing increased T_H/T_{SC} ratios (3.9 vs 2.1). The MS patients had increased T_H levels in CSF (62%) when compared to OND patients (49%) but the T_{SC} subset was not different. Comparisons of the subset values in blood versus CSF from the same patients showed no correlation for the T_H and T_{TOTAL} subsets and a weak correlation for the T_{SC} subset.

Although most (> 70%) of the CSFs in these patients with early neurologic problems had low cell counts (<3 cells/mm^3), several had increased cellularity. The patients with elevated cell counts had significant increases in T_{TOTAL} (88% vs 61%) and T_H (72% vs 46%) subsets, but no changes in the T_{SC} subset versus patients with <3 cells/mm^3. Additionally, the T_H but not the T_{SC} subset in CSF increased concomitantly with increases in the T_{TOTAL} subset ($p<0.0001$). Finally, as expected from the previous findings, changes in the T_H/T_{SC} ratio in CSF were related to changes in the percent of total T cells.

DISCUSSION

The results presented above suggest that changes in T-cell subsets in the CSF of neurologic disease patients are not reflected by evaluations of blood. However, the CSF shows significant increases in T_{TOTAL} and more specifically, the T_H subpopulation as the number of cells in the CSF increases. Since the T_{SC} subpopulation contributes little to the increase in total T-cells, it is not surprising that the increase in T_H/T_{SC} ratio observed is mostly accounted for by selective increases in the T_H subpopulation. This observation does not agree with previous reports concerning CSF T-cell subpopulations[1,12], probably because these reports do not include data from CSFs with low cell numbers. Comparison of CSFs with elevated cell numbers presented here does in fact show great similarity with comparable patient groups reported previously[1,12]. The assessment of CSF from patients with low cell counts has been made feasible by reading the entire preparation of CSF cells stained directly with fluorescein-conjugated monoclonal antibodies (to minimize washes) on a precalibrated cytofluorograph. The results presented here support the idea that the CSF compartment represents a special environment where T_H/T_{SC} ratios are often higher than in blood. Furthermore, processes which increase the cellularity in CSF are likely to result in further elevated T_H/T_{SC} ratios, caused primarily by increases in the T_H subset. This in turn may lead to the observed increases in antibody synthesis and production of oligoclonal bands, as well as cell-mediated immune responses directed in part to self antigens (see Chapters 5, P10 and P15).

ACKNOWLEDGEMENTS

The authors wish to thank Agnes Delsaer for typing the manuscript, and Tony Van Galen for preparing the graphics for presentation at the 25th Anniversary Symposium of the Belgian Research Group for MS, Brussels, Belgium which this manuscript describes.

This work was supported by the Paul J. Cams Foundation of Belgium, the Wetenschappelijk Onderzoek MS Organization of Belgium and the United States Veterans Administration.

References

1. Cashman, N., Martin, C., Eizenbaum, J. F., Degos, J. D. and Bach, A. M. (1982). *J. Clin. Invest.*, **70**, 387
2. Reinherz, E. L., Weiner, H. L., Hauser, S. L., Cohen, J. A., Distaso, J. A. and Schlossman, S. L. (1980). *N. Engl. J. Med.*, **303**, 125
3. Bach, M. A., Phan-Dhin-Tuy, F., Tournier, E. *et al.* (1980). *Lancet*, **2**, 1221
4. Huddlestone, J. R. and Oldstone, M. B. A. (1979). *J. Immunol.*, **123**, 1615
5. Merril, J. E., Biberfeld, G., Landin, S., Siden, A. and Norrby, E. (1980). *Clin. Exp. Immunol.*, **42**, 345
6. Santoli, D., Moretta, L., Lisak, R., Gilden, D. and Koprowski, H. (1978). *J. Immunol.*, **4**, 1369
7. Arnason, B. G. W. and Antel, J. (1978). *Ann. Immunol. (Paris)*, **129c**, 159

8. Gonzales, R.L., Dav, P.C. and Spitler, L.E. (1979). *Clin. Exp. Immunol.*, **36**, 78
9. Wallen, W.C., Houff, S.A., Iavanainen, M., Calabrese, V.P. and De Vries, G.H. (1981). *Neurology*, **31**, 668
10. Goust, J.M., Hoffman, P.M., Pryjma, J., Hogan, E.L. and Fudenberg, H.H. (1980). *Ann. Neurol.*, **8**, 526
11. Antel, J.P., Richman, D.P., Oger, J.J.F., Noronha, A.B.C., Medof, E.M. and Arnason, B.G.W. (1980). In Davison, A.N. and Cuzner, M.L. (eds.). *Suppression of experimental allergic encephalomyelitis and multiple sclerosis.* pp. 261–275 (London: Academic Press)
12. Panitch, H.S. and Francis, G.S. (1982). *N. Engl. J. Med.*, **307**, 60

Poster 7
Laboratory test for hyperactivity (HA) in children: is childhood HA related to multiple sclerosis?

E. J. FIELD and G. JOYCE

SUMMARY

The syndrome of the 'Hyperactive Child' (HA) is far from universally recognized, but diagnosis can now be established by a laboratory test which eliminates subjective assessment. The latter, however, made by the mother, turns out to be nearly always correct. The test involves no more than taking a few ml of blood and depends upon electrophoretic mobility changes induced in red blood cells (RBC) by linoleic and arachidonic acids and by PGE_2.

INTRODUCTION

Many general practitioners and indeed some paediatric consultants convey to harassed parents of hyperactive (HA) children a sense of disbelief in the existence of the condition as a clinical entity, and so generate bewilderment and frustration. In this way they continue the tradition in which one of us (EJF) was brought up, that it is the parents rather than the child who are in need of treatment. Educational psychologists and social workers are much less sceptical but recognize the difficulty of drawing a line between the merely 'lively' child and the clinically 'hyperactive' with excessive thirst, sleeplessness at night, possibly with 'head banging', inattention and lack of concentration at school leading to poor progress. In practice the mother turns out to be the best judge of a truly hyperactive child, and this is especially striking when she positively distinguishes between her offspring. The present work offers an objective laboratory test for the diagnosis of hyperactivity, dependent upon some anomaly in the red blood cell (RBC) membrane brought out by electrophoretic studies. It must be confessed that one of us (EJF) entered this study with considerable scepticism, our attention being drawn to it by the Hyperactive Children's Support Group who, amongst a gallimaufry of other treatments, employed essential fatty acids in which we had a long standing interest[1].

PATIENTS AND METHODS

36 children have been referred through the HACSG, local social workers and distracted mothers. They have extended in age from 1.5 years to 14 years. 25 were male and 11 females. Mothers, especially when able to compare their HA with other children, were emphatic in maintaining the existence of HA. School teachers (who complained of fidgeting, inattention, distractions etc. in class) and social workers were also clear about it, and some children had been to Educational Psychologists and even Child Psychiatrists. (It is interesting that two negative children we saw had also been so judged by the above.) The majority of children showed in addition to hyperkinesia, with disregard for dangers involved, an abnormal thirst and disturbed sleep, some with 'head banging' and their condition in general appeared to become less pronounced on ageing. No predominance of blond children was noted as has been reported by some workers. Most mothers claimed that orange juice made matters worse and some had used the Feingold diet.

The E-UFA test[2], has been confirmed in its original form by double blind tests[3,4] or as modified by Seaman's group[5-7] (reference 7 is especially interesting as its senior author concerned had emphatically denied the validity of the test in the columns of the *Lancet*[8]. Seaman *et al*[5] have outlined the reasons for failure). In addition, Seaman *et al*[9] found that a labile factor responsible for the special properties of the MS-RBC resided in the plasma (and not serum) of MS subjects. This we have substantiated and have gone on to elaborate and 'Office Test' for MS[10] using fresh plasma from the subject to be tested on normal RBCs. The results show a very high correlation with the immediate E-UFA test itself (unpublished). Some of our tests were carried out by the plasma method (PL-EUFA).

RESULTS

With either the E-UFA test or the PL-EUFA (Plasma E-UFA test) 24/36 children gave a clearly abnormal result when the electrophoretic mobility of RBC was measured in the presence of 0.08 mg/ml, 0.02 mg/ml linoleic acid (LA) and arachidonic acid (AA)[11], whilst the PGE_2 test was always normal[12]. Astonishingly, the results were different for the 17 boys and 7 girls (Table 1). It will be noted that:

(1) The result in boys approximates that in MS, *but the PGE_2 test is normal* – differentiating the HA condition clearly from MS. The actual magnitude of the mobility change with LA and AA was less in HA males than in MS ($p = 0.005$–0.001).

(2) Observations in girls are quite different from boys.

(3) We have studied many hundreds of normal children in the course of our MS work.

We have reported that the results of the E-UFA test on MS-RBC (but not on non-MS RBC) could be markedly magnified by allowing the sterile washed RBC to stand at 4 °C for up to 3 weeks[13]. The 'MS Type' reaction displayed by

Table 1 Electrophoretic mobility of RBC from children exhibiting hyperactivity. 12 of 36 showed multiple sclerosis type reaction. Figures indicate mobility in $\mu m\,s^{-1}\,V^{-1}\,cm^{-1} \pm$ SD. All mobility changes shown are highly significant ($p \ll 0.001$)

	CON*	LA 0.08 mg/ml	AA 0.08 mg/ml	LA 0.02 mg/ml	AA 0.02 mg/ml	CON* (no alcohol)	PGE₂ 31.25 pg/ml
HA Males n = 17	0.98 ± 0.03†	0.91 ± 0.03†	0.91 ± 0.03	1.07 ± 0.03	1.07 ± 0.03	0.99 ± 0.03	1.07 ± 0.03
% change in mobility		− 7.1	− 7.1	+ 9.2	+ 9.2		+ 9.2
HA Females n = 7	0.98 ± 0.03	1.06 ± 0.03	1.07 ± 0.03	1.07 ± 0.03	1.07 ± 0.03	0.98 ± 0.03	1.08 ± 0.03
% change in mobility		+ 8.2	+ 9.2	+ 9.2	+ 9.2		+ 10.2
HA + MS n = 12	0.93 ± 0.03†	0.87 ± 0.03†	0.87 ± 0.03	1.06 ± 0.03	1.07 ± 0.03	0.98 ± 0.03	0.87 ± 0.03
% change in mobility		− 11.2	− 11.2	+ 8.2	+ 9.2		− 11.2

* Control – for LA and AA contains 10 μl alcohol
for PGE₂ 10 μl medium TC 199

† $p = 0.005$–0.001 (Student's t-test)

405

the boys was *not* increased in six cases tried, so that in this, as in the PGE_2 result (S in MS), the male HA reaction differed from the MS result.

However, 12/36 of the referred children gave a full MS result. This was so unexpected that in five available cases it was repeated on a different specimen of blood (as is our custom when feasible). Great care was taken to carry out tests only on children who were not on drug therapy, though some mothers had been following a Feingold diet, and had a special antipathy to orange juice or other anthracene derived dye-stuff containing materials. In addition, amongst the 24 children who gave a pure 'HA' reaction one boy had a mother who gave a positive MS reaction and on clinical examination showed unmistakable signs of the disease; and one girl had a brother, who had been labelled 'HA', but gave a true MS result, the mother of these children herself had MS. Of the 13 children who were both 'HA' and 'MS' nine had mothers who showed an 'MS' result (three with a clinical picture: others not examined); the remaining four had mothers who were 'red circles', i.e. showed decreased RBC mobility with LA and increased mobility with AA – a feature we have learned to associate with the mothers of definite MS subjects in more than 300 consecutive cases examined.

DISCUSSION

We believe we have established:

(1) A laboratory test for the diagnosis of hyperactivity in children deserving of further study.
(2) That the results of the test are sex associated.
(3) The HA picture might, in about one third of cases, be a manifestation in childhood of an already extant MS diathesis or, indeed, a manifestation of the disease itself at this age. French neurologists have recognized that MS in childhood may present in aberrant forms and 'classical' MS in childhood is uncommon. Indeed, it would be remarkable if it were not so, for the malfunctioning of regions not yet properly developed in the unripe brain could hardly give a deficiency picture. There is some hitherto unsuspected association between clinical HA in children and MS, and a prospective study is required to establish how frequently HA leads into MS in later life.

The association of MS with a 'functional' HA (we are ruling out cases associated with birth injury etc.) would surprise no-one who has read Curtius[14] on the subject of the 'neuropathic family', although he himself appears to have been oblivious of Charcot's[15] previous introduction of the concept, itself based on still earlier work (*loc. cit*). A striking modern example of '*une famille neuropathologique*' is recorded by Cameron and Crawford[16]. Amongst 131 members of the family there were six cases of MS, three of cerebellar atrophy; one of spino-cerebellar degeneration; five insane and three showed presenile dementias.

The test we have described, if confirmed by workers who conform to the standard laid down by Seaman *et al*[5], will no doubt aid in further research into the genetics of HA. We ourselves have already begun this, and have picked up anomalies (not of MS character) in the RBC of mothers of HA children, but consideration of this is complicated and outside the scope of the present preliminary report.

Finally, the totally unexpected high proportion of positive MS diathesis (not actual MS) results amongst children presenting as 'hyperactive' has alerted us to ask about the childhood of patients (when mothers are available). Already we have heard descriptions very suggestive of childhood HA from several mothers. It is astonishing that while there are many papers dealing with the psychological make-up and characteristics during the decade or so before MS develops, we are unable to find any work on the childhood (prior to 10 years) character of children who later develop MS. Clearly there is a case here for a prospective study of true HA.

ACKNOWLEDGMENTS

We would like to thank Mrs Colquhoun and Mrs Bundy of the Hyperactive Children's Support Group for putting us in touch with many patients. This work was supported by the Naomi Bramson Trust.

References

1. Colquhoun, G., Bundy, S. (1981). A lack of essential fatty acids as a possible cause of hyperactivity in children. *Med. Hypoth.*, **7**, 63
2. Field, E. J., Joyce, G., Smith, B. M. (1977). Erythrocyte – UFA (E-UFA) Mobility Test for Multiple Sclerosis: Implications for Pathogenesis and Handling of the Disease. *J. Neurol.*, **214**, 113
3. Bisaccia, G., Caputo, D., Zibetti, A. (1977). E-UFA test in Multiple Sclerosis. *Boll Ist Sieroter*, **56**, 583
4. Caputo, D., Zibetti, A., Ghezzi, A., Cazzullo, C. L., Frosio, C., Bertoni, G. (1979). Erythrocyte unsaturated fatty acid test (E-UFA); A biological test to detect optic neuritis as initial feature of multiple sclerosis. *J. Neurol.*, **221**, 53
5. Seaman, G. V. F., Swank, R. L., Tamblyn, C. H., Zukoski, C. F. (1979). Simplified red cell electrophoretic mobility test for Multiple Sclerosis. *Lancet*, **ii**, 1138
6. Tamblyn, C. H., Swank, R. L., Seaman, G. V. F., Zukoski, C. F. (1980). Red cell electrophoretic mobility test for early diagnosis of Multiple Sclerosis. *Neurol. Res.*, **2**, 69
7. Jones, R., Capildeo, R., Rose, C. F., Forrester, J. A., Luckman, N. P., Preece, A. W. (1981). A diagnostic test for multiple sclerosis using glutaraldehyde fixed erythrocytes and laser cytophotometry. In Preece, A. W. and Light, P. A. (eds.). *Cell Electrophoresis in Cancer and other Clinical Research*, pp. 189–195. (Amsterdam: North Holland/Elsevier)
8. Forrester, J. A., Smith, W. J. (1977). Screening children at risk of Multiple Sclerosis. *Lancet*, **ii**, 453
9. Seaman, G. V. F., Swank, R. L. Zukoski, C. F. (1979). Red-cell membrane differences in Multiple Sclerosis are acquired from plasma. *Lancet*, **i**, 1139
10. Field, E. J., Joyce, G. (1982). An office test for Multiple Sclerosis. *IRCS Med. Sci.*, **10**, 560
11. Field, E. J. (1980). *Multiple Sclerosis in Childhood*, pp. 19–21. (Springfield, Illinois: Charles C. Thomas)
12. Field, E. J., Joyce, G. (1977). Prostaglandin (PGE_2) and human erythrocyte mobility: a specific test for Multiple Sclerosis? *IRCS Med. Sci.*, **5**, 158
13. Field, E. J., Joyce, G. (1981). Simplified E-UFA Test for Multiple Sclerosis (MS): Some sources of 'False' Results. *J. Neurol.*, **226**, 149

14. Curtius, F. C. (1933). *Multiple Sklerose und Erbanlage*, pp. 215 (Leipzig: George Thieme Verlag)
15. Charcot, J. M. (1882). *Leçons du Mardi a la Salpètrière*. p. 410. (Paris: Louis Bataille)
16. Cameron, E., Crawford, A. D. (1974). A familial neurological disease complex in a Bedfordshire community. *J. R. Coll. Gen. Pract.*, **24,** 435

Poster 8
Isoelectric focusing of the CSF gamma-globulins in 2594 patients

R. E. GONSETTE, Y. De SMET and P. DELMOTTE

Due to its concentrating effect, isoelectric focusing (IEF) makes possible the detection of very low concentrations of oligoclonal IgG fractions in the cerebrospinal fluid (CSF).

The aim of the study was to investigate the possible influence of the increased sensitivity of this technique on the percentage of CSF oligoclonal patterns (OP) in various neurological diseases.

2594 IEF have been performed, 632 in multiple sclerosis (MS) patients and 1962 in other neurological diseases (OND). The highest incidence of OP was observed in MS: 90% when the diagnosis was definite, 51% when probable and 22% when possible.

Acute and chronic infectious diseases of the CNS were frequently associated with an OP of the CSF and, with the exception of a transient OP in acute aseptic meningitis, it seems that, when present, OP remains detectable for many years. The high incidence of OP in CNS tumours is interesting and particularly marked in patients with brain metastases from a pulmonary origin. The OP was definitely infrequent in vascular disorders (30 out of 496 patients).

These observations will be discussed extensively in a further publication, but, due to the high sensitivity of the method and its reproducibility, IEF is a reliable diagnostic tool for the neurologist.

Poster 9
Modulation of immunity in multiple sclerosis: a double-blind levamisole–placebo controlled study in 85 patients

R. E. GONSETTE, L. DEMONTY, P. DELMOTTE, J. DECREE,
W. DE COCK, H. VERHAEGHEN and J. SYMOENS

Levamisole seems to regulate cell-mediated immunity by restoring T-cell function. Since a deficiency of T lymphocytes has been described by various authors in multiple sclerosis patients, an investigation was carried out on the possible effect of levamisole, a thymomimetic agent, on multiple sclerosis patients.

Of the 85 patients involved in the trial, evaluation of functional and neurological scores was possible in 54 (32 with placebo and 22 with levamisole). The mean follow-up period was 2 years. This double-blind controlled study indicates that both neurological function and disability significantly deteriorated in the placebo-treated patients, but remained fairly stable in the levamisole-treated group. Since the difference between both groups was not significant, no levamisole effect was demonstrated on progression in multiple sclerosis.

With the exception of one case of granulocytopenia (which had no clinical effect), no drug-related changes could be demonstrated. This contrasts with the general impression that this immunomodulator agent might be harmful to patients with multiple sclerosis.

The fact that during this blind study both annual relapse rate and disability score remained more stable in treated patients with severe disability suggests that, while waiting for a more effective treatment, long-term levamisole therapy could be useful in patients with a shorter evolution and a lower disability score at entry in the treatment.

Poster 10
Brain antigens detected by cerebrospinal fluid from multiple sclerosis patients

H. HEYLIGEN, F. VAN ROMPAEY, D. NIJST, J. RAUS
and A. A. VANDENBARK

ABSTRACT

Increased levels of antibodies against both multiple sclerosis (MS) and control brain extracts were observed in the cerebrospinal fluid of MS patients using a sensitive assay (Enzyme Linked Immunosorbent Assay, ELISA). The possibility that antibodies in MS CSF can detect 'MS associated' brain antigens was examined by testing various CSFs for reactivity against chromatofocused fractions obtained from MS or control brain extracts. The MS CSF showed increased reactivity against many of the chromatofocused fractions, indicating the presence of a broad spectrum of antigens in the various brain extracts. However, quantitative differences in reactivity against various fractions were observed, resulting in reproducible reactivity patterns of CSF against various brain extracts. A comparison of these reactivity patterns revealed that the same MS CSFs recognized the same regions (roughly nine in all) in the separation profile of two MS brain extracts. The MS CSFs showed significantly less reactivity against five of these regions from normal brain, but against only three regions from a Huntingtons brain extract. Reactivity to two regions of the MS brain extracts was significantly reduced to both normal and Huntingtons brain extracts. Whether these quantitative differences in the reactivity patterns reflect qualitative differences in the fractions will be analysed further by preabsorbing reactive CSFs on normal brain fractions to remove antibodies directed against identical or cross reactive antigens.

INTRODUCTION

Cerebrospinal fluid (CSF) from most patients with multiple sclerosis (MS), and a lower percentage of patients with other neurologic diseases (OND), contains antibodies which react with crude brain extracts[1]. The specificity of the antibody is largely unknown, although some of the immunoglobulin is clearly directed at myelin basic protein (MBP). The CSF antibody in MS patients shows similar levels of reactivity (measured by the enzyme linked immunosorbent assay, ELISA) to extracts prepared from different areas of the same brain, from plaques and the surrounding periplaque tissue, and from different brains[1]. The extraction techniques that solubilized the greatest amount of reactive antigen (3 mol/l KCl and -butanol) are somewhat selective in extracting membrane associated molecules[2,3]. Indeed, Van Rompaey et al[1] and Offner et al[5], could detect MBP in the cathodic regions of brain but not synovial tissue extracts. Since total reactivity of CSF antibodies to crude extracts cannot distinguish differences in reactivity to individual components, we separated the crude extracts from several brains by chromatofocusing and gel filtration, and compared the pattern of reactivity of a single MS CSF versus the individual fractions.

METHODS

CSFs were obtained by lumbar puncture from patients with MS and OND. Cells were sedimented at $200g$ and the CSFs stored at $-20\,°C$ until use. Brains were obtained at autopsy from two MS patients, a patient with Huntingtons disease (HD) and an accident victim without neurologic disease. Brain specimens were collected $<12\,h$ after death and were frozen at $-80\,°C$ until use. Extracts were prepared from unselected areas of each brain by 3 mol/l KCl[2]. Chromatofocusing (CF) was carried out by adding 25 mg (protein) of extract to a $1 \times 20\,cm$ column containing polybuffer (Pharmacia PBE 94) and eluted with a 7.4–3.8 pH gradient, followed by washing with 1 mol/l NaCl. The resulting fractions were analysed for absorbance at 280 nm and by SDS polyacrylamide gel electrophoresis using a flatbed system (LKB) and silver staining to detect protein. Some CSF fractions were pooled, concentrated, and separated further by exclusion chromatography using a $2.5 \times 100\,cm$ Sephacryl S 300 column. Crude extracts and fractions obtained above were evaluated for antigenic content by ELISA. The extracts (5 mg protein/ml) or $10\,\mu l$ of each fraction were coated onto a 96 well polyvinyl chloride (PVC) plate overnight at $4\,°C$. Reactive binding sites on the PVC plates were saturated with a buffer containing both 1% bovine serum albumin (BSA) and 0.1% histones[6]. After washing, $20\,\mu l$ of CSF from the MS patient was added for $2\frac{1}{2}\,h$ at $4\,°C$ (in saturation buffer). Antibody which adhered to the plate was detected using peroxidase-conjugated α-human IgG and substrate (orthophenyldiamine) read for absorbance at OD 450 nm. Results of 2–4 replicate wells were compared with background reactions (wells containing no CSF and wells containing no α-IgG).

RESULTS

Chromatofocusing of crude 3 mol/l KCl extracts of MS brain produced a number of 280 nm absorbing peaks, including cathodic fractions (column pass) and fractions which eluted at pH 7.1, 7.0, between 4 and 4.8, and 3.8

Table 1 Reactivity of MS CSF with chromatofocused 3 mol/l KCl extracts from MS, HD, and
normal brains

Elution pH	Reactivity to brain extract		
	MS	HD	Normal
> 7	+ +	+ +	+
6.8	−	−	+
6.7	+	+	+
6.6	−	−	+
6.4	+	−	+
6.2	−	+	−
6.0	+	+	−
5.7	+ +	+ +	+
5.5	+ +	−	+
5.2	+	+ +	+
4.8	+ +	+	−
4.3	+ +	+ +	−
4.0	+ +	+	−
3.8	−	+ +	−
NaCl	+ + +	+ +	+

- −   <0.06
- +   >0.06
- + +   >0.10
- + + +   >0.14

CSF was (−) vs polybuffer in all fractions

with 1 mol/l NaCl. Analysis of selected fractions by SDS polyacrylamide electrophoresis and silver staining revealed many smaller molecular weight components (<50 kD) in the neutral fractions (pH 5-7.5), and both large and small MW components in the more acidic fractions (pH 3.8-5). Similar fractionation and analysis of the HD and normal brain revealed remarkably similar elution profiles. Analysis of MS CSF antibody reactivity against the chromatofocused fractions from two different MS brains revealed reproducible patterns of reactivity. The most reactive peaks were in the cathodic region (containing MBP), and at elution pHs of 6.8, 6.5, 5.6, 4.3-4.8, 4.0 and with 1 mol/l NaCl. Similar comparisons of MS brain extract versus the HD and normal brain extract revealed several quantitatively different reactivities present in each extract (Table 1). Notably the MS brain had increased reactivity relative to both HD and normal brain at pH 5.5, 4.8, 4.0 and in the NaCl elution. HD brain had increased reactivity at pH 5.2 and 3.8, and normal brain slightly increased reactivity at pH 6.8 and 6.6.

Further fractionation of the MS brain fraction at pH 4.0 by Sephacryl S 300 chromatography revealed virtually no OD 280 absorbance in any fraction, but significant ELISA reactivity with the MS CSF in regions with molecular weights of $> 10^6$; 800 000, 150 000, 100 000, 60 000, and 40 000 Daltons. No reactivity of OND CSF was detected to either the chromatofocused fractions or the S 300 fractions.

DISCUSSION

The data presented above clearly show that the MS CSF recognized distinct regions in chromatofocused fractions of different brain extracts, even though the total ELISA reactivity to the unfractionated extracts was the same. The CSF reactivity to the brain fractions was not related to the protein concentration (measured by absorbance at 280 nm) of the fractions, and was unaffected by the presence of the polybuffer. These data suggest that the reactivity pattern is not due to nonspecific adsorbance of CSF IgG to different concentrations of protein present in each of the fractions. Further fractionation by exclusion chromatography of a reactive peak (pH 4.0) from the chromatofocused MS extract revealed additional heterogeneity of ELISA reactive components, including a major reactive peak at 150 000 MW. This fraction may contain IgG which could be present as an antigen (i.e. rheumatoid factor), or as part of an immune complex.

The differences observed between comparable chromatofocused fractions from different brains are at best quantitative, and without adsorptions, no conclusions concerning qualitative differences in extracts can be made. Some differences in reactivity can be attributed to quantitative variations in extracted components from the unselected sections of the different brains. (The total ELISA reaction is dependent upon the antigen coating concentration[6].) Such a variation was not observed when comparing extracts from two separate MS brains, however. The antibody used was not a variable since the same CSF was utilized in all experiments.

Taken together, these data suggest that at least quantitative differences in brain antigens exist among MS, HD and normal brains. These molecules may be membrane associated, are eluted predominantly at acidic pHs, and may represent altered products of normal molecules produced by the disease processes, or perhaps even disease-associated antigens. The range of antibody specificities in the MS CSF appears extremely broad, and may represent the products of unregulated clonal expansion within the CSF (see accompanying chapters by Offner et al[5], and De Saedeleer et al[7]).

ACKNOWLEDGEMENTS

The authors wish to thank Agnes Delsaer for typing the manuscript and Tony Van Galen for preparing graphics for presentation at the 25th Anniversary Symposium of the Belgian Research Group for MS, Brussels, Belgium which this manuscript describes.

This work was supported by the Paul J. Cams Foundation of Belgium, the Wetenschappelijk Onderzoek MS Organization of Belgium and the United States Veterans Administration.

References

1. Vandenbark, A. A., Van Rompaey, F., Nijst, D., Heyligen, H. and Raus, J. (1983). Cerebrospinal fluid antibodies detect brain antigens. In Gonsette, R. E. and Delmotte, P. (eds.). *Immunological and Clinical Aspects of Multiple Sclerosis*, Chap. 5. (Lancaster: MTP Press)
2. Meltzer, M. S., Leonard, E. J., Rapp, J. J. and Bersos, T. (1971). *J. Natl. Cancer Inst.*, **47**, 103
3. Le Grue, S. J., Kahan, B. D. and Pellis, N. R. (1980). *J. Natl. Cancer Inst.*, **65**, 191
4. Van Rompaey, F., Nijst, D., Raus, J. and Vandenbark, A. A. (1983). Antibrain antibody adsorption on microtiter plates. In Gonsette, R. E. and Delmotte, P. (eds.). *Immunological and Clinical Aspects of Multiple Sclerosis*, Chap. P21. (Lancaster: MTP Press)
5. Offner, H., Van Rompaey, F., Nijst, D., Raus, J. and Vandenbark, A. A. (1983). Shared antibrain specificities of cerebrospinal fluid and synovial fluid antibodies. In Gonsette, R. E. and Delmotte, P. (eds.). *Immunological and Clinical Aspects of Multiple Sclerosis*, Chap. P15. (Lancaster: MTP Press)
6. Vandenbark, A. A., Van Rompaey, F., Heyligen, H., Nijst, D. and Raus, J. (1982). In Peeters, H. (ed.). *Protides of the Biological Fluids*, Vol 30 (Oxford: Pergamon)
7. De Saedeleer, J., Dom, R., Raus, J., Stragier, J., Carton, H. and Vandenbark, A. A. (1983). Increased T helper cell levels in cerebrospinal fluid. In Gonsette, R. E. and Delmotte, P. (eds.). *Immunological and Clinical Aspects of Multiple Sclerosis*, Chap. P6. (Lancaster: MTP Press)

Poster 11
Cell-mediated immunity in progressive forms of multiple sclerosis treated by lympho-plasmapheresis

B. KENNES, C. P. LEROY, J. P. DUMONT, D. FAVERLY, D. BROHÉE,
J. JACQUY, G. NOËL and P. NÈVE

Static and dynamic cell mediated immunities (CMI) were investigated in 22 progressive forms of no drug-treated multiple sclerosis (PFMS) and compared to sex and age cross matched controls.

There were no changes in blood total, helper, suppressor/cytotoxic T-cells, nor in B (Ia$^+$) and IgA, IgG, IgM bearing lymphocytes. Only the proportion of late T-rosette forming cells decreased, but not significantly, due to very low levels in some isolated cases of PFMS.

Proliferative responses (PR) to T (PHA, ConA) or to T- and B-mitogens (PWM) declines ($p \leqslant 0.01$) and T-suppressor activity showed normal values. Owing to the pattern of histogram PR distribution, PFMS were separated into Low Responders (LR) or into Normal Responders (NR).

At 6 months lympho-plasmapheresis programme (LP) abolished the PR deficiency in LR, did not modify PR in NR and significantly increased the proportion of some suppressor T-cells and B-cells ($p \leqslant 0.005$) in both categories of patients.

No relationship could be observed between PR and sex, neurological scores, duration of the disease or clinical response to LP.

The data indicate that CMI abnormalities found in some PFMS do not play a role in the evolution of the disease.

Poster 12
Myelin basic protein in cerebrospinal fluid, detected by an enzyme-immunoassay, and its diagnostic value

J. C. KOETSIER, G. J. VAN KAMP, L. LUYENDIJK and
J. O. MISPELBLOM BEYER

ABSTRACT

A non-radioactive technique for the detection of myelin basic protein (MBP) was developed and used for the estimation of MBP in the cerebrospinal fluid (CSF) of neurological patients. The sensitivity of the test is less than 1 ng/ml. MBP concentration was measured for a number of neurological diseases and a control group. Normal values for MBP in CSF appeared to be less than 4 ng/ml. Higher values were found in CSF from patients with active multiple sclerosis (exacerbations and chronic progressive course), infectious diseases of the central nervous system, traumatic brain damage and cerebral infarction.

INTRODUCTION

Thirty per cent of the proteins in the myelin fraction of the central nervous system consists of myelin basic protein (MBP), a linear polypeptide of approximately 170 amino-acid residues. MBP in Freund's adjuvant may cause, on injection into animals, e.g. guinea pigs, rabbits, monkeys etc., experimental allergic encephalomyelitis. MBP has been demonstrated in the cerebrospinal fluid (CSF) of patients with demyelinating diseases and other neurological diseases, accompanied by breakdown of myelin[1]. A non-radioactive technique for the detection of MBP was developed on the basis of an earlier described technique[2], and applied to the analysis of cerebrospinal fluid from different categories of neurological patients.

417

MATERIALS AND METHODS

(1) Human myelin basic protein was prepared according to Deibler et al[3].
(2) Antibodies against MBP have been raised in rabbits by injection of MBP with Freunds Incomplete Adjuvant[4].
(3) The titre of the antibodies was determined by the Complement Fixation Test[5].
(4) Conjugate: swine anti-rabbit-serum IgG horseradish peroxidase (HRP) conjugated (Dako).
(5) 96-Well flat-bottom microtitre plates (Greiner).
(6) 0.1 mol/l $NaHCO_3$, pH 9.6 as coating buffer.
(7) Substrate solution: 20 mg 1,2 phenylenediamine (OPD) and 0.3 ml 3% H_2O_2 in 40 ml citric acid phosphate buffer (0.1 mol/l citric acid adjusted to pH 5.5 with 0.2 mol/l Na_2HPO_4).
(8) Washing buffer: phosphate buffered saline (PBS) + 1% bovine serum albumin (BSA) + 0.05% Tween 20.
(9) Plate-cover: self-adhesive labels (Avery, 10 × 11.5 cm).
(10) Micro elisa reader system

 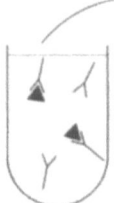 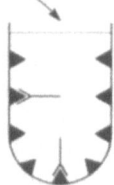 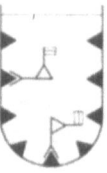 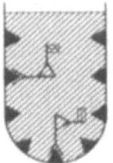

| coating of MBP on microtiterplate (plastic) | mix standards or sample with antiserum (glass) | binding of unreacted antibody to coated MBP | binding with HRP-labeled antibody | reaction with colour producing substrate measure extinction |

Figure 1

Procedure (Figure 1)

(1) microtitreplates were coated with 200 μl human MBP solution per well (30 ng/ml in coating buffer) 16 h at 37 °C
(2) wash procedure: 3 × 220 μl washing buffer for 5 min
(3) *standards and samples: 150 μl, incubate 2 h at 37 °C
(4) wash procedure as above
(5) 200 μl conjugate dilution (1:5000 in PBS): incubate 30 min at 37 °C
(6) wash procedure as above but without BSA
(7) 200 μl substrate, 30 min at room temperature in the dark
(8) stop reaction by addition of 50 μl HCl 4N
(9) measure intensity of colour at 492 nm in photometer.

* note: standards (MBP dilutions in PBS + 1% BSA) and samples CSF were mixed with anti-MBP-antiserum (diluted 1:2000 in PBS + 1% BSA); proportion: 450 μl + 50 μl, respectively. Reaction time: 16 h at 4 °C in glass tubes. From this mixture 150 μl was pipetted into the MBP-coated microtitreplate-wells.

Patients

CSF was obtained from patients admitted to the neurological ward. The control group was composed of patients with lumbar disk herniation. Samples were collected in plastic sample tubes (Beckman) and immediately frozen and stored at $-70\,°C$.

RESULTS

A typical standard curve for the described technique is depicted in Figure 2. The sensitivities of this test and the radio-immunoassay described by Cohen *et al* are comparable.

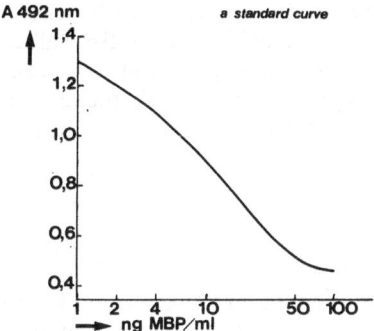

Figure 2

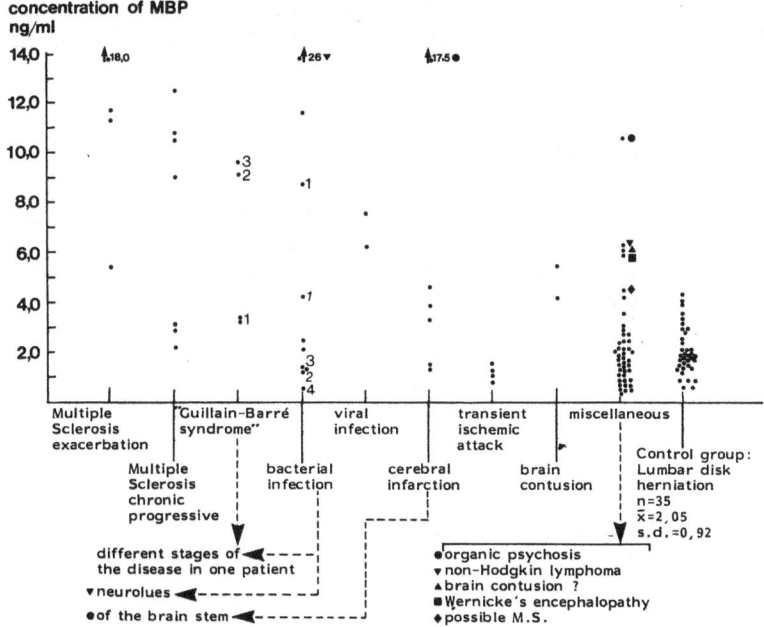

Figure 3

We have estimated the MBP content in the CSF of controls and neurological patients as shown in Figure 3.

The control group contained 35 samples, in which values ranged from less than 1.0 to 4.3 ng/ml MBP. The 95th percentile was at 4.0 ng/ml MBP. In the CSF of patients with an exacerbation of multiple sclerosis we have found high values. In the CSF of MS-patients with a chronic progressive course we found values higher than 4 ng/ml in only some cases. High values were also found in the group of patients with infections of the central nervous system, especially in a case of neurolues. Treatment of these patients resulted in a decrease in the MBP content in the CSF corresponding with the improvement of the clinical condition. The highest MBP value in the group of patients with a cerebral infarction was in the CSF of a patient with an infarction of the brainstem. The miscellaneous group consisted of patients with other neurological diseases, including two cases of optic neuritis with MBP values lower than 1 ng/ml. MBP values higher than 4 ng/ml were found in a case of organic psychosis, non-Hodgkin lymphoma of the brain, Wernicke's encephalopathy and in cases of brain contusion, possible multiple sclerosis and Guillain–Barré syndrome.

CONCLUSION

By using an enzyme immunoassay we have found high values of myelin basic protein in the cerebrospinal fluid of patients with different neurological diseases. Not only in the active phase of multiple sclerosis, but also in other diseases in which myelin breakdown occurs, values higher than 4 ng/ml have been found. These findings are compatible with the results of other investigators[1,6].

ACKNOWLEDGEMENTS

We are indebted to Dr Theo Out and members of the Dutch WOMS for supplying us with CSF and stimulating discussions; the department of Histology, Free University, for hospitality and handling of the immunized rabbits and to the Princess Beatrix Fund for financial support.

References

1. Cohen, S. R., Brooks, B. R., Herndon, R. M. and McKhann, G. M. (1980). *Ann. Neurol.*, **8**, 25
2. Kamp, G. J. van, Koetsier, J. C., Luyendijk, L., Mispelblom Beyer, J. O. and Verwey, C. L. (1983). In Peeters, H. (ed.), *Protides of the biological fluids*. Proceedings of the 30th coll. (1982). pp. 227–229 (Oxford: Pergamon Press)
3. Deibler, G. E., Martenson, R. E. and Kies, M. W. (1972). *Prep. Biochem.*, **2**, 139
4. Kohlschütter, A. (1978). *Eur. J. Pediatr.*, **127**, 155
5. Hudson, L. and Hay, F. C. (1980). *Practical Immunology*. 2nd Edn. pp. 149–152. (Oxford: Blackwell)
6. Jacque, C., Delasalle, A., Rancurel, G., *et al.* (1982). *Arch. Neurol.* **39**, 557

Poster 13
Onset-related values of serotonin, ceruloplasmin and 5-HIAA in patients with MS

V. VOICULESCU, N. LUCA, D. HATEGAN and C. ALECU

Serotonin (S) and ceruloplasmin (C) blood levels and urine excretion of 5-hydroxyindoleacetic acid (5-HIAA) were determined in 25 patients with multiple sclerosis (MS) and in 10 healthy controls. The data showed decreased C values in patients in whom the disease onset occurred 1 month to 2 years ago, and increased C values (up to 40%) in patients with disease onset over 5 years. Likewise, 5-HIAA excretion values were very low in patients with recent onset and high in those with older onset. In eight chronic patients 5-HIAA excretion was correlated with C activity. Unlike the obvious C and 5-HIAA alterations mentioned above, no correlation was found between the S blood level and the time elapsed since onset, possibly because of the wide limits of S normal values.

Poster 14
Visual evoked potentials: a contribution in the assessment of multiple sclerosis

A. GHEZZI, R. MONTANINI and C. L. CAZZULLO

INTRODUCTION

Visual evoked potentials (VEPs) are widely used in several laboratories for assessment of multiple sclerosis (MS). A large number of papers report (for a review see Sokol[1] and Montanini and Ghezzi[2]) the diagnostic aid of the VEP test in MS for the demonstration of a multifocal involvement within CNS, in patients with clinically unaffected optic pathways[3]. Data collected from different laboratories, using similar procedures, are reported[2] in Table 1. Furthermore, VEPs are useful in monitoring MS patients, MS suspected cases[4] and patients who suffered from optic neuritis (Ghezzi *et al*, Chapter P3), in the assessment of optic pathway damage by an objective method.

Table 1 Results collected from literature reports (from Montanini and Ghezzi[2])

Total number of abnormal responses	950/1412	67.2%
Abnormal responses in possible or suspected cases	225/480	46.8%
Abnormal responses in subjects with no visual symptoms or signs	366/654	55.9%

Our paper summarizes our experience with VEPs recording in MS (data from optic neuritis are reported in another paper in this volume), in connection with clinical findings and different methods of stimulation.

VEPs in definite and probable cases

VEPs were recorded in 63 definite and 29 probable cases, according to McDonald and Halliday[5], in response to a LED pattern reversal (total field 5.5°, single check 55′, reversal rate 0.8 Hz: for further details see Ghezzi and Orsini[6]): responses were considered abnormal for a delayed $P_2 > 113.5$ ms, corresponding to the upper confidence limit of 99%, or for an abnormal interocular difference (> 8 ms). VEPs were abnormal respectively in 84% and 65% of cases (Table 2).

Table 2   Incidence of abnormal visual evoked responses in relation to clinical findings

	No	Abnormal VEPs
Definite MS	63	84%
Probable MS	29	65%
Progressive spastic paraplegia	48	68%
Suspected MS (excluding optic neuritis)	19	31%
MS patients with no history of optic neuritis	97	53%

VEPs in progressive spastic paraplegia and in suspected cases

The above mentioned criteria of McDonald and Halliday[5] were used; cases with optic neuritis were excluded. Responses, recorded with the method described above, were abnormal in 33 out of 48 cases with spastic paraplegia and in 9 out of 19 suspected cases (Table 2).

Comparison of VEPs with ophthalmological findings

Results are reported in Table 2, in relation to the anamnestic report of a previous attack of optic neuritis, and in Table 3, in relation with ophthalmological findings, in a subgroup of 40 cases. The colour vision was tested with Forworth 100 Hue and Hardy Rand Ritter tests.

Table 3   VEPs results in relation to ophthalmological findings

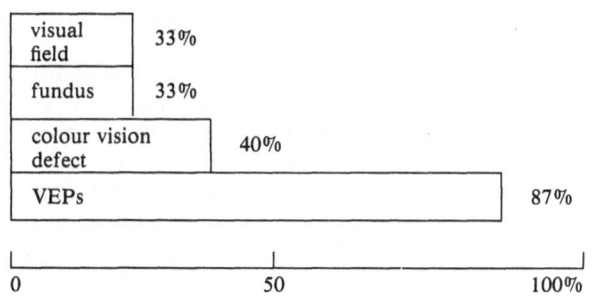

Comparison of different stimuli

Responses from a LED pattern reversal (see above), a Led pattern onset–offset (obtained with the same LED matrix; the averager was triggered by the onset of a pattern which was presented for 400 ms, stimulation rate 0.8 Hz) a flash (reddish light, 0.6 joules, stimulation rate 1 Hz)[6,7] were compared in 46 cases: normative data and results are reported in Tables 4 and 5.

VEPs were finally compared in a restricted group of 20 MS patients in response to a LED pattern reversal, a foveal stimulus (a square subtending

Table 4   The normal response in relation to different stimuli (latency in ms, amplitude in μV)

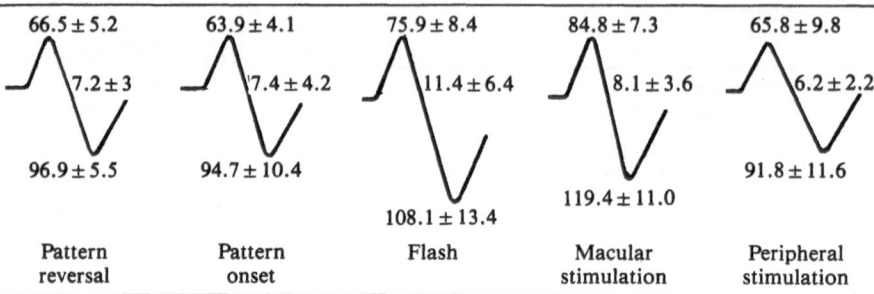

| Pattern reversal | Pattern onset | Flash | Macular stimulation | Peripheral stimulation |

Table 5   % incidence of abnormal responses in relation to different stimuli

	Pattern reversal	Pattern onset	Flash	Macular stim.	Peripheral stim.
Abnormal responses					
+ 2 SD	93	74	61	57	75
+ 3 SD	80	57	22	38	50

90', duration 400 ms, stimulation rate 0.8 Hz) a peripheral stimulus (external edge 17°, internal one 13°): results are reported in Tables 4 and 5.

COMMENT

The frequent involvement of optic pathways in MS is well known from pathological studies[8,9]. VEPs studied in our series confirm the high incidence of optic pathway lesions in MS: the percentage of abnormality varies among different series[1], probably reflecting differences of techniques and of selection of cases. Our figure of 84%, in definite cases, completely agrees with the available literature data (see Table 1), and further demonstrates that the optic nerve is an elective site of lesion in MS. However, the diagnostic helpfulness of VEPs depends on the possibility of detecting a second subclinical site of lesion in patients with objective signs and symptoms outside the optic nerve. In patients with progressive spastic paraplegia we obtained abnormal responses in 68% of cases and in 31% of suspected cases. In such instances, when neuroradiological investigations are negative, diagnosis of MS can be assessed with sufficient reliability, especially if confirmed by CSF examination[4,10]. A similar point of view is substained by Trojaborg et al[11], who reclassified his series, namely possible cases, in the light of neurophysiological and CSF findings.

The effectiveness of VEPs in detecting subclinical lesions of optic pathways is emphasized by the high incidence of abnormal responses with respect to ophthalmological data, similar to that observed by Lowitzsch[12] and Nikoskelainen[13].

In recent years many efforts have been made to investigate the most appropriate method of stimulating; comparing different pattern reversals[14],

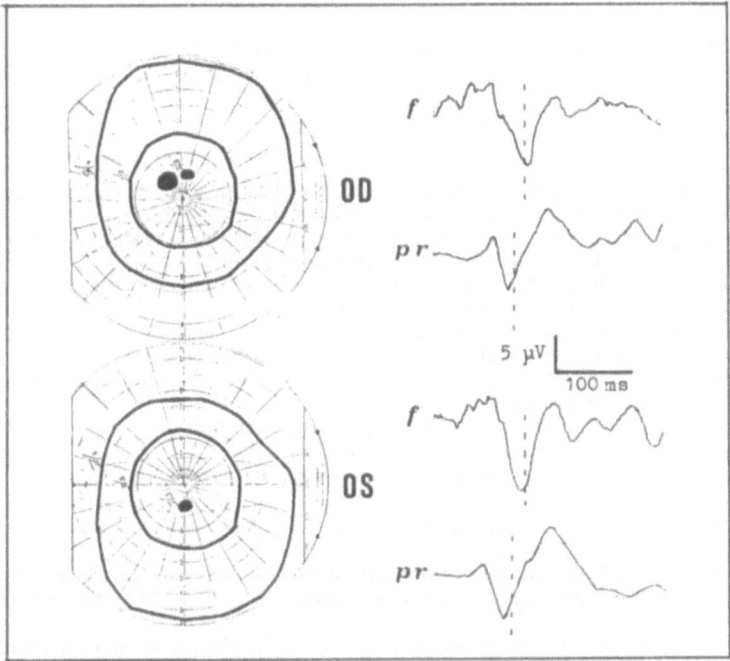

Figure 1 Flash (f) and pattern visual evoked responses (pr) in relation to visual field. Dashed line indicates upper confidence limit of 99%

patterned and unpatterned stimuli[15], foveal and peripheral stimuli and/or pattern reversal[16,17], pattern reversal and pattern onset[18], with different and non-conclusive results. In our material, the stimulation with a pattern reversal produced the highest percentage of abnormal responses. Pattern onset–offset does not seem to give important results, differing from that observed by Aminoff[18]: the incidence of abnormality is lower, the variability in healthy subjects quite high.

Flash VEPs, as known, present a great variability in normal subjects and are less frequently delayed in MS patients. Nevertheless, in a few cases flash may be helpful: when PRVEPs are not well defined and are doubtful to interpret, when visual defects are in extrafoveal regions (see Fig. 1, with a normal PRVEP, but a delayed flash VEPs): in our series this occurred in two cases. Hennerici[17] and Rossini[16] pointed out the usefulness of foveal stimuli, which appear to elecit abnormal responses in higher percentage than pattern reversal and peripheral stimuli. In our experience a small square of 90′ was used, compared with a peripheral stimulus (from 13° to 17°) and with a pattern reversal: our data seem only to indicate a complementary role of peripheral and foveal stimuli in the assessment of the site of lesion with respect to pattern reversal.

Acknowledgement

This investigation was supported by a CNR grant for: 'Progetto Finalizzato Medicinia Preventiva e Riabilitativa - Malattie S.N.C. - OB.26'.

References

1. Sokol, S. (1980). Visual evoked potentials. In Aminoff, M. J. (ed.). *Electrodiagnosis in Clinical Neurology*, (Edinburgh: Church Livingstone)
2. Montanini R., and Ghezzi, A. (1981). Contributo dei potenziali evocati visivi alla diagnosi di laboratorio di sclerosi multipla. *Proceedings of Congress S.I.N.*
3. Halliday, A. M., McDonald, W. and Mushin, J. (1973). Visual evoked response in diagnosis of multiple sclerosis. *Br. Med. J.*, **4**, 661
4. Bottcher, J. and Trojaborg, W. (1982). Follow up of patients with suspected multiple sclerosis: a clinical and electrophysiological study. *J. Neurol. Neurosurg. Psych.*, **45**, 802
5. McDonald, W. I. and Halliday, A. M. (1977). Diagnosis and classification of multiple sclerosis. *Br. Med. Bull.*, **33**, 4
6. Ghezzi, A. and Orsini, O. (1981). Confronto tra stimoli patterned e unpatterned nella sclerosi multipla. *Riv. Ital. EEG Neurofis. Clin.*, **1**, 157
7. Ghezzi, A. (1979). Visual evoked potentials in multiple sclerosis. *Acta Neurol.*, **XXXIV**, 387
8. Cazzullo, C. L. (1956). Le encefalomieliti demielinizzanti. *Atti XII Congr. Soc. Ital. Neurol.*, pp. 201–278 (Padova: S. I. N.)
9. Lumsden, G. E. (1970). The neuropathology of multiple sclerosis. In Vinker, P. J. and Bruyn, G. W. (eds.). *Handbooks of clinical neurology, Vol. 9*, pp. 217–309, (Amsterdam: Elsevier)
10. Ghezzi, A., Caputo, D., Montanini, R., Procaccia, S., Zibetti, A. and Cazzullo, C. L. (1981). Multiple tests in diagnosis of multiple sclerosis. *Ital. J. Neurol. Sci.*, **3**, 297
11. Trojaborg, W., Bottcher, J. and Saxtrup, O. (1981). Evoked potentials and immunoglobulin abnormalities in multiple sclerosis. *Neurology*, **31**, 866
12. Lowitzsh, K. (1980). Pattern reversal visual evoked potentials in 251 MS patients. In Bauer, H. J., Poser, S. and Ritter, G. (ed.). *Progress in MS research* (Basel: Springer Verlag)
13. Nikoskelainen, E. and Falck, B. (1982). Do visual evoked potentials give relevant information to the neuroophthalmological examination in optic nerve lesion? *Acta Neurol. Scand.*, **66**, 42
14. Nilsson, B. Y. (1978). Visual evoked responses in multiple sclerosis: comparison of two methods for pattern reversal. *J. Neurol. Neurosurg. Psych.*, **41**, 499
15. Wilson, W. B. and Keyser, R. B. (1980). Comparison of the pattern and diffuse light visual evoked responses in definite multiple sclerosis. *Acta Neurol.*, **37**, 30
16. Rossini, P. M., Pirchio, M., Sallono, D. and Caltagirone, G. (1979). Foveal vs. peripheral retinal response: a new VEP for the early diagnosis of multiple sclerosis. *Electroenceph. Clin. Neurophys.*, **47**, 515
17. Hennerici, N., Wenzel, D. and Freund, H. J. (1977). The comparison of small size rectangle and checkerboard pattern reversal stimulation for the evaluation of delayed visual evoked response of multiple sclerosis. *Brain*, **100**, 119
18. Aminoff, M. J. and Ochs, A. L. (1981). Pattern onset visual evoked potentials in suspected multiple sclerosis. *J. Neurol. Neurosurg. Psych.*, **44**, 608

Poster 15
Shared antibrain specificities of cerebrospinal fluid and synovial fluid antibodies

H. OFFNER, F. VAN ROMPAEY, D. NIJST, J. RAUS
and A. A. VANDENBARK

ABSTRACT

Both the cerebrospinal fluid (CSF) from multiple sclerosis (MS) patients and synovial fluid (SF) from rheumatoid arthritis (RA) patients demonstrate increased lymphocyte infiltration and production of immunoglobulin of multiple specificities. To explore the possibility that antibodies present in these widely separated compartments share similar or identical specificities, reactions of CSF and SF with extracts of brain and synovial tissue or with purified antigens were compared by the enzyme linked immunosorbent assay (ELISA). CSF and SF showed significant reactivity to both of the tissue extracts as well as to myelin basic protein (MBP) and keyhole limpet haemocyanin (KLH). The reactivity to MBP of CSF and SF was inhibitable by preincubation with specific rabbit antibody, suggesting that the same or closely associated determinants were recognized by antibodies in both fluids and by the rabbit antibodies. In additional experiments, reactivity of pooled CSF or SF to chromatofocused fractions of brain or synovial tissue extracts revealed similar reaction patterns, although each fluid reacted distinctly with at least one fraction of each extract. These results support the suggestion that a common deregulation process in MS and RA stimulates non-selectively a large repertoire of B-cell clones to produce 'nonsense' immunoglobulins to many antigens, including some presumably not found in the respective tissue compartments. Responses to disease-associated 'target' antigens are difficult to discern, but may be detectable in CSF or SF reactions to fractions of crude tissue extracts.

INTRODUCTION

Cerebrospinal fluids (CSF) from patients with multiple sclerosis (MS) and other neurologic diseases (OND), and synovial fluid (SF) from patients with rheumatoid arthritis (RA), often have increased cellularity and antibody levels[1,2].

In CSF, the increase in cells appears to be due to a selective migration of the T-helper subset[3] which may lead to imbalances in T-cell regulation of antibody production by B-cells.

Such a process raises the possibility of a non-selective clonal expansion of B-cells, including the production of antibodies against antigens not present in the respective tissue compartments. This study sought to detect and compare antibody specificities in CSF and SF to antigens prepared from the central nervous system, the synovium, and to a non-self antigen, keyhole limpet haemocyanin (KLH), to which humans are usually unreactive[4].

MATERIALS AND METHODS

Patient samples

CSF samples were pooled from the following groups:

(1) MS : eight patients with confirmed MS.
(2) (+) OND : three patients with OND, in which neat CSF contained significant antibrain antibody reactivity
(3) (−) OND : five patients with OND, in which neat CSF contained no significant antibrain antibody reactivity,
(4) SF : samples from six patients with rheumatoid arthritis were pooled. The fluids were collected fresh, spun to remove cells and stored frozen until use.

Brain and synovial tissue extracts were prepared by extraction with 1-butanol[5] from unselected sections of brain (obtained <12 hours after autopsy from an MS patient, and stored at −80 °C) and synovium (obtained surgically from a rheumatoid arthritis patient and stored at −80 °C).

Procedures

The ELISA was carried out as described previously[6,7] using as antigen the extracts described above, purified whole myelin[8], myelin basic protein, MBP[9], cerebrosides (Sigma) and KLH[4].

In one set of experiments, plates coated with MBP or KLH were pretreated with rabbit α-MBP or α-KLH (at 1/1000, 1/2000 and 1/10000 dilutions of antiserum, raised by injection of MBP or KLH first in Freund's complete adjuvant and repeatedly in Freund's incomplete adjuvant) before the addition of CSF or SF samples, and finally rabbit α-human IgG antiserum.

Chromatofocusing was carried out as described elsewhere in this book[10].

RESULTS

CSF and CF have similar antibody recognition to brain and synovial tissue antigens

In initial experiments, CSF and SF were tested for antibody recognition to a range of antigens. Pooled CSF from eight MS patients, three (+) OND patients, and five (−) OND patients, and pooled SF from six rheumatoid arthritis patients were adjusted to the same IgG concentration (10 μg/ml) and tested by ELISA for reactivity to brain extract, synovial tissue extract, whole myelin, MBP, cerebrosides and KLH. Significant reactivity was observed in the MS, (+) OND, and RA pools to all antigens except cerebrosides; the (−) OND pool was less reactive than the other pools to brain extract and was unreactive to the other antigens.

Rabbit antibody inhibits CSF and SF reactivity to MBP and KLH

In order to establish the specificity of the antibody reactions against MBP and KLH, rabbit α-MBP and α-KLH were used to inhibit CSF and SF recognition. Plates coated with MBP or KLH were treated first with various dilutions of rabbit α-MBP and α-KLH to block reactive sites, and then with CSF or SF. Finally, antihuman IgG was used to detect CSF and SF antibody reactivity. The results indicate that pretreatment with rabbit α-MBP blocked both the CSF and SF reactivity to MBP in a dose dependent fashion relative to α-KLH. Conversely, rabbit α-KLH blocked both CSF and SF reactivity to KLH relative to α-MBP.

CSF and SF show similar patterns of antibody reactivity to chromatofocused fractions of brain or synovial tissue extracts

To evaluate further the antibody reactivities in CSF and SF the pooled fluids were tested versus chromatofocused fractions of butanol extracts prepared from brain and synovial tissue. The reactivity pattern of CSF was very similar to that of SF to both extracts, although different patterns of reactivity were detected to brain versus synovial tissue. Most strikingly, both CSF and SF were reactive to most cathodic brain fractions (which contain MBP) but were unreactive to similar fractions of cationic molecules extracted from synovial tissue. Slight differences in reactivity between CSF and SF were noted in the fractions eluting between pH 6.3 and 6.7, where CSF was more reactive to brain extracts and SF was more reactive to synovial tissue extracts.

DISCUSSION

These data show clearly the similarities in antigen recognition shared by CSF and SF antibodies. Quantitatively, CSF from MS patients and (+) OND patients and SF from rheumatoid arthritis patients show similar ELISA reactivity when tested at the same IgG concentration to brain extract, synovial tissue extract, myelin, MBP, and KLH and no significant reactivity to cerebrosides. OND CSF without antibrain activity when tested neat (− OND) had approximately half the antibrain antibody activity as the other pooled fluids when concentrated to the same IgG levels, but showed no reactivity to any of the other antigens. These data suggest that CSF and SF from patients with significantly elevated total IgG and antibrain antibody also share similar antibody specificities to other self (whole myelin, MBP) and non-self (KLH) antigens.

To further document the specificity of the α-MBP and α-KLH responses, rabbit antibody to each of these antigens was used to block reactivity of the human CSF or SF antibody. The inhibition observed was reciprocally specific for the antigen–rabbit antibody combination, and was dose dependent, suggesting that similar epitopes are recognized in immunized rabbit antibody and in human CSF and SF.

The recognition of MBP was further demonstrated when CSF and SF were tested versus chromatofocused fractions obtained from brain or synovial tissue extracts. Both fluids reacted strongly to the most cathodic fractions of brain extract (which have been shown to contain MBP[11]), but were unreactive to the corresponding cations focused from synovial tissue. Further comparisons of CSF and SF reactivity indicate similar reaction profiles versus each chromatofocused extract, although the CSF was more reactive than SF to brain fractions eluting in the pH 6.3–6.7 region, and SF more reactive to similar synovial tissue fractions.

In general, the CSF and SF antibody reactivity pattern versus brain extract differed from that versus synovial tissue extract. Not only were ELISA readings greater versus brain, but the neutral and basic fractions also appeared to be more reactive in the brain extract.

The demonstration of antibody to brain antigen in CSF has been documented previously by us[6,7,10] and others[12], and are increased in CSFs with oligoclonal bands and elevated IgG[6,7]. SF also has greatly elevated IgG, probably associated with increased cellularity in the synovium[2]. The presence of antibrain antibodies in SF and antisynovial tissue antibodies in CSF, suggest that non-specific activation of B-cell clones occurs similarly in both tissue compartments. This expansion apparently occurs without antigen, since MBP is a myelin specific protein and since KLH is an uncommonly encountered non-self antigen (to which normal humans have a low precursor frequency[13], and no demonstrable immunity[4]).

The results showing antibrain antibody in SF extend our previous observations[14,15] showing increased active E rosettes to brain antigens in patients with juvenile and adult onset RA.

Taken together, these observations suggest a common process in MS and RA in which the balance of regulatory T-cells is altered in CSF and SF, leading to deregulation of B-cell clones and the non-specific expression of a wide range of antibodies to self and non-self antigens.

ACKNOWLEDGEMENTS

The authors wish to thank Agnes Delsaer for typing the manuscript, and Tony Van Galen for preparing graphics for presentation at the 25th Anniversary Symposium of the Belgian Research Group for MS, Brussels, Belgium which this manuscript describes.

This research was supported by a grant from the Jacob and Olga Madsen

Foundation of Denmark, the Paul J. Cams Foundation of Belgium, the Wetenschappelijk Onderzoek MS Organization of Belgium and United States Veterans Administration.

References

1. Iivanainen, M. V. (1981). The significance of abnormal immune responses in patients with multiple sclerosis. *J. Neuroimmunol.,* **1,** 141
2. Janossy, G., Panyi, G., Duke, O., Bofill, M., Poulter, L. W. and Goldstein, G. (1981). Rheumatoid arthritis: a disease of T lymphocyte/macrophage immunoregulation. *Lancet,* 839
3. De Saedeleer, J., Dom, T., Raus, J., Stragier, J., Carton, H. and Vandenbark, A. A. (1983). Increased T helper cells levels in cerebrospinal fluid. In Gonsette, R. E. and Delmotte, P. (eds.). *Immunological and Clinical Aspects of Multiple Sclerosis,* Chap. P6. (Lancaster: MTP Press)
4. Vandenbark, A. A., Yoshihara, P., Carveth, L. and Burger, D. R. (1981). All KLH preparations are not created equal. *Cell. Immunol.,* **60,** 240
5. LeGrue, S. J., Kahan, B. D. and Pellis, N. R. (1980). Extraction of a murine tumor-specific transplantation antigen with l-butanol. 1. Partial purification by isoelectric focusing. *J. Natl. Cancer Inst.,* **65,** 191
6. Vandenbark, A. A., Van Rompaey, F., Heyligen, H., Nijst, D. and Raus, J. (1982). CSF autoantibodies detect brain antigens. In Peeters, H. (ed.). *Protides of the Biological Fluids.* Vol. 30. (Oxford: Pergamon)
7. Vandenbark, A. A., Van Rompaey, F., Nijst, D., Heyligen, H. and Raus, J. (1983). Cerebrospinal fluid antibodies detect brain antigens. In Gonsette, R. E. and Delmotte, P. (eds.). *Immunological and Clinical Aspects of Multiple Sclerosis,* Chap. 5. (Lancaster: MTP Press)
8. Konat, G. and Clausen, J. (1980). Suppressive effect of triethyl lead on entry of proteins into the CNS myelin sheath in vitro. *J. Neurochem.,* **35,** 382
9. Diebler, G. E., Martenson, R. E. and Kies, M. W. (1972). Large scale preparation of myelin basic proteins from central nervous system tissues of several mammalian species. *Prep. Biochem.,* **2,** 139
10. Heyligen, H., Van Rompaey, F., Nijst, D., Raus, J. and Vandenbark, A. A. (1983). Brain antigens detected by cerebrospinal fluid from multiple sclerosis patients. In Gonsette, R. E. and Delmotte, P. (eds.). *Immunological and Clinical Aspects of Multiple Sclerosis,* Chap. P10. (Lancaster: MTP Press)
11. Van Rompaey, F., Nijst, D., Raus, J. and Vandenbark, A. A. (1983). Antibrain antibody absorption on microtiter plates. In Gonsette, R. E. and Delmotte, P. (eds.). *Immunological and Clinical Aspects of Multiple Sclerosis,* Chap. P21. (Lancaster: MTP Press)
12. Ryberg, B. (1978). Multiple specificities of antibrain antibodies in multiple sclerosis and chronic myelopathy. *J. Neurol. Sci.,* **38,** 357
13. Ford, D. M. and Burger, D. R. (1982). Evidence that primary sensitization of human T-cells to KLH *in vitro* increases the KLH-specific precursor frequency. *Fed. Proc.,* **41,** 797
14. Offner, H., Pedersen, F. K. and Konat, G. (1981). Lymphocyte stimulation by ganglio-sides cerebrosides and basic protein in juvenile rheumatoid arthritis. *J. Clin. Lab. Immunol.,* **6,** 35
15. Offner, H., Konat, G., Legg, N. J., Raun, N. E., Winterberg, H. and Clausen, J. (1980). Antigenic stimulation of active E rosette-forming lymphocytes in multiple sclerosis, systemic lupus erythematosus, and rheumatoid arthritis.

Poster 16
Eye movement disorders in multiple sclerosis and optic neuritis

J. P. H. REULEN, E. A. C. M. SANDERS and L. A. H. HOGENHUIS

Horizontal saccadic and smooth pursuit eye movements were studied in 84 patients with multiple sclerosis (MS) and 21 patients with optic neuritis (ON). The registration and computation of saccadic latency, maximal saccadic velocity, saccadic accuracy and smooth pursuit velocity gain were performed using a newly developed, portable, test battery. The chief methodological improvements introduced in our procedure were the following: placing of electrodes on both canthi of both eyes for more comprehensive following of eye movements, random presentation of stimuli for saccadic eye movements to avoid response anticipation effects, comparison of both reaction time and accuracy of eye movements on the one hand and maximal saccadic velocity on the other, and addition of smooth pursuit investigation to the test battery.

The MS patients were clinically classified as 'definite', 'probable' or 'possible'. Subclinical eye movement disorder was found in 80% of the definite, 74% of the probable and 60% of the possible category. Five of the ON patients (25%) showed a subclinical eye movement deficit; these five were young patients with a recent history of ON.

In a group of 11 probable and possible MS patients with symptoms of spinal cord involvement only, seven showed subclinical oculomotor disorder indicating the involvement of cerebral structures in the demyelination process.

The findings confirm the value of standardized, objective, examination of eye movements in the detection and clarification of subclinical lesions in the central nervous system of patients with an early diagnosis of MS or ON.

Detailed results of this study are published in *Brain*, (1983). **106**, 121–140

Poster 17
Do venous refluxes hurt the brain in MS? The fundamental problem

F. SCHELLING

In a valvular insufficiency of an internal jugular vein[1] repeated elevations of the central venous pressure exceeding the arterial pressures[2] may reach the thin-walled cerebral veins.

The extent of the intracranial vascular expansion (ΔV) at a given pressure gradient from the thoraco–abdominal to the cranio–vertebral veins depends mainly on:

(1) the compliance of the engorged veins and of their surrounding tissues,
(2) the momentary levels of the cerebrospinal fluid (CSF) pressure (Figure 1) and of
(3) the compliance of the dura mater and of the posterior wall of the vertebral channel.

Velocity and extent of the cerebral venous expansions in an individual valvular insufficiency will be raised in a consecutive phlebosclerosis of the struck internal jugular vein as in a narrow delimitation of the reflux (Figure 2).

The width of the sigmoid sinus acts on a reflux in the cerebral veins in a double way: (1) the resistance of the sinus directly involved hampers the reflux in its competition with arterial pulsations as with an eventual reflux in other, namely lumbar, epidural veins. (2) Both terminal sigmoid sinuses together are the bottle neck in the venous drainage of the brain, they dam up the blood in all cerebral vessels. So they influence the cerebrospinal fluid pressure by the intravascular pressure in relation to the osmotic pressure-gradients between the blood and the cerebrospinal fluid and according to the different vascular permeabilities.

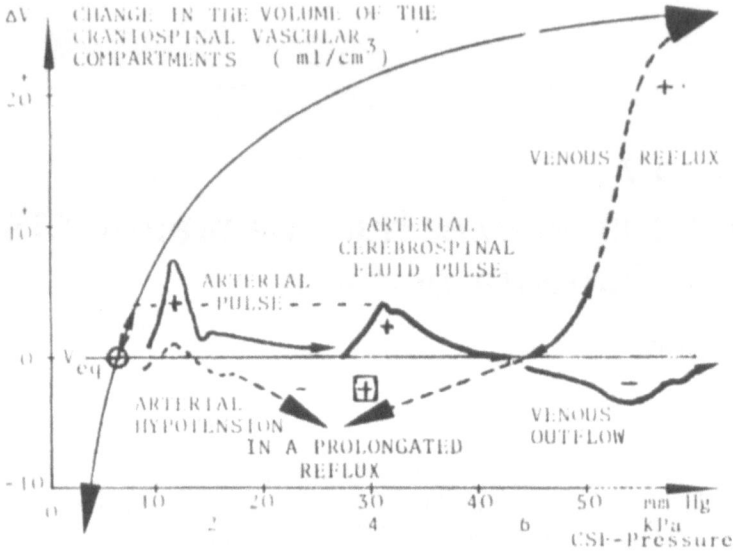

Figure 1 The short-term changes in the volume of the craniospinal vessels in their mutual limitation according to the volume-pressure relationship of the cerebrospinal fluid[3]

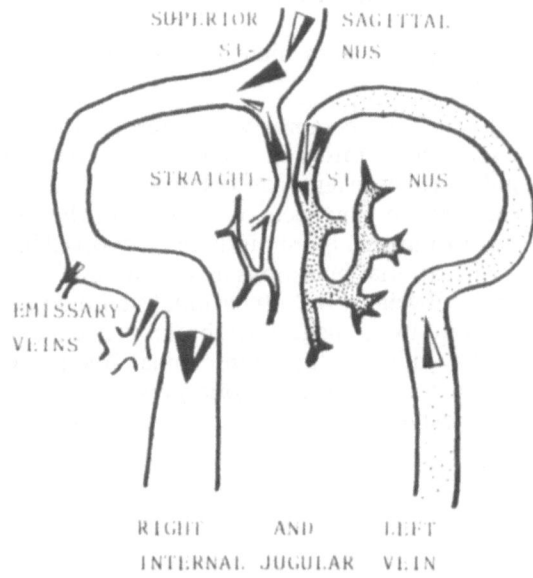

Figure 2 Delimitation of a reflux into the left internal jugular vein to the left internal cerebral veins by complete splitting of the straight sinus[4]

MATERIAL AND METHODS

To explore the individual range in the relation of the conductivity of both the sigmoid sinus to the volume of the skull (V) 116 human skulls were examined at the Institute of Anatomy in Innsbruck.

For the evaluation of the conductivity of the sigmoid sinus the diameters (D, D) of its short terminal part entering the jugular foramen proved the most revealing[5], whereas the differences in its length are to be neglected. So the 'terminal conductivity' of the sigmoid sinus (C_T) was calculated according to the formula:

$$C_T = D^3 \times D^3/8 \, (D^2 + D^2)$$

The volume of the skulls (V) was measured with rice.

In 3000 radiographs of the skull examined in the archive of the Institute of Neuroradiology at Salzburg, the diameters needed for the calculation of C_T and of V were used without a correction of the magnification figure. V (the volume) of these skulls was estimated by the formula:

$$V = L \times B \times H/2 \text{ (Figure 3)}$$

which was stated by Martin in 1928[6].

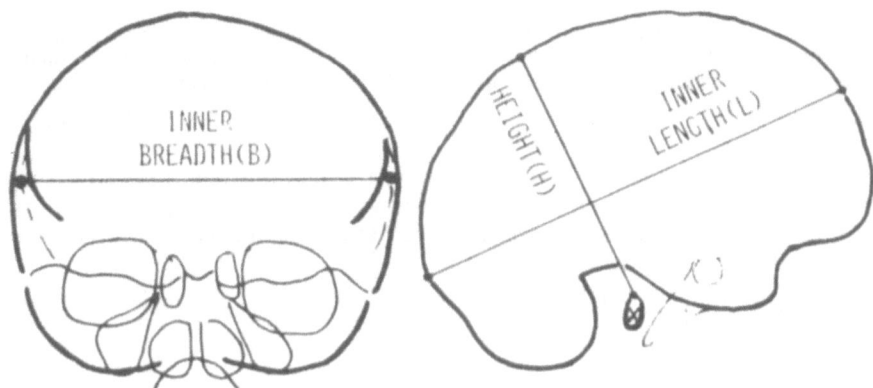

Figure 3 The diameters measured in the radiographs for the estimation of the volume of the skull in patients (x = External Auditory Meatus)

RESULTS

Some human skulls show a striking disproportion between their volume and the width of their sigmoid sinus (Figure 4, top). In an attempt to become acquainted with the effects of such disproportions the revision of 3000 radiographs of the skull pointed to an elevation of the relative width of the sigmoid sinus (C_T/V) in patients with multiple sclerosis. This discrepancy between the statements in the patients with multiple sclerosis and those in the

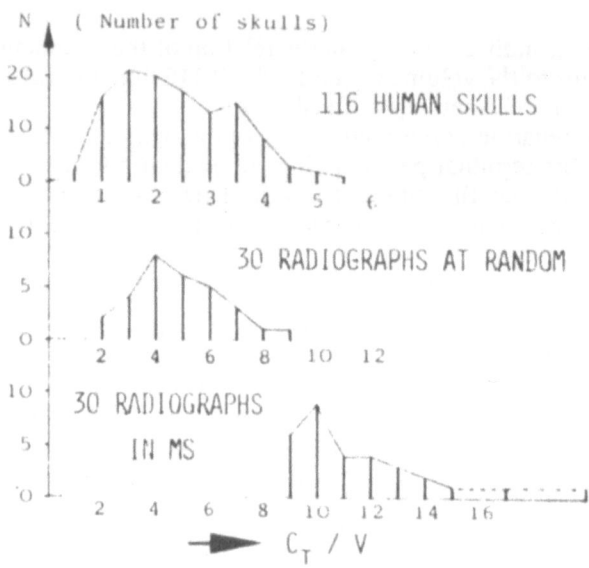

Figure 4 The individual relations between the conductivity of the terminal sigmoid sinus (C_T) and the volume of the skull in 116 human skulls (top), in 30 radiographs selected at random (middle) and in 30 radiographs of patients with multiple sclerosis (bottom)

radiographs of the skulls selected at random is documented in the confrontation of 30 controlled values of either group (Figure 4, middle and bottom).

The diameters measured for the evaluation of the conductivity in the terminal sigmoid sinus were:

(1) In the human skulls

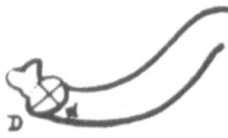

(2A) In the radiographs of the skulls selected at random

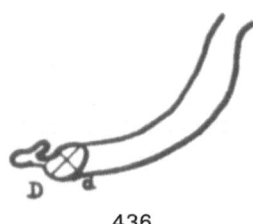

(2B) In the radiographs of the patients with multiple sclerosis

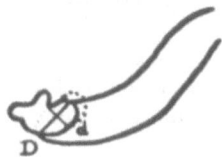

COMMENT

Venous reflux into the brain will expand its veins and their perivascular spaces where the surroundings give way[7-11] until the wave of a reflux is stopped in capillaries, or until the cerebrospinal fluid pressure is adjusted, or until there is no cerebrospinal fluid or venous blood to be displaced any more (Figure 5).

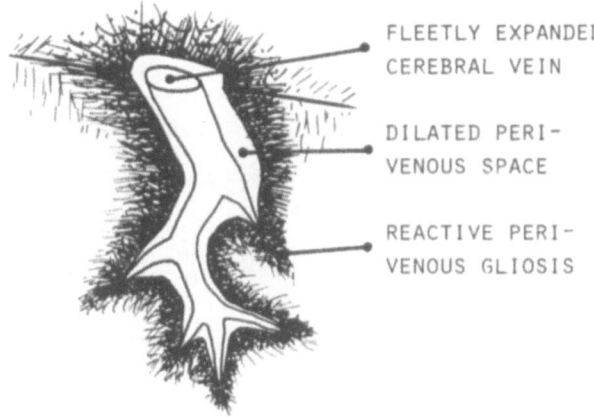

FLEETLY EXPANDED
CEREBRAL VEIN

DILATED PERI-
VENOUS SPACE

REACTIVE PERI-
VENOUS GLIOSIS

Figure 5   The alterations in the loose white matter of the brain produced by repeated fleeting expansions of a cerebral vein

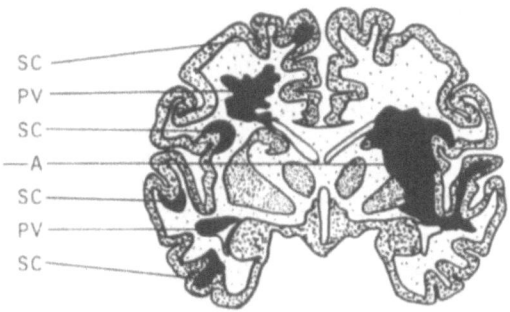

SC
PV
SC
—A—
SC
PV
SC

Figure 6   Zones of reduced resistance against extravasations from veins (PV – periventricular, SC – subcortical zone) and from arteries (A – area of predilection for arterial haemorrhages)

437

For comparison see the distribution of the perivenous bleedings in obstructions of the venous outflow, in the agonal and postmoral extravasation (Figure 6)[12-15]

Cerebrospinal fluid pressed by sudden periventricular venous expansions may bulge the partitions between the ventricles of the brain and subarachnoid cisterns. Resulting strains especially can wear out the dorsal contour of the optic chiasm[16] (Figure 7).

All the cerebrospinal fluid pushed out from the cranial cavity tries to drag the spinal cord, the nerve roots and prominent vessels with it, which will strain at their anchoring tissues[17,18] (Figure 8).

In the spinal cord the lesions of multiple sclerosis[18,19] should not be confused with the damages by virtual vascular or meningeal diseases[20].

If the membranes (pia mater and membrana limitans gliae) enclosing the nervous structures are ruptured, myelin fragments may be flushed out into the cerebrospinal fluid[21].

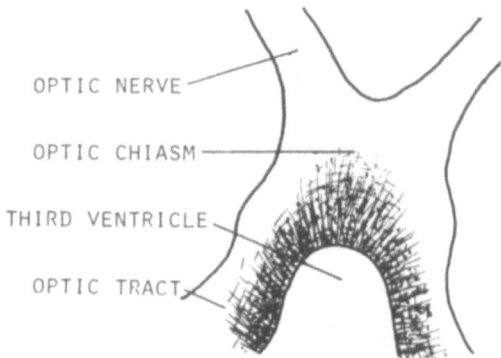

Figure 7 The dorsal contour of the optic chiasm – a spot especially exposed to ventriculo-cisernal pressure gradients

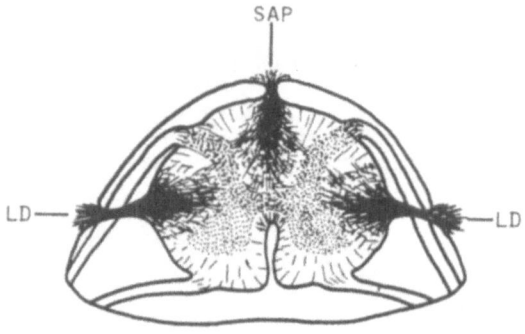

Figure 8 The trajectories of augmented tensions within the spinal cord in its cranio-caudal displacements along the vertebral channel

Short excessive pressure-gradients at the optic disc can contribute to the development of a papilloedema; in the retinal veins, jets of venous blood can cause a periphlebitis retinae[22].

Inflammatory infiltrations of the dural[23], meningeal and cerebral veins[24], the meninges, glial structures or vessels supporting the spinal cord[25] and of the retinal veins[22] are no proof of the involvement of a material agent in a morbid process, as shown by equivalent changes in the hypertensive arteriolopathy or arteriolonecrosis[26,27].

The assumption of a material cause of multiple sclerosis will explain either the persistence of certain myelin-sheaths amidst a large, active destruction[28] or the long, slender runners of lesions unswervingly crossing tracts of white matter as the tight textures of glial fibres or grey matter[29].

The peculiar mechanical vulnerability of the myelin sheaths[30,31,32] seems often to be neglected. In the postulated pathomechanisms one would expect an initial sparing of neuronal structures, whereas glial as mesenchymal tissues should be involved from the beginning[5].

SUGGESTIONS

It seems of the utmost importance to examine the function of the valves in the internal jugular veins, the course of a possible reflux and the width of the main venous outlets from the skull, especially in patients with multiple sclerosis, other neurological diseases and functional mental disorders.

The substitution of venous valves might be of eminent therapeutic as well as prophylactic value in these patients.

References

1. Gruber, W. (1847). 4 Abhandlungen aus dem Gebiete der medicinisch-chirurgischen Anatomie. (Berlin: Förstner) Hamernjk, J. (1847). Physiol.-patholog. Untersuchungen über die Erscheinungen an Arterien und Venen. (Prag: Ehrlich) Weathersby, H. T. (1956). The valves of the axillary, subclavian and int. jugular veins. Anat. Rec. (Phil.) 124, 379 Anderhuber, F. (1983). Venenklappen in den großen Venenstämmen der Vena cava sup. Acta anta. (Basel) (In press)
2. Rollet, E. (1877). Über den Einfluß der Körperlage auf die Ergebnisse der Brustuntersuchung. Dtsch. Arch. klin. Med. 19, 295 Hamilton, W. F. et al (1944). Arterial, CSF and venous pressures in man during cough and strain. Am. J. Physiol., 141, 42 Sharpey-Schafer, E. P. (1953). The mechanism of syncope after coughing. Brit. Med. J., 2, 860 McIntosh, H. D. et al (1956). The mechanisms of cough syncope. Am. Heart J., 52, 70
3. Avezaat, C. J. J. et al (1979). CSF pulse pressure and intracranial volume-pressure relationships. J. Neurol. Neurosurg. Psychiat., 42, 687 Avezaat, C. J. J. et al (1980). Effects of hypercapnia and arterial hypotension and hypertension on CSF pulse pressure and intracranial volume-pressure relationships. J. Neurol. Neurosurg. Psychiat., 43, 222 Fuhrmeister, U. (1980). Spinaler Infusions test und verwandte Methoden lumbaler Druckmessung. In Dommasch, D., and Mertens, H. G. (eds.). Cerebrospinalflüssigkeit, pp. 242 (Stuttgart: Thieme) Gaab, M. R. et al (1981). Pressure-volume Test and pulse-amplitude analysis of ICP. Ref. 32. Jahrestagung dtsch. Ges. Neurochir. Tübingen
4. Saxena, R. C. et al (1973). Double straight sinus. J. Neurosurg., 39, 540
5. Schelling, F. (1978). Die Emissarien des menschlichen Schädels. Anat. Anz., 143, 340
6. Martin, R. (1928). Lehrb. d. Anthropologie, Vol. II, pp. 648 2nd Edit. (Jena: Fischer)

7. Gauer, O.H. (1972). Kreislauf des Blutes. In Gauer, O.H, Kramer, K. and Jung, R. (eds.). *Physiologie des Menschen*. pp. 174 (München: Urban & Schwarzenberg)
8. Fog, T. (1965). The topography of plaques in MS. *Acta Neurol. Scand.*, (Copenh.) (Suppl. 15), **41**, 1
9. King, L.S. (1937). The connective tissue reaction in MS and in diffuse sclerosis. *Arch. Pathol.* (Chic.), **23**, 338
10. Fog, T. (see 8)
11. Steiner, G. (1931). *Krankheitserreger und Gewebsbefund bei MS*. **108**, 120 (Berlin: Springer)
12. Schwartz, P. and Fink, L. (1926). Morphologie und Entstehung d. geburtstraumat. Blutungen in Gehirn u. Schädel d. Neugeborenen. *Zschr. Kinderheilk.*, **40**, 427
13. Wollschlaeger, G. *et al* (1971). Die cerebrale Venenthrombose. *Radiologe,* **11**, 419
14. Dahl, B. (1938). Pathol.-anat. und exp. Untersuchungen über die sogenannten Duret-Bernerschen Blutungen etc. *Dtsch. Z. ges. gerichtl. Med.*, **29**, 366
15. Pfeifer, R.A. (1930). *Grundlegende Untersuchungen für die Angioarchitektonik des menschlichen Gehirns*. (Berlin: Springer)
16. Zimmerman, H.M. and Netsky, M.G. (1950). *The pathology of MS*. Res. Publ. Assoc. Res. Nerv. Ment. Dis., **28**, 271
17. Ziehen, T. (1903). Makroskop. Anat. des Rückenmarks. In Bardeleben, K.v. and Eggeling H.v. (eds.). *Handb. d. Anat. d. Menschen.*, pp. 64–68 (Jena: Fischer)
18. Fot, T. (1950). Topographic distribution of plaques in the spinal cord in MS. *Arch. Neurol.*, **63**, 382
19. Oppenheimer, D.R. (1978). The cervical cord in MS. *Neuropath. Appl. Neurobiol.*, **4**, 151
20. Schneider, H. (1980). Kreislaufstörungen u. Gefäßprozesse des Rückenmarks. In Schneider, H. (ed.) *Pathologie des Nervensystems I. Cervós-Navarro J.*, pp. 512 (Berlin: Springer)
21. Herndon, R.M. and Johnston, M. (1970). A method for electron microscopic study of cerebrospinal fluid sediment. *J. Neuropath. Exp. Neurol.*, **29**, 320
22. Doden, W. (1957). Einscheidungen der Netzhautvenen bei MS. *Dtsch. Med. Wschr.*, **28**, 1866
23. Margulis, M.S. (1933). Uber die patholog. Anatomie u. Pathogenese d.MS. *Dtsch. Z. Nervenheilkd.*, **131**, 125
24. Adams, C.W.M. (1975). The onset and progression of the lesion in MS. *J. Neurol. Sci.* (Amsterdam), **25**, 165
25. Falkiewicz, T. (1926). Zur Pathogenese der Multiplen Sklerose. *Arb. Neurol. Inst. Wien.*, **28**, 172
26. Scheinker, I.M. (1947). *Neuropathology*. (Springfield, Illinois: Thomas)
27. Ule, G. (1974). In Doerr, W. (ed.). *Organpathologie III*, pp. 9–35 (Stuttgart: Thieme)
28. Strötker, S. (1969). Quantit. morpholog.-klin. Studien an 15 Fallen akuter, subakuter u. subchron. diss. Entmarkungsenzephalomyelitis. Diss. Göttingen: Abb. 1
29. Falkiewicz, T. (see 25) – 30) Scheinker, I.M. (see 26)
31. Bunge, R.P. and Settlage, P.H. (1957). Neurological lesions in cats following cerebrospinal fluid manipulation. *J. Neuropath. Exp. Neurol.* (Baltimore) **16**, 471
32. Broser, F. (1981). Topische u. klin. Diagnostik neurolog. Krankheiten. (Munich: Urban & Schwarzenberg)

Poster 18
Blood–CSF barrier permselectivity and measurement of intrathecal IgG synthesis in multiple sclerosis

P.LIVREA, I. L. SIMONE, M. TROJANO, G. B. ZIMATORE, R. PISICCHIO and G. C. LOGROSCINO

A slight blood-CSF barrier (BCB) damage can be found in about 20% of multiple sclerosis (MS) patients[1,2].

In acute experimental encephalomyelitis protein leakage from vessels has been observed only in areas with perivascular inflammation[3], and the loss of restriction of BCB in MS could be related to increased permeability of capillary in newly formed lesions. The increased entry of serum proteins into interstitial fluid and CSF occurs through unknown routes[4,5] (increased vesicular transport in capillary endothelial cells; opening of tight junctions; damage of capillary basement membrane), and in acute experimental encephalomyelitis it does not seem related to emperipolesis because it occurs before the tissue infiltrate formation[3]. The role that the barrier damage can play in the pathogenesis of demyelination is still a matter of speculation.

The passage of serum proteins in CSF is inversely related to the protein hydrodynamic radius (R)[6]. In normal conditions a linear positive regression

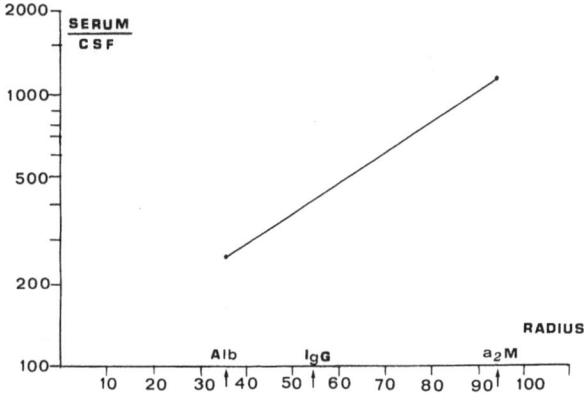

Figure 1 Regression line of log serum/CSF of individual proteins vs radius

exists between the log serum/CSF ratio of individual proteins and the R^6 (Figure 1).

Changes in albumin quotient can be regarded as a measure of BCB restriction, but the slope of the regression line obtained by quotients of larger proteins can be assumed as a measure of BCB selectivity[7] (Figure 1). It is not known if changes in BCB restriction are accompanied by changes in BCB selectivity[7].

This paper reports preliminary results about changes in BCB permselectivity in MS, obtained by laser nephelometric measurement[8,9] of albumin, IgG, α_2-macroglobulin levels in serum and CSF (CSF/serum $\times 10^3 = Q$).

All CSF and serum samples were examined by isoelectric focusing in thin layer polyacrilamide gel (pH range 3.5–9.5)[10]. The presence of abnormally increased IgG fractions in CSF without corresponding increase in serum was considered as sign of intrathecal IgG synthesis. All MS patients had such an abnormality.

Table 1 Blood–CSF barrier (BCB) restriction in multiple sclerosis

	Neurological controls (65)	Multiple sclerosis (77)
*Q-Albumin (mean ± SD)	4.13 ± 1.1	5.49 ± 2.7†
Q-Albumin > mean ± 2 SD in neurological controls	—	15 (19.5%)

* $Q = CSF/serum \times 10^3$
† t-test $p < 0.01$

Mean Q-Albumin was significantly higher in MS patients than in neurological controls (Table 1).

In 15/77 (19.5%) MS patients, Q-Albumin was higher than mean ± 2 SD of neurological controls (Table 1). This finding is in agreement with reports indicating a loss of restriction of BCB in about 20% of MS patients. No correlation was found between clinical parameters (age, duration, acute or stationary phase of disease) and BCB damage.

A significant linear regression was found in neurological controls between Q-α_2-macroglobulin and Q-Albumin (Figure 2 and Table 2). A significant linear regression was found in MS patients between Q-α_2-macroglobulin and

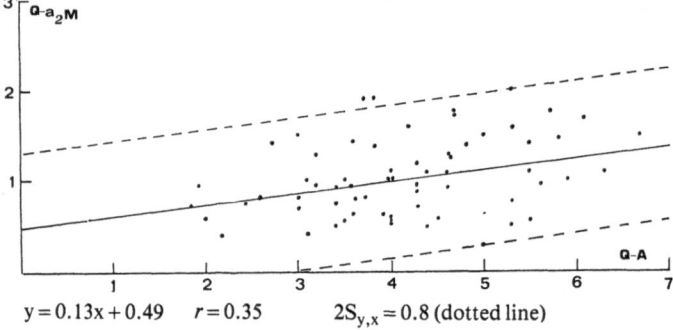

$y = 0.13x + 0.49$ $r = 0.35$ $2S_{y,x} = 0.8$ (dotted line)

Figure 2 Linear regression of Q-α_2-M vs. Q-A in neurological controls (65)

Table 2 Blood—CSF barrier (BCB) selectivity evaluated by Q-α_2-macroglobulin (Q-α_2M) regression vs. Q-Albumin (Q-A) in neurological controls and multiple sclerosis patients

Q-α_2M vs. Q-A*	Regression	$S_{y,x}$	T	R	p
Controls ($n = 65$)	$0.49 + 0.13x$	0.41	2.9	0.35	<0.05
Multiple sclerosis ($n = 77$)	$-0.1 + 0.31x$†	1.15	6.4	0.6	<0.01

* $Q = CSF/serum \times 10^3$
† t-test for difference between regression coefficients $p > 0.05$ n.s.

Q-Albumin (Table 2); the regression coefficient was not significantly different from controls (Table 2).

In 11/62 (17.7%) MS patients with normal BCB restriction to albumin and in 9/15 MS patients with loss of BCB restriction to albumin, Q-α_2-macroglobulin was higher than expected from the regression line ($+2S_{y,x}$) obtained in controls (Figure 3).

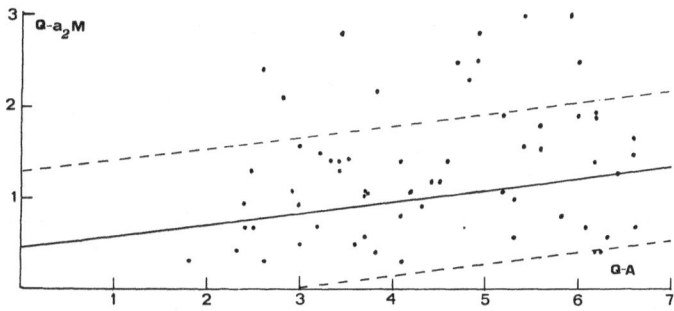

Figure 3 Blood-CSF barrier (BCB) selectivity evaluated by Q-α_2-macroglobulin (Q-α_2M) regression vs Q-Albumin (Q-A) in multiple sclerosis patients with normal BCB restriction. Heavy line = regression in neurological controls. Dotted line = $2S_{y,x}$ of regression line in controls

Increase in α_2-macroglobulin levels is normally found in inflammatory reactions. High α_2-macroglobulin levels in CSF could be related to an increase in proteinase inhibitory activity[11]. Cultured human monocytes can synthesize and secrete α_2-macroglobulin[12], and electrophoretically abnormal α-macro-globulin can be found in the serum of MS patients, likely related to binding of α_2-macroglobulin with proteinases[13]. Nevertheless, the significant correlation of Q-α_2-macroglobulin vs Q-Albumin in MS suggests that the BCB function is the main factor regulating α_2-macroglobulin levels in CSF in MS.

The high α_2-macroglobulin levels found in CSF indicate that besides a loss of BCB restriction, a change in BCB selectivity can be found in MS, irrespective of clinical signs of activity of the disease. An increased demyelina-tion linked proteinase activity could affect capillary basement membrane, and basement membrane can play a role in protein sieving process or in regulation of pinocytotic activity of endothelial cells[14].

Methods which are commonly used to calculate the amount of intrathecal

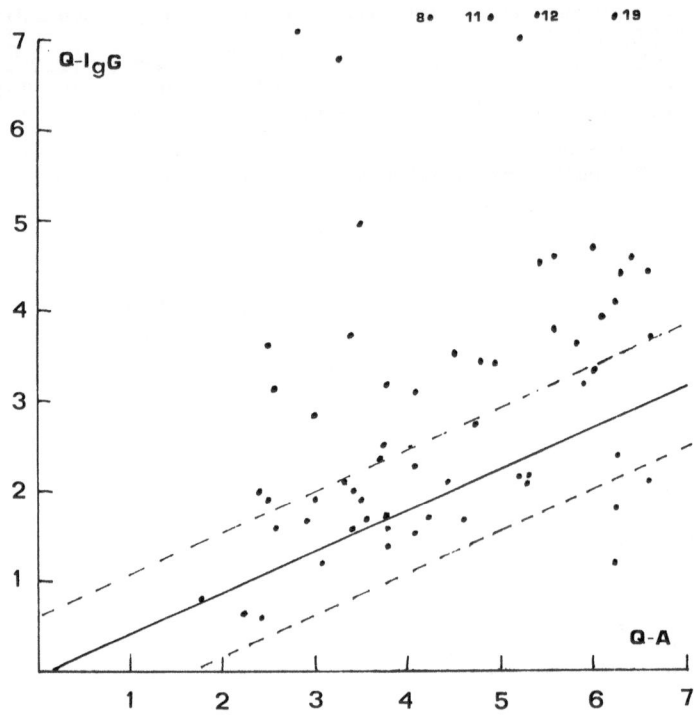

Figure 4 BCB restriction to albumin and estimate of serum derived CSF IgG in multiple sclerosis patients with intrathecal IgG synthesis demonstrated by isoelectric focusing. Heavy line = regression line in neurological controls. Dotted line = $2S_{y,x}$ of regression line in controls

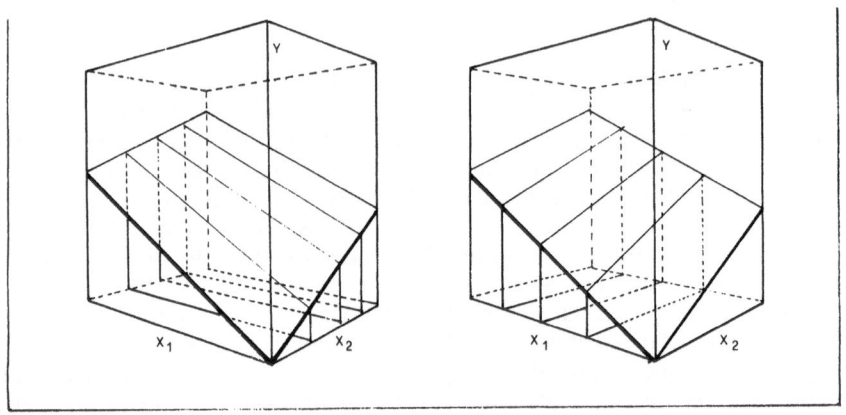

Figure 5 Multiple regression of a dependent variable vs 2 variables. Left: Regression y vs. x_1 with constant x_2. Right: Regression y vs. x_2 with constant x_1

Table 3 Multiple regression of Q-IgG vs. Q-albumin and Q-α_2-macroglobulin in neurological controls, acute idiopathic polyneuropathy and acute meningo–encephalitis

Multiple regression	Sy, x_1, x_2	T_1	T_2	R
Controls (n=65) Q-IgG $= -0.22 + 0.45\ Q$-alb $+ 0.14\ Q$-α_2M	0.36	10.3	1.27	0.83
Acute idiopathic polyneuropathy $(n=27)$ Q-IgG $= -2.5 + 0.86\ Q$-alb $- 0.47\ Q$-α_2M (*)	7.4	7.8	1.3	0.92
Acute meningo–encephalitis $(n=17)$ Q-IgG $= -7.2 + 0.66\ Q$-alb $+ 0.28\ Q$-α_2M (*)	8.2	8.2	1.72	0.97

All patients with acute meningo–encephalitis and acute idiopathic polyneuropathy had a loss of restriction of BCB (Q—alb higher than 6.9)
(*) Significantly different (ANOVA Test) $p < 0.01$

IgG synthesis in MS assume a constant ratio between permeability of BCB for albumin and IgG[2,5,16]. About 60% of MS patients show intrathecal IgG synthesis when Q-IgG is plotted against Q-Albumin and compared with the regression line obtained in controls[16] (Figure 4).

Preliminary results obtained by multiple linear regression (Figure 5) of Q-IgG vs. Q-Albumin and Q-α_2-macroglobulin indicate that significantly different partial regression coefficients can be found in neurological controls and in conditions of BCB damage (Table 3), and suggest that different types of changes in BCB permselectivity can occur in inflammatory diseases[17].

Changes in BCB permeability in MS indicate that the actual permeability of BCB to IgG cannot be carefully evaluated but only by the permeability to albumin.

If multiple regression Q-IgG vs. Q-Albumin and Q-α_2-macroglobulin obtained in controls ($+2S_{y,x_1,x_2}$) was used to estimate the serum derived IgG in MS, high Q-IgG values, indicating intrathecal IgG synthesis, were obtained only in 50% of patients. A protein which is not synthesized within BCB and with an R similar to IgG[7] (for example, ceruloplasmin, $R = 4.68$ nm) could be used to assess the effective BCB area for diffusion of serum IgG when an alteration of BCB permselectivity is suspected[7].

ACKNOWLEDGEMENT

Supported by CNR grants 82.02259.83, 81.00859.83 and 82.02212.56.

References

1. Tourtellotte, W. W. (1970). On cerebrospinal fluid IgG quotients in Multiple Sclerosis and other diseases. A review and a new formula to estimate the amount of IgG synthesized per day by central nervous system. *J. Neurol. Sci.,* **10**, 279
2. Tourtellotte, W. W. and Ma, B. I. (1978). Multiple Sclerosis: blood–brain barrier and the measurement of the *de novo* central nervous system IgG synthesis. *Neurology,* **28**, 76
3. Behan, P. O. and Currie, S. (1978). Experimental Allergic Encephalomyelitis. In Behan, P. O. and Currie, S. (eds.). *Clinical Neuroimmunology.* Vol. 8, pp. 97–112. (London: W. B. Saunders)
4. Brightman, M. W., Klatzo, I., Olsson, Y. and Reese, T. S. (1970). The blood–brain barrier to proteins under normal and pathological conditions. *J. Neurol. Sci.,* **10**, 215
5. Felgenhauer, K. (1974). Protein size and cerebrospinal fluid composition. *Klin. Wochenschr.,* **52**, 1158
6. Felgenhauer, K., Schliep, G. and Rapic, N. (1976). Evaluation of the blood–CSF barrier by protein gradients and the humoral immune response within the central nervous system. *J. Neurol. Sci.,* **30**, 113
7. Felgenhauer, K. (1980). Protein filtration and secretion at human body fluid barriers. *Pflügers Arch.,* **384**, 9
8. Felgenhauer, K. (1981). The laser nephelometric evaluation of the humoral immune response in the central nervous system. *Vortrag auf dem. XI. Internationalen KongreB für Klinische Chemie.* Vienna.
9. Felgenhauer, K., Hanssen, Chr. and Remy, A. (1982). Laser nephelometric evaluation of the humoral immune response in the central nervous system. *Med. Lab.,* **11**, 48
10. Livrea, P., Trojano, M., Simone, I. L., Zimatore, G. B., Lamontanara, G. and Leante, R. (1981). Intrathecal IgG synthesis in Multiple Sclerosis. Comparison between Isoelectric Focusing and quantitative estimation of cerebrospinal fluid IgG. *J. Neurol.,* **224**, 159

11. Price, P. and Cuzner, M. L. (1979). Proteinase inhibitors in cerebrospinal fluid in Multiple Sclerosis. *J. Neurol. Sci.,* **42,** 251
12. Hovi, T., Mosher, D. and Vaheri, A. (1977). Cultured human monocytes synthesize and secrete alpha$_2$-macroglobulin. *J. Exp. Med.,* **145,** 1580
13. Rastogi, S. C., Clausen, J. and Fog, T. (1981). Abnormal serum alpha$_2$-macroglobulin in Multiple Sclerosis. *Eur. Neurol.,* **20,** 33
14. Robert, A. M., Miskulin, M., Maati, F. and Godeau, G. (1978). Role of the basement membrane collagen in the blood–brain barrier permeability. In Kefalides, N. A. (ed.). *Biology and chemistry of basement membranes,* pp. 195–203. (New York: Academic Press)
15. Link, H. and Tibbling, G. (1977). Principles of albumin and IgG analysis in neurological disorders. Evaluation of IgG synthesis within the central nervous system in Multiple Sclerosis. *Scand. J. Clin. Lab. Invest.,* **37,** 397
16. Reiber, H. (1979). Quantitative bestimmung der lokal im zentralnervensystem synthesierten Immunoglobulin G-fraktion des liquors. *J. Clin. Chem. Biochem.,* **17,** 587
17. Livrea, P., Trojano, M., Simone, I. L., Zimatore, G. B., Pisicchio, R. and Solazzo, A. (1983). Barriera emato-liquorale e sintesi intratecale di IgG. In Tavolato, B. and Livrea, P. (eds.). *L'anelisi diagnostica del liquor.* pp. 55–78. (Padova: Piccin)

Poster 19
Azathioprine vs. transfer factor in multiple sclerosis patients: preliminary data

S. STECCHI, R. PIPERNO, M. FRANCESCHINI, G. A. MAGAGNI,
C. G. MONTAGNA and G. MICCOLI

The authors report data obtained from the comparison of two basic thera-peutical trials in patients affected by multiple sclerosis.

The two therapeutical trials compared are:

(1) Immunodepressive trial[1]: using azathioprine, $2 \, mg \, kg^{-1} \, day^{-1}$
(2) Immunostimulating trial[2]: using transfer factor, a dose every 15 days. A dose of transfer factor is obtained from 2×10^8 mononuclear cells of human peripheral blood, taken from a pool of at least 10 donors chosen from the patient's relatives.

The following preliminary data concern nine patients observed during an 18 month follow-up period (Table 1). One more patient, belonging to the azathioprine group, had to discontinue the treatment at the second month, because of side-effects.

Table 1 Patient data

	Average age (years)	Range	Average age at onset	Range	Average duration	Range	Male	Female
Transfer factor (5 patients)	36.6	28–42	25.0	19–37	11.6	3–19	3	2
Azathioprine (4 patients)	35.7	24–46	27.7	17–37	8.0	4–15	2	2

The complete study provides for a 36 month follow-up period of 20 patients. Patients chosen at random included in the study have the following features[3].

(1) They are between 18 and 50 years of age, onset age between 17 and 40 years,
(2) clinically confirmed neurological diagnosis of MS according to Schumacher et al[4],

(3) presence of oligoclonal bands noticeable with IEF in the α-globulin CSF region,
(4) course of the disease with clinical evidence of exacerbations and remissions, and
(5) mild or moderate disability: subjects with a disability degree up to and including five, according to the Kurtzke scale[5], have been included.

Sex has not been regarded as a discrimination criterion.
None of the chosen patients had previously been submitted to immuno-depressive or immunostimulating therapeutical treatment, nor prolonged steroid therapy.
No treatment interfering at the immunologic level had been carried out during the trial.
The two therapeutical trials are tested in reference to:

(1) Exacerbation rate variations,
(2) changes in disability according to Kurtzke scale,
(3) modifications of the immunological reactivity parameters: E, EAC, E activated rosettes; lymphocyte populations activated with phyto-haemagglutinin (PHA) and concanavalin A (Con A).

RESULTS

The changes in disability during the follow-up period and the average increase of disability during intercurrent bouts (Table 2), do not show any significant difference between the two groups compared.

Table 2 Patients' disability status

	Transfer factor (5 patients)	Azathioprine (5 patients)
Average disability before starting trial	1.8	3.5
Range	1–3	2–5
Average disability after 18 months trial	1.6	3.5
Range	1–3	2–6
Average disability in intercurrent bouts	2.6	4.8
Range	1–4	3–6
Difference between follow-up start and stop	− 0.2	0.0
Difference between bout and stationary phase	+ 1.0	+ 1.3

The apparently surprising decrease of the average disability in the transfer factor (TF) group is well explained by a good result of the rehabilitative treatment in two cases.
In six patients the disability is substantially unchanged after 18 months; in two cases they improved (one in TF group and one in Az group), whereas the disability increased in one case (Az group).
The exacerbation rate (Table 3) decreased in parallel in the two compared groups. This result is clearly not significant.
The decrease registered is, in our opinion, due to the discrepancy between

the evaluation of bouts without direct clinical survey during the 18 months before starting the trial, and the clinical assessment carried out during the follow-up period.

The monitoring of the immunological reactivity has been carried out with the following parameters:

(1) Lymphocyte cultures in autologous serum, stimulated with PHA (at 0.1 and 3 μg/ml) and Con A. They have been carried out also in a control AB serum, in order to evaluate a possible depressing effect of the serum.

(2) Rosettes E, EAC, E activated: in Tables 4 and 5 the data obtained by the check effected at the beginning of the trial are compared to the last results. For each case in the two groups the plus and minus variations are expressed both as absolute values (cells/mm^3) and as relative percentages.

Table 3   Exacerbation rate

	Transfer factor (5 patients)	Azathioprine (5 patients)
Exacerbation rate 18 months before starting trial	1.33	1.33
Exacerbation rate 18 months after starting trial	0.80	0.83
Difference in exacerbation rate	− 0.53	− 0.50

Table 4   Azathioprine group: rosette forming variations between first and last control (18th month)

Patient	E % Variation	Absolute variation	EAC % Variation	Absolute variation	E act. % Variation	Absolute variation
A.S.	+ 6	ND	+ 10	ND	+ 8	ND
L.M.	− 24	− 2590	+ 5	− 375	− 3	− 380
P.R.	− 24	− 194	+ 15	+ 384	− 1	+ 63
A.A.	− 27	− 897	− 7	+ 314	− 22	− 417
Average values	− 25	− 1227	− 7	− 375	− 8	− 398
Subjects with decreased values	3/4	3/3	1/4	1/3	3/4	2/3

Table 5   Transfer factor group: rosette forming variations between first and last control (18th month)

Patient	E % Variation	Absolute variation	EAC % Variation	Absolute variation	E act. % Variation	Absolute variation
B.B.	− 26	− 188	− 11	− 106	+ 4	+ 228
I.B.	− 21	− 149	− 5	− 57	− 31	− 552
G.B.	− 16	+ 560	− 3	− 327	− 10	− 26
F.G.	− 21	− 667	− 3	− 115	− 18	− 443
A.G.	− 8	− 232	+ 19	+ 169	+ 5	+ 70
Average values	− 18.4	− 309	− 5.5	− 151	− 19.6	− 340
Subjects with decreased values	5/5	4/5	4/5	4/5	3/5	2/3

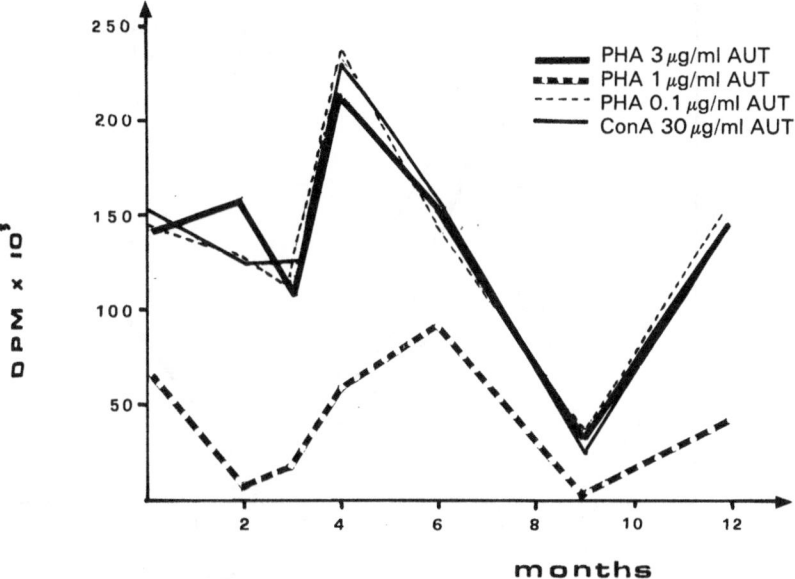

Figure 1a Lymphocyte populations activated with PHA and ConA, in autologous serum. Azathioprine group

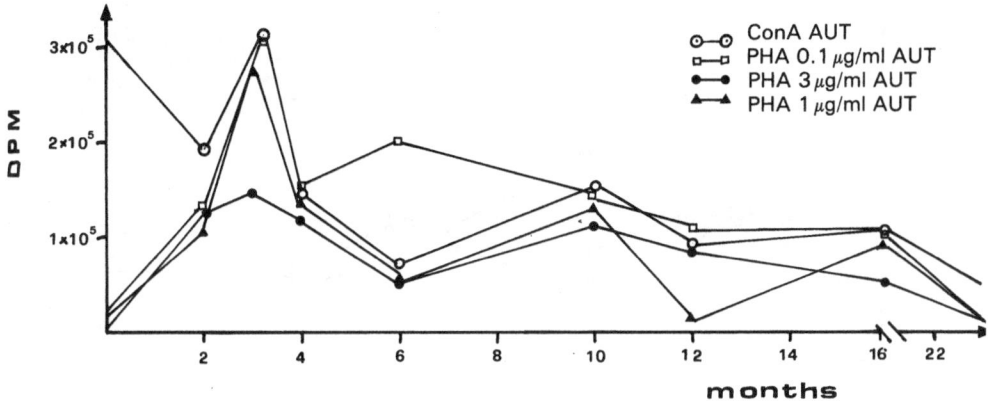

Figure 1b Lymphocyte populations activated with PHA and ConA, in autologous serum. Transfer factor group

In both examined groups a reduction of studied immunological parameters is noticed.

There isn't any significant difference between the values found in the two compared groups, except for some differences statistically not significant concerning EAC rosettes.

Likewise, the abrupt falls in lymphocyte reactivity which have been observed in some cases have no apparent explanation (Figures 1a, b and 2a, b).

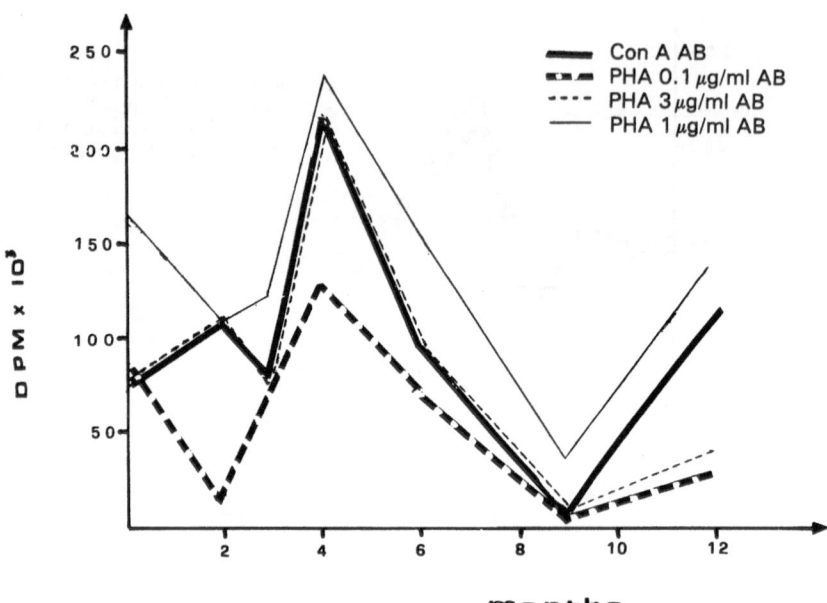

Figure 2a Lymphocyte populations activated with PHA and ConA, in AB serum. Azathioprine group

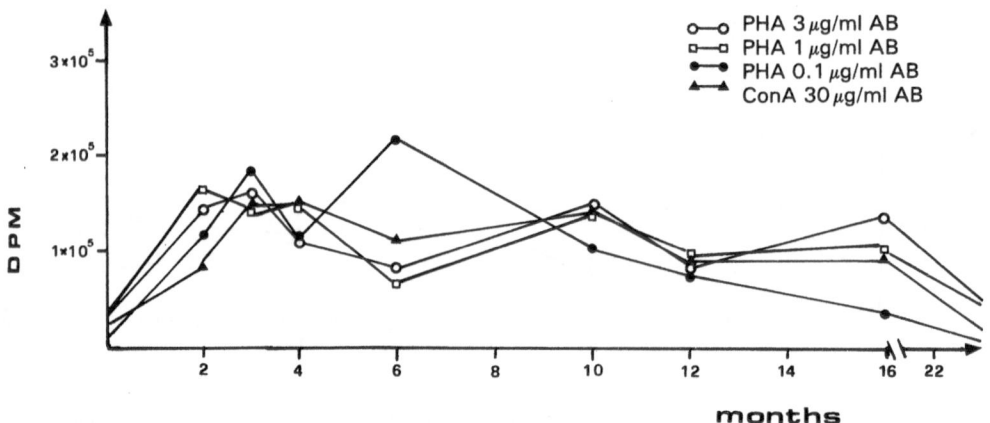

Figure 2b Lymphocyte populations activated with PHA and ConA, in AB serum. Transfer factor group

CONCLUSIONS

In both examined groups a reduction of studied immunological markers with no significant difference between the values found in the two tested therapeutical trials is noticed.

Likewise, the clinical data so far collected do not suggest any significant difference.

Side effects have been noted in the azathioprine group, whereas the TF group shows a very good tolerance.

According to the authors it is not yet possible to draw a final conclusion. At this stage the two treatments do not show differences such that a choice of either therapy can safely be made.

References

1. Aimard, G., Confaveux, C., Trouillas, P. and Devic, M. (1978). L'Azathioprine dans le traitement de la Sclérose en Plaques. *Rev. Neurol.*, **134**, 215
2. Basten, A., Pollard, J. D. *et al* (1980). Transfer factor in treatment of multiple sclerosis. *Lancet*, 931
3. Brown, J. R., Beebe, G. W., Kurtzke, J. F., Loewenson, R. B., Silberberg, D. H. and Tourtellotte, W. W. (1979). The design of clinical studies to assess therapeutic efficacy in M. S. *Neurology*, **20**, Suppl.
4. Schumacher, G. A. *et al* (1965). Problems of experimental trials of therapy in multiple sclerosis. *Ann. NY Acad. Sci.*, **122**, 552
5. Kurtzke, J. F. (1961). On the evaluation of disability in MS. *Neurology*, **11**, 686

Poster 20
Epidemiology of multiple sclerosis in Italy. A further descriptive study in Barbagia, Sardinia

E. GRANIERI, R. TOLA, L. PINNA, M. MANCA and P. DE BASTIANI

SUMMARY

Italy is currently regarded as a medium-frequency area for MS. This opinion is based on the results of 30 prevalence studies undertaken on large populations exceeding 300000. Recently, however, it has been stated that the surveys of large populations in Italy do not provide reliable figures comparable to those found in northern-central Europe. In fact, current public health organization in Italy is inadequate for epidemiologic search, and accurate estimates of MS frequency are possible only as a result of intensive surveys of small populations. To date, eight studies of this sort are available, which suggest that Italy also falls into the high-risk zone. However, more accurate investigations of this kind are needed. For this reason, we carried out a second survey of MS in Barbagia, Sardinia, an appropriate area for descriptive investigation. On prevalence day, October 24, 1981, 32 subjects (18 women and 14 men) living in the study area were found to be suffering from probable MS. The patients were classified according to the diagnostic criteria of Allison and Millar. As the total population was 49022, the crude prevalence rate was 65.3 per 100000 (95% CI:44–93). The rate, age- and sex-adjusted to the Italian population, was 78. These results, higher than those found in a previous study in the same area, give further support to the possibility that the risk for MS in Italy is similar to that in northern-central Europe, and, therefore, cast doubt on the widely accepted opinion that MS prevalence is a function of geographic latitude.

INTRODUCTION

The current hypothesis that Italy and the Mediterranean areas are medium-frequency zones for multiple sclerosis (MS) is based on the results of about 30

454

prevalence studies, which have appeared in literature in the years from 1962 to 1980[1,2]. All these studies, which report prevalence figures varying from 7.2 to 27.1 probable MS cases per 100000, have been undertaken on large populations, generally exceeding 300000.

Recently, however, it has been emphasized that the surveys of large populations in Italy do not allow us to obtain reliable figures, comparable to those found in northern-central European countries, which have a greater tendency to epidemiological research[3,4]. In fact, current public health organization in Italy has several defects, which can lead to a severe underestimation of the prevalence especially when large populations are studied.

In the light of these considerations, some authors have recently decided to verify the prevalence of MS in Italy by using relatively small communities, with the view to minimizing biased data. Based on this approach, much higher prevalence figures have been reported in the most recent literature, which would seem to contradict the opinion of a drop of MS frequency in Mediterranean Europe, strengthening the possibility that Italy, too, falls into the high-frequency area[3,5-11]. Nevertheless, these results can also be open to criticism. In fact, owing to the size of the populations investigated, the high prevalence rates in the intensive surveys show very wide confidence limits, which could reduce the precision rates in measuring the true frequency of MS in Italy. Moreover, studies carried out on small populations are still too few to be considered indicative of the true frequency of MS in Italy and, therefore, other numerous investigations of this sort are needed before any definitive conclusion can be drawn.

For this reason, we undertook a further descriptive survey of MS in Barbagia, Sardinia, to identify patients overlooked in the first study in 1975[11]. We have previously reported that in Barbagia on December 31, 1975, the prevalence of MS was 40.7 per 100000 (95% confidence limits: 26-62). Having previously verified the suitability of this area for epidemiological studies, we decided to maintain Barbagia as our study area.

METHODS

Area of investigation

Barbagia covers an area of 1242 square km in the east-central part of Sardinia (40°13' and 39°54' North, and 8°58' and 9°39' East). The geographic, climatic and socio–economic characteristics have been described in detail in the previous epidemiologic investigation on MS in the same area. In recent years, medical organization has become more efficient, and three rehabilitation facilities for handicapped people as well as various other institutions have been provided for the whole territory.

Case collection and ascertainment

The patients found to have probable and possible MS in 1975 (21 and 3 respectively) formed the basis of this second study. Additional potential MS cases were identified from the following sources: archives of the hospitals of Nuoro and Ozieri and from the Sassari and Cagliari University Hospitals, records of the National Health Insurance scheme, archives of the National Pension Institute, local section of the Italian Association for MS, telephone surveys of most neurologists and ophthalmologists in Nuoro, and directly from neurologists, general practitioners, chemists, physiotherapists and social workers employed in the territory. Excellent cooperation was obtained from physicians working in the territory. Hospital archives were studied for a 20 year period, from 1960 to 1981 inclusive. Patients with a diagnosis of MS, optic neuritis, myelopathy, encephalitis, spastic ataxia and spinocerebellar ataxia were reviewed. All the patients, previously contacted by phone or letter, were examined at home in the summer of 1982. The standard inquiry included a detailed interview, a neurologic examination and a further analysis of personal medical charts of each patient. Not all patients were known to the local medical facilities, since a few attended neurological or rehabilitation centres outside their district. However, it must be emphasized that all patients interviewed had already been diagnosed during previous admissions to neurological centres of Sardinia or continental Italy.

For inclusion in the present material, residency qualifications were required: seven patients who had emigrated and two who had died before the prevalence day were excluded from prevalence computation. All were born in the study area and also lived there until the onset of the disease.

In this manner, 32 probable and 4 possible MS patients were considered for prevalence estimation, since they were alive and residing in Barbagia on prevalence day, October 24, 1981.

The prevalent cases satisfied both the diagnostic criteria of Allison and Millar[12] and the Schumacher Committee criteria[13]. The possible cases were excluded from further treatment in the present study.

RESULTS

On prevalence day, October 24, 1981, 32 patients (18 women and 14 men) living in Barbagia were found to be suffering from probable MS. The mean age was 40.7 ± 13.7 y for women and 41.1 ± 3 y for men, and the average was 40.8 ± 11.7 y.

As the total population on prevalence day was 49022 (24832 women and 24190 men), the crude prevalence rate for probable MS was 65.3 per 100000 (95% confidence limits: 44–93). If this rate is standardized for both age and sex from the Barbagia population to the Italian population at the 1981 general Census (October 24, 1981), the expected rate for Italy is 77.9. The prevalence rates for women and men were 72.5 and 57.9 respectively (87.2 and 68.3 if age-adjusted to the Italian population), a non-significant difference. MS appeared to be uniformly distributed in the 22 communes included in the study area.

The mean age at onset, ranging from 13 to 49 years, was 27.1 ± 9.0 years, 26.5 ± 10.4 for women and 27.4 ± 5.2 for men. The mean duration of MS on the prevalence day was 15.2 ± 9.9 years: 15.8 ± 11.2 for women and 14.5 ± 8.2 for men. Paraparesis was the first symptom in 14 patients (43 per cent), and diplopia and visual impairment in 12 patients (37 per cent). Of all the patients, 31 had at least partial remission, and only one had a non-remitting course from the onset. Among all cases, two were familial siblings, giving a familial frequency of 6.2 per cent.

DISCUSSION

This second descriptive study in Barbagia has confirmed that the disease occurs there more frequently than expected on the basis of previous epidemiologic surveys in a Mediterranean area. In fact, the prevalence rate of 65.3 per 100 000 found in Barbagia (77.9 if standardized to the Italian population) is the highest figure that has yet been estimated from any community in Italy.

However, caution may be required regarding several factors when evaluating the results of this survey as indicators of the frequency of MS in Italy. Foremost is the possibility that Barbagia is a focus of high frequency owing to a particular concentration in this area of unspecified factors, both genetic and environmental, associated with the disease. In our opinion, at present we do not believe that Barbagia's population is exposed to risk factors any different from those of communities in other parts of Italy. Secondly, the relatively small number of cases, from which rates are calculated, tends to have wide confidence limits surrounding the prevalence rate, but in our study the reported rate has both lower and upper 95% confidence limits which support the idea that Barbagia also falls into the high-risk zone for MS.

The excess of MS cases in this further study is no doubt partly due to the fact that many of the problems which make it difficult to obtain valid epidemiologic data in Italy have been greatly reduced in Barbagia, even more so than during our first study. Since our group has been using this small population for years for other neuro-epidemiologic studies, we have achieved an active cooperation with physicians as well as a willingness on the part of both the community and the public medical organization to collaborate. Moreover, full collaboration was obtained this time from the physiotherapists engaged in the recently instituted socio–sanitary services. This enabled us to trace four probable MS patients, with onset of the disease before the prevalence day of the previous study and living in Barbagia, who are presently taking part in rehabilitation programmes in the territory. These four patients were not included in the previous study, but in 1975 they would have been eligible for inclusion in prevalence estimation. In this connection, it is noteworthy that the revised prevalence of probable MS in 1975 in retrospect is 48.4 per 100 000, a rate that more accurately reflects the occurrence of MS in Barbagia than the figure we previously found at that time.

In addition to the present survey, eight prevalence studies have been carried out in Italy using small population groups[3,5-11]. Taken together, these studies indicate that the prevalence of MS in Italy is higher than 30 per 100 000 and, therefore, would seem to question the current opinion that Italy falls into the medium-frequency zone. On the contrary, they suggest that the risk for MS in Italy is similar to that found in most communities in central and northern Europe. In our opinion, this is a likely suggestion. The studies so far considered as a basis for drawing conclusions on the risk for MS in Italy have established much lower figures, but it must be emphasized that all these studies have been carried out on populations exceeding 300000[1,2]. In our previous study[11], we pointed out that in Italy there are many reasons for believing that the use of large populations and the many difficulties involved in obtaining complete data, no doubt provide serious underestimates of MS frequency. In other words, accurate prevalence estimates in Italy can be achieved only by means of limited population groups. Although studies of this sort are still too few to permit definitive conclusions, all are convergent in indicating that Italy falls into the high-risk zone for MS and not into the medium-risk zone as currently reported.

ACKNOWLEDGEMENT

This work was supported by the Bank of Sardinia and by the Ministero della Pubblica Istruzione.

References

1. Kurtzke, J. F. (1975). *Acta Neurol. Scand.,* **51,** 110
2. Kurtzke, J. F. (1980). *Acta Neurol. Scand.,* **62,** 65
3. Dean, G., Grimaldi, R., Kelly, R. and Karhausen, L. (1979). *J. Epidemiol. Commun. Health,* **33,** 107
4. Rosati, G. (1981). *Proceedings of the 22nd National Congress of the Italian Society of Neurology,* Scalea (Italy), November 5-7, pp. 173-178
5. Rossi, G., Ferrari, G. and Dalri, E. (1980). *Proceedings of the 2nd Italian Meeting of Neuroepidemiology,* Milan (Italy), December 12-13, pp. 149-152
6. Rosati, G., Granieri, E., Carreras, M. and Tola, R. (1981). *Acta Neurol. Scand.,* **62,** 244
7. Rosati, G., Granieri, E., Carreras, M., Pinna, L., Tola, R. and Paolino, E. (1980). *Proceedings of the Italian Meeting of Neuroepidemiology,* Milan (Italy), December 12-13, pp. 157-161
8. Savettieri, G., Daricello, D., Giordano, D., Ventura, A., Karhausen, L. and Dean, G. (1981). *J. Epidemiol. Commun. Health,* **35,** 114
9. Savettieri, G., Grimaldi, G., Giordano, D., Ventura, A., Karhausen, L. and Dean, J. (1981). *Proceedings of the 22nd National Congress of the Italian Society of Neurology,* Scalea (Italy), November 5-7, pp. 355-356
10. Dean, G., Savettieri, G., Taibi, G., Morreale, S. and Karhausen, L. (1981). *J. Epidemiol. Commun. Health,* **35,** 118
11. Granieri, E. and Rosati, G. (1982). *Neurology,* **32,** 466
12. Allison, R. S. and Millar, J. H. D. (1954). *Ulster Med. J.,* **23,** 1
13. Schumacher, G. A., Beebe, G. and Kibler, R. F. (1965). *Ann. NY Acad. Sci.,* **122,** 552

Poster 21
Antibrain antibody adsorption on microtitre plates

F. VAN ROMPAEY, D. NIJST, J. RAUS and A. A. VANDENBARK

ABSTRACT

Low concentrations of antibrain antibody can be detected in cerebrospinal fluid (CSF) from most patients with multiple sclerosis and a few patients with other neurologic diseases.

The CSF antibody specificities, detected by the sensitive enzyme-linked immunosorbent assay (ELISA), have been utilized to characterize brain 'target' antigens in chromatofocused fractions of brain extracts. In order to compare the antigenic composition of extracts and fractions which are recognized by antibrain antibodies, without wasting limited quantities of CSF or serum, a versatile method for specific absorption of antibody on the ELISA plates was developed. Polyvinyl chloride (PVC) plates, pretreated with glutaric dialdehyde (to bind antigens irreversibly), were coated with the adsorbing antigen and the antibody mixture was incubated to remove specific reactivity before transfer to a second PVC plate coated with the test antigen. Under optimal conditions this method could remove specifically more than 80% of anti-myelin basic protein (MBP) reactivity with a single absorption. By comparing reactive and preabsorbed rabbit anti-MBP antiserum, both native MBP and MBP fragments or complexes could be detected in chromatofocused fractions of MS brain extracts.

INTRODUCTION

Immunoabsorption techniques which remove unwanted antibody specificities often reduce desired antibody reactivity due to non-specific adsorption of antibody to the supporting matrices or manipulation of the antibody after separation. These problems become critical when the concentration of the desired antibody is limited. In order to achieve efficient immuno-absorption without wasting limited resources, a versatile method for specific removal of antibody on ELISA plates was developed.

METHODS

For the experiments described below, antiserum was obtained from rabbits immunized with human myelin basic protein (MBP[1]) in Freund's complete adjuvant, or with keyhole limpet haemocyanin (KLH[2]) given intradermally. The basic method involved coating polyvinyl chloride (PVC) plates with saturating antigen concentrations (30–40 μg/ml of MBP, KLH, or 3 mol/l KCl extracts of brain or kidney), followed by incubation with antiserum under various conditions. The absorbed antiserum was then transferred to a second PVC plate coated with 1 μg/ml MBP or KLH or 5 μg/ml 3 mol/l KCl-extract[3]. After further incubation and washes, the reactive antibodies were detected by ELISA[4] using peroxidase labelled goat α-rabbit IgG and substrate (orthophenylenediamine, OPD). Reactions (absorption at 450 nm) were quantitated and replicate wells (usually four wells) were averaged for statistical comparisons. Chromatofocusing of 3 mol/l KCl extracts of brain was performed as described earlier[4], and individual fractions were evaluated for the presence of MBP as described below.

RESULTS

Preliminary experiments using MBP-α-MBP and KLH-α-KLH reactions established the following characteristics for absorption.

(1) Pretreatment of the PVC plates with 2% polymerized glutaraldehyde[5] to irreversibly bind the antigens to the wells resulted in a more efficient absorption of specific antibody.

(2) The efficiency of the absorption of α-MBP and α-KLH increased from 44% at the highest antibody concentration (10^{-2} dilution) to 92% at the lowest concentration (10^{-5} dilution). Sequential absorptions resulted in further reduction of antibody reactivity.

(3) Overnight absorption at 4 °C, with shaking, was slightly more efficient than overnight absorption at room temperature (20 °C), but both procedures were more efficient than overnight incubation at 4 °C without shaking, or $2\frac{1}{2}$ hour incubation at 37 °C or 4 °C. Shaking at temperatures above 4 °C resulted in condensation and mixing of wells.

(4) Efficiency of absorption increased with increasing absorbing antigen concentrations used to coat the PVC plate.

In order to establish the specificity of the absorption, α-MBP or α-KLH was absorbed on PVC plates coated with MBP, KLH or no antigen, and transferred to a second plate coated with MBP or KLH. The absorption of α-MBP on MBP resulted in a 90% reduction of α-MBP reactivity relative to absorption on KLH or PVC. Similarly, α-KLH reactivity was removed specifically after absorption on KLH coated plates.

An extension of these experiments showed that plates coated with both MBP and KLH were equally efficient at removing specific antibody as plates coated with only one antigen. Conversely, plates coated with one antigen could remove specific antibody reactivity from a mixture of α-MBP and α-KLH as efficiently as from a single antiserum. In order to determine if a complex mixture of brain antigens (3 mol/l KCl extract) contained detectable amounts of MBP, α-MBP was absorbed on MBP, brain extract, or kidney extract, and reacted with MBP, brain extract, or kidney extract. Both MBP and brain extract, but not kidney extract could absorb α-MBP reactivity resulting in 50–70% reduced reactivity to both MBP and brain extract.

In further experiments, the elution pH of MBP and MBP fragments or complexes was evaluated in chromatofocused fractions of brain extracts. Anti-MBP antiserum which had been preabsorbed on MBP or an empty plate was reacted with each fraction: fractions containing reactive MBP fragments would show significant ELISA reactivity with antiserum absorbed on an empty plate, and a significant reduction with antiserum absorbed on whole MBP. The results showed two major MBP reactive regions with a pH > 7 and 10 minor regions containing MBP with an elution pH between 3 and 7.

DISCUSSION

The results presented above show clearly that preabsorption of antibody on antigen coated microtitre plates offers an efficient (90% reduction in one step) antigen specific method for removing antibody activity. The optimal conditions for removal occur when the antibody is incubated overnight at 4 °C with shaking on PVC plates pretreated with polymerized glutaraldehyde, and then coated with a saturating concentration ($> 40\,\mu g/ml$) of antigen. The method has been utilized to detect a specific antigen within a complex mixture (i.e. MBP in 3 mol/l KCl extracts of brain tissue).

Additionally, comparison of BP absorbed and control antiserum has allowed identification of MBP in a number of chromatofocused fractions of the crude brain extract. The major reactive peaks elute in the column pass fractions (pH > 7) as expected, and probably represent native MBP and its major cleavage fragments. Additional MBP reactivity was detected in more acid fractions (eluting between pH 3 and 7) and probably represents either minor cleavage fragments, or MBP complexed with other more acidic molecules (perhaps including cerebrosides as suggested earlier by Raine and Traugott[6]).

ACKNOWLEDGEMENTS

The authors wish to thank Agnes Delsaer for typing the manuscript, and Tony Van Galen for preparing graphics for presentation at the 25th Anniversary Symposium of the Belgian Research Group for MS, Brussels, Belgium which this manuscript describes.

This research was supported by the Paul J. Cams Foundation of Belgium, the Wetenschappelijk Onderzoek MS Organization of Belgium and the United States Veterans Administration.

References

1. Diebler, G. E., Martenson, R. E. and Kies, M. W. (1972). *Prep. Biochem.*, **2**, 139
2. Vandenbark, A. A., Yoshihara, P., Carveth, L. and Burger, D. R. (1981). *Cell Immunol.*, **60**, 240
3. Meltzer, M. S., Leonard, E. J., Rapp, J. J. and Bersos, T., (1971). *J. Natl. Cancer Inst.*, **47**, 103
4. Vandenbark, A. A., Van Rompaey, F., Heyligen, H., Nijst, D. and Raus, J. (1982). In Peeters, H. (ed.). *Protides of the Biological Fluids*, Vol. 30 (Oxford: Pergamon)
5. Place, J. D. and Schroeder, H. R. (1982). *J. Immunol. Meth.*, **48**, 251
6. Raine, C. S. and Traugott, U. (1982). *J. Neuroimmunol.*, **2**, 83

Poster 22
Search for viral nucleic acid sequences in the human central nervous system

W. W. TOURTELLOTTE, P. SHAPSHAK, S. NAKAMURA, M. DARVISH,
G. C. FAREED, K. SIDHU, P. SCHMID, M. C. GRAVES and K. BERRY

ABSTRACT

We have commenced a comprehensive systematic study of central nervous
system (CNS) tissue derived from patients with a variety of chronic neurologic
diseases and controls to detect and localize viral nucleic acid sequences in
affected areas of the CNS. We use *in situ* hybridization in cryosections of
frozen tissue and ^{3}H-labelled viral DNA probes. The tissues analyzed include
optic nerves, spinalcords, brainstem, and cerebral tissues selected from individuals who died from subacute sclerosing panencephalitis (SSPE), progressive
multifocal leukoencephalopathy (PML), Alzheimer's, Parkinson's, and
Huntington's Diseases. The controls include individuals who died from traffic
accident and heart attack with no evidence of psychiatric or neurologic
disease. Virus infected and uninfected cell cultures are also used as controls.
The viral probes were labelled to high specific activity with ^{3}H and include
SV40 viral DNA, subgenomic cloned HSV-1 DNA, and cloned cDNA to the
measles nucleocapsid (NP) mRNA. We find strong hybridizations for measles
in SSPE cerebrum and for SV40 in PML cerebrum. We are continuing these
studies focusing on the use of measles cloned probes in MS tissues.

INTRODUCTION

The discovery of measles nucleotide sequences in cryosections of plaque edges
in MS brain by Haase *et al*[1] using *in situ* hybridization of ^{3}H-labelled measles
randomly initiated cDNA probes has provided a new powerful tool for the
investigation of the viral pathogenesis of MS and other neurological diseases.
This finding comes 20 years after Adams and Imagawa[2] first reported elevated
measles titres in MS patients, implicating measles virus in the aetiology of MS.
The involvement of viruses in chronic neurological disorders has been
extensively reviewed[3-5].

Prior to the Haase *et al*[1] report, liquid nucleic acid hybridization techniques were used, and measles could not be detected in MS tissues[6]. Some additional searches for viruses in other neurological diseases have also been made. HSV-1 nucleotide sequences were detected in brain cells from dementia patients using *in situ* hybridization[7]. Using liquid hybridization techniques, poliovirus nucleic acid sequences were detected in motor neurones of two patients with amyotrophic lateral sclerosis (ALS)[8,9].

We present the results of our search for viral nucleotide sequences in CNS cryosections from patients with several neurological diseases and controls using *in situ* hybridization with ^{3}H-labelled viral probes.

MATERIALS AND METHODS

Specimens

Postmortem quick-frozen optic nerves, spinalcords, brainstems and cerebral tissue mentioned in Table 1 were obtained from the National Neurological Research Bank. Cryosections were made in a Harris Cryostat.

Cell and virus cultures

Virus infected Vero cells were grown as previously described[10]. At maximum cytopathic effect the virus infected cells were trypsinized, rinsed three times in phosphate buffered saline (PBS) and then deposited on slides treated for *in situ* hybridization[11]. The Edmonston measles virus laboratory strain used was originally obtained from R. T. Johnson. D. Carrigan provided the SSPE virus isolate and M. Cook and J. Stevens provided the Patton strain of HSV-1.

Probes

Growth of the bacteria containing recombinant plasmids, and purification of the plasmids was done according to the literature[12]. ^{3}H-isotopic labelling was performed according to Rigby *et al*[13]. Measles total genome ^{3}H-cDNA was a gift from A. Haase. The measles nucleocapsid (NP) clone was a gift from S. Rozenblatt[14] The HSV-1 subgenomic clone, pdHSV12-7 contained 10% of the HSV-1 genome consisting of the replication origin and packaging sites[15]. We received several nick translated probes from C. Winchell and A. Tobin.

In situ hybridization and tissue staining

The methods of Brahic and Haase[11] and Haase *et al*[1] were followed in detail.

RESULTS

Using both total genome measles cDNA obtained from Dr A. Haase as well as NP gene cloned cDNA obtained from Dr S. Rozenblatt, we have found

Table 1 *In situ* hybridization in cryosections and cell cultures. The ratios represent the number of different cases with positive hybridization over the number of cases tested

		Tissues					Homologous virus infected cell cultures
³H probes	SSPE cerebrum	Huntington's Disease optic nerve	Parkinson's Disease optic nerve	Alzheimer's Disease optic nerve	Non-neurological controls optic nerve	PML (JC type) cerebrum	
Measles cDNA (entire genome)	1/1	—	—	—	—	—	+
Measles NP clone	2/2	0/2	0/2	0/2	0/1[a]	—	+
HSV-1 clone	—	0/2	0/2	0/2	0/2[b]	—	+
SV-40	—	—	0/3	0/2	0/2[b]	1/1	+

[a] traffic accident
[b] traffic accident and heart attack

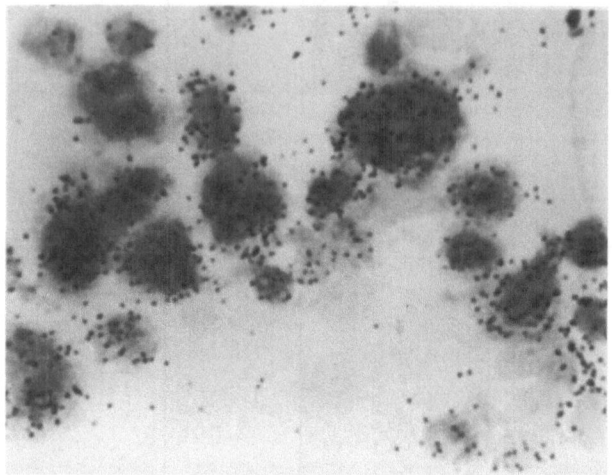

Figure 1 Measles virus infected Vero cells. *In situ* hybridization with ³H-NP probe (specific activity 7×10^7/dpm/μg) Autoradiography was done for 16 days. Giemsa stain. Magnification × 980.

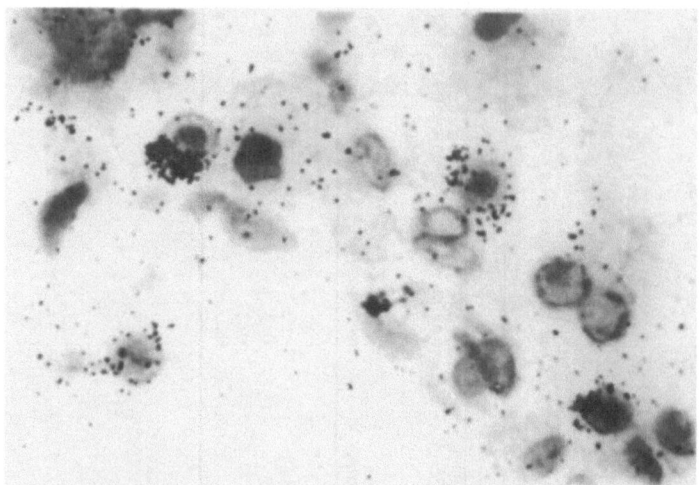

Figure 2 SSPE (NNRB #300). The probe was the same as in Figure 1. Autoradiography was for 23 days. Hematoxylin–eosin stain. Magnification × 1500.

hybridized measles nucleotide sequences in SSPE cerebral tissue, but not in Huntington's, Parkinson's, and Alzheimer's diseases nor in non-neurological control tissue. The HSV-1 cloned probe did not hybridize in any tissues examined. SV40 viral probe *in situ* hybridization detected viral sequences only in PML cerebrum. All probes gave positive hybridization in homologous virus

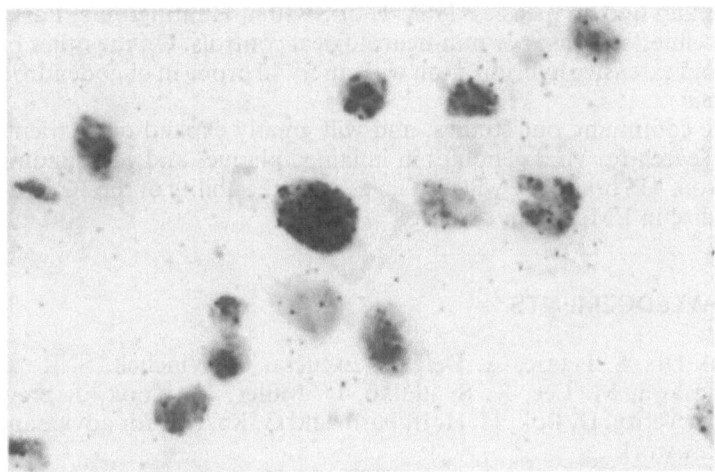

Figure 3 PML (NNRB #120) cerebrum. ^{3}H-SV40 probe (specific activity 10×8 dpm/μg). Autoradiography was for 21 days. Giemsa stain. Magnification $\times 1500$

infected Vero cells and no hybridization in non-homologous combinations. Several examples of our hybridizations are shown in Figures 1 and 2. About 50 grains are present per measles infected Vero cell in Figure 1, as is the case with SSPE measles positive cells shown in Figure 2. Uninfected Vero cells show up to four grains per cell, and the uninfected cells in SSPE tissues show two grains on average. Figure 2 shows infected oligodendroglia cells with nuclear inclusion bodies, but surprisingly without any grains over these inclusion bodies. We have found that SV40 hybridized in oligodendrocytes of PML, shown in Figure 3. There was an average of 44 grains per infected cell but 3 grains per uninfected cell in PML tissue. The cryosections cut for the SV40 hybridizations were from a brain cryopreserved at the NNRB for 13 years and had been shown to harbour the JC type virus[16,17].

DISCUSSION

In situ hybridization is a highly sensitive technique to search for viral genomes in the CNS. When the procedure is optimized, it is possible to detect about one viral genome equivalent per infected cell both in cell culture and in CNS tissue[1,2]. This was done in MS tissue using a randomly initiated measles ^{3}H-cDNA probe[18]. In our *in situ* hybridization studies using a cloned NP gene cDNA probe we were readily able to detect measles nucleotide sequences in cryosections of SSPE cerebral tissue. However, we did not detect any measles hybridization in the SSPE nuclear inclusions; a possible explanation could be that our experimental conditions were not sufficiently vigorous to allow the measles probe to penetrate to the tightly packed nucleocapsids in the inclusions.

We have commenced a search for viral sequences in several neurological disorders and find no measles, HSV-1, or SV40 in Huntington's, Parkinson's and Alzheimer's diseases or non-neurological controls. On the other hand we have found extensive hybridization with an SV40 probe in oligodendrocytes of PML brain.

We are continuing our studies, and will greatly expand our patient series, and will search for viral genomes in inflamed plaques and surrounding white matter from MS brain. We will also investigate the ability of the JC virus probe to hybridize in PML brain tissues.

ACKNOWLEDGEMENTS

We thank Drs A. Haase, A. Delgado-Escueta, C. Winchell, S. Rozenblatt, D. T. Imasawa, M. Lee, K. Syndulko, C. Miller, M. Cook, J. Stevens, J. Brown, A. Verity, D. Bok, H. H. Itabashi and G. Kazekis for advice and effort during this work.

We have been supported by a research grant from the Kroc Foundation and in part by VA Merit Funds, VA Southwest Regional Epilepsy Center funds, and a travel fellowship (to KB) from the Canadian Medical Research Council.

References

1. Haase, A. T., Ventura, P., Gibbs, C. J. Jr. and Tourtellotte, W. W. (1981). Measles virus nucleotide sequences: detection by hybridization *in situ. Science*, **212**, 672
2. Adams, J. M. and Imagawa, D. J. (1962). Measles antibodies in MS. *Proc. Soc. Exp. Biol. Med.*, **8**, 562
3. Johnson, R. T. (1982). *Viral Infections of the Nervous System.* (New York: Raven Press)
4. Timakov, V. D. and Zuev, V. A. (1980). *Slow Virus Infections.* (Moscow: Mir Publishing)
5. Norrby, E. (1978). Viral antibodies in MS. *Prog. Med. Virol.*, **24**, 1
6. Stevens, J. G., Bagstone, V. B. Ellison, G. W. and Myers, L. W. (1979). No measles information detected in MS derived brains, *Ann. Neurol.*, **8**, 625
7. Sequiera, L. W., Carrasco, L. H., Curry, A., Jennings, L. C., Lord, M. A. and Sutton, R. N. P. (1979). Detection of HSV genome in brain tissue, *Lancet*, 609
8. Kohne, D. E., Gibbs, C. J., White, L., Tracy, S. M., Meinke, W. and Smith, R. A. (1981). Virus detection by nucleic acid hybridization: examination of normal and ALS tissues for the presence of poliovirus. *J. Gen. Virol.*, **56**, 223
9. Viola, M. V., Lazarus, M., Antel, J. and Roos, R. (1982). Nucleic acid probes in the study of ALS. *Adv. Neur.*, **36**, 317
10. Shapshak, P., Graves, P. and Imagawa, D. T. (1982). Polypeptides of CDV strains derived from dogs with chronic neurological diseases. *Virology*, **122**, 158
11. Brahic, M. and Haase, A. T. (1978). Detection of viral sequences of low reiteration frequency by *in situ* hybridization. *Proc. Nat. Acad. Sci.*, **12**, 6125
12. Bolivar, F. and Backman, K. (1979). Plasmids of *E. coli* as cloning vectors, In Wu, R. (ed.). *Methods in Enzymology, vol. 68; Recombinant DNA*, pp. 245–267. (New York: Academic Press)
13. Rigby, P. W. J., Dieckmann, M., Rhodes, C. and Berg, P. (1977). Labeling DNA to high specific activity *in vitro* by nick translation with DNA polymerase, *J. Mol. Biol.*, **113**, 237
14. Gorecki, M. and Rozenblatt, S. (1980). Cloning of DNA complementary to the measles virus mRNA encoding the nucleocapsid protein. *Proc. Nat. Acad. Sci.*, **77**, 3686
15. Denniston, K. J., Madden, M. J., Enquist, L. W. and van de Woude, G. (1981). Characterization of coliphage lambda hybrids carrying DNA fragments from HSV-1 DI particles. *Gene*, **15**, 365

16. Weiner, L. P., Herndon, R. M., Narayan, O., Johnson, R. T., Shah, K., Rubinstein, L. J., Preziosi, T. J. and Conley, F. K. (1972). Isolation of virus related to SV40 from patients with PML, *N. Engl. J. Med.*, **286,** 385
17. Weiner, L. P., Narayan, O., Penney, J. B., Herndon, R. M., Feringa, E. R., Tourtellotte, W. W. and Johnson, R. T. (1973). Papovavirus of JC type in PML. *Arch Neurol.*, **29,** 1
18. Haase, A. T., Swoveland, P., Stowring, L., Ventura, P., Johnson, K. P., Norrby, E. and Gibbs, C. J. Jr. (1981). Measles virus genome in infections of the CNS. *J. Inf. Dis.*, **144,** 154

Poster 23
Ultrastructural study of virus-like particles in an acute case of multiple sclerosis

G. F. WALTER, Y. DE SMET, R. E. GONSETTE and J. M. BRUCHER

SUMMARY

The present report concerns an ultrastructural investigation in a severe acute case of multiple sclerosis (MS); the patient died during a relapse. Four types of virus-like or mycoplasma-like particles were observed, and compared to similar alterations previously described in three other acute cases and even in chronic cases of MS. The significance of those lesions is discussed, but most of them can be considered as artefacts or aspecific and non-viral. Looking for virus particles, even in brains of patients with a fulminating evolution, seems, therefore, the least promising approach to the possible viral aetiology of MS.

INTRODUCTION

It is generally believed that viruses could be related, to some extent, to the pathogenesis of multiple sclerosis (MS), but until now extensive search of brain tissue has failed to clearly demonstrate infectious organisms (see reviews[1-7]). Most of those investigations have been carried out in patients with a chronic evolution but, if MS is the result of a virus infection, it is likely that virus particles will be found more easily in the brain of patients experiencing acute forms of the disease. In those cases indeed, inflammatory reactions are particularly pronounced.

We had the opportunity to examine, by ultramicroscopy, the brain obtained within 4 h of death from a patient with acute MS, who died during a final relapse with severe brainstem involvement, $2\frac{1}{2}$ years after the onset of the disease.

CASE REPORT

In January 1973, following a 'flu-like illness, this 16 years old female student (case no. 3058) developed diplopia and a marked weakness of both legs. At the same time she became urinary incontinent. The CSF analyses revealed a sharp rise in the IgG content (20.5 mg%) and an oligoclonal pattern with the electro-focusing technique. The patient was diagnosed as probable MS and had a course of adrenocorticotropic hormone with definite improvement. Six months later she developed a left hemiplegia for 6 weeks, and the diagnosis was clinically confirmed. During the year 1974 she experienced two more relapses and developed cerebellar symptoms, in addition to a spastic para-plegia requiring support at all times when walking.

In November 1975 she became bedridden and was admitted to the Belgian National Centre for MS. At that time she experienced signs of brainstem involvement with paralysis of III, IV and VII cranial nerves, intermittent hyperthermia and impairment of consciousness. Approximately 6 weeks after admission a coma vigil and a drug-fast hyperthermia had developed. Despite a course of ACTH she developed bulbar symptoms and died some $2\frac{1}{2}$ years after her first attack.

MATERIAL AND METHODS (CASE A 3122, E 1157)

The unfixed brain was cut at early autopsy (4 h) in frontal slices and several parts from macroscopically visible MS plaques and surrounding tissue were taken for electron microscopic preparation. Then the slices were fixed in 10% formaldehyde and, after embedding in paraffin, large sections were stained with haematoxylin–eosin, Masson-trichrome, Nissl's cresyl violet and with the methods of Spielmeyer and Holzer, for light microscopy. For electron micro-scopy, the taken specimens were fixed in 3% buffered glutaraldehyde, post-fixed in 1% osmium tetroxide and, after dehydration in graded alcohols, embedded in Araldite. The ultrathin sections were double-stained with uranyl-acetate and lead citrate and examined with a Zeiss EM 9A electron microscope.

RESULTS

External examination of the cerebrum revealed atrophy. On coronal sections the cerebrum displayed multiple, well-demarcated greyish areas essentially concentrated around the lateral ventricles. Small white foci were seen in the periaqueductal grey and in the sub-pial areas of the pons and the medulla. No lesions were found in the other areas of the cerebrum, brainstem and cerebellum.

Histological study of lesions showed typical active plaques. In electron microscopy various kinds of intranuclear changes in the MS lesions have been observed which might be discussed as possible virus-like particles while only a few cytoplasmic alterations of questionable viral origin could be found.

(1) Some nuclei of ependymal cells contained *bundles of fine filaments* which were sometimes arranged in angles. At high magnifications these fibrils appeared to be thin tubules with an external diameter of approximately 4 nm (Figure 1).

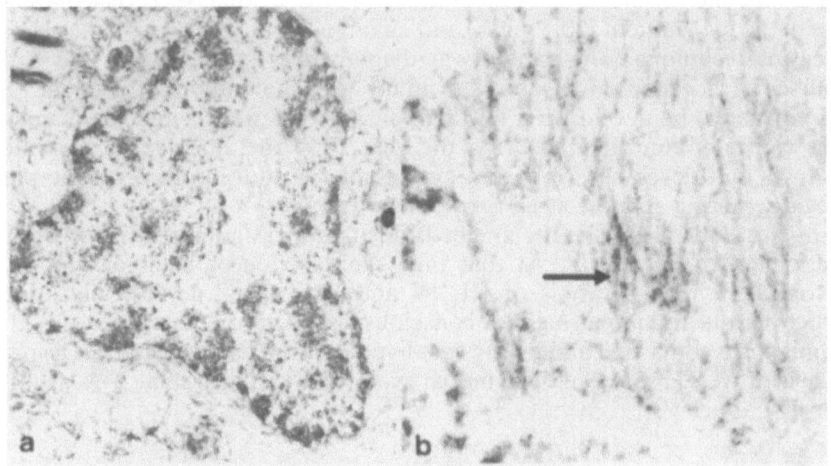

Figure 1
  a. Nuclear bundles of filaments in an ependymal cell. × 9000
  b. Part of a. showing the tubular structure (arrow) × 111 000

(2) *Dense granules* of about 20–24 nm in diameter laid either freely in the karyoplasm of many different glial cells (Figure 2a), or in cytoplasmic vesicles surrounded by a thin unit membrane (Figure 2b). It was not quite clear if they might be transversally cut filaments.

(3) Different nuclear bodies were widely spread in nuclei of oligodendrocytes, astrocytes and even endothelial cells. The most common form consisted of *heterogenic nuclear bodies* with a diameter of approximately 600 nm. These bodies were formed by either an all over membranous spiral-like or concentric structure (Figure 2c) or by a more or less central amorphous core surrounded by a less dense halo and a thin membranous ring (Figure 2a). Sometimes only degenerated shadows of these bodies were present, particularly in endothelial cells (Figure 3b). They occurred mostly, but sometimes with some few (2–5) within the same nucleus. They were found in different cell types, especially in oligodendrocytes (Figure 3a).

(4) Another form of *globular nuclear body* with an electron dense granular or floccular map-like core was surrounded by filamentous rings and appeared in different types of glial cells. These bodies were always single within the nucleus and did not occur as frequently as the smaller membranous globules. They reached a diameter of about 800–1600 nm. Some of them seemed to have a granular relatively regu-

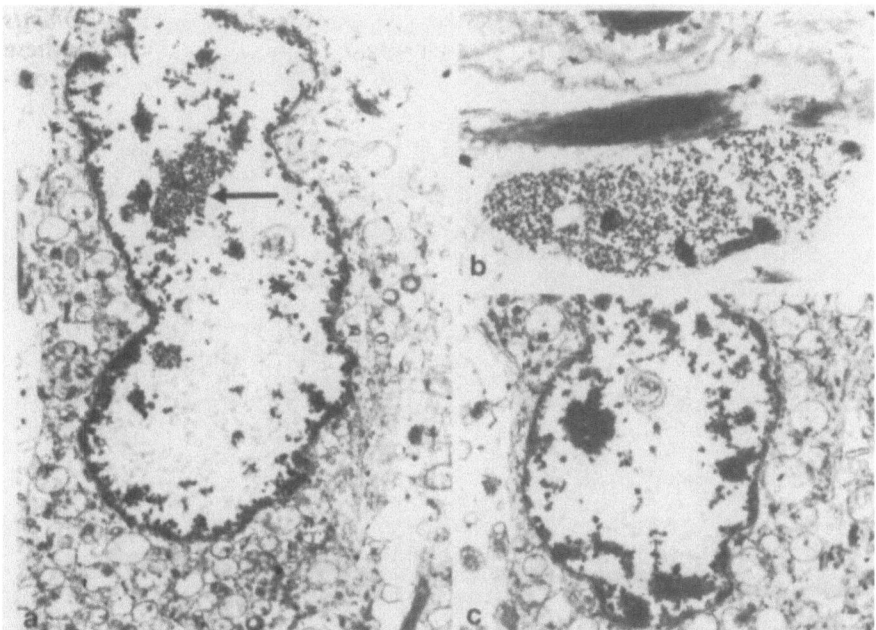

Figure 2
   a. Nuclear dense granules (arrow) and nuclear body consisting of core and halo surrounded by a membrane. × 9000
   b. Granules within a cytoplasmic vesicle. × 17 000
   c. Intranuclear membranous globule. × 9000

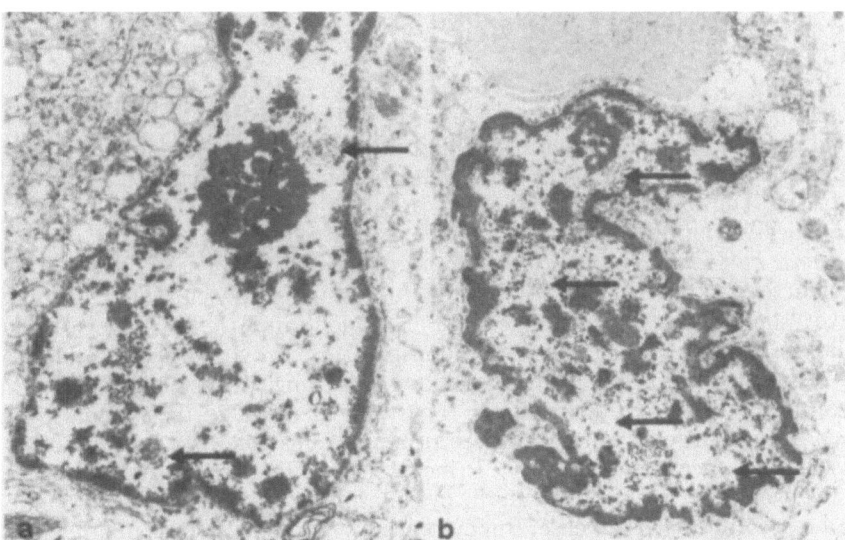

Figure 3
   a. Two heterogenic nuclear bodies in the nucleus of an oligodendrocyte (arrows). × 9000
   b. Several possibly degenerated nuclear bodies in the nucleus of an endothelial cell. × 9000

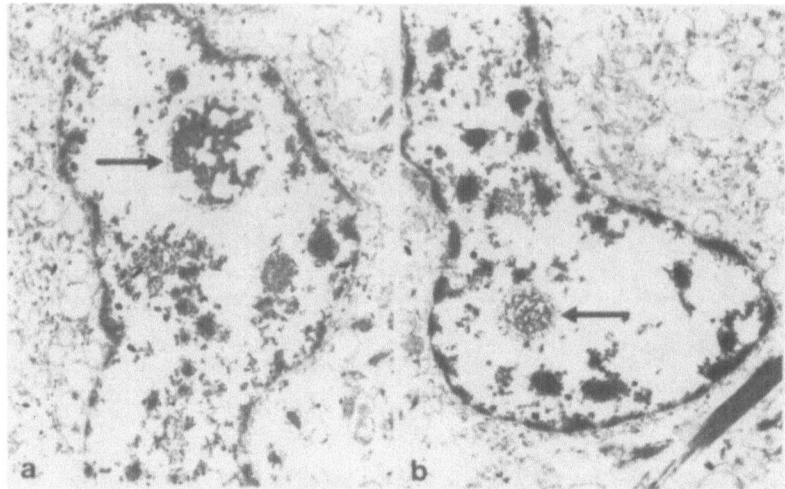

Figure 4
a. and b. Mycoplasma-like globular nuclear bodies (arrows). Both × 9000

larly arranged 'corona radiata' (Figure 4b). It was not possible to decide definitely if the larger forms without 'corna radiata' were identical alterations (Figure 4a).

DISCUSSION

Nuclear filamentous bundles may appear in both normal and pathological conditions in brain cells as shown by Hirano and Zimmerman[8] in rats, and by Popoff and Stewart[9] in ependymal cells and oligodendrocytes of the golden hamster. The authors regarded their presence within the normal range of biological variation.

Dense nuclear and cytoplasmic granules of the same size as in our case have been described by many authors. Sometimes transversally cut filaments might have a similar appearance. Raine and Field[10] mentioned the constancy of their relationship with MS. Bauer *et al*[1] described similar cytoplasmic granules of 18-20 nm in diameter resembling papova-virus nucleocapside, but either in size, morphology and distribution, they were identical to the reticulosomes and related particles which occur as proteinaceous artefacts in a variety of tissues and subcellular fractions[12]. Prineas[6] showed them in the nuclei, but also in the cytoplasm in MS cases. In the cytoplasm the granules were surrounded by a membrane as in our case. But cytoplasmic granular vesicles might simply consist of β-glycogen with a diameter of 15-30 nm.

In chronic MS patients[5,7,13-21] as well as in three 'acute' cases who died during a relapse[22-25], hollow-cored vesicles have been observed in the cytoplasm or nucleus as well as granular, tubular or filamentous inclusions resembling papova-, corona-, parainfluenza- or paramyxo-viruses. Their viral nature remained questionable and they were even identified as non-viral subcellular structures[26]. As a matter of fact the intranuclear 'paramyxovirus-like' material is not specific for MS[27] and might be due to autolysis[28] or unusual organization of chromatin microfibrils[2,6,29,30].

Heterogenic nuclear bodies were found in cases of subacute sclerosing panencephalitis (SSPE)[31] and in neoplasms[32]. But Büttner and Horstmann[33], who called those formations 'sphaeridions', considered them as a functional differentiation of the karyoplasm of normal cells proved in different animal species. They admitted that the 'sphaeridions' might be more numerous in virus diseases and under experimental and pathological circumstances.

The larger *globular nuclear bodies* resemble mycoplasma-like membrane-bound bodies shown by Andrews and Andrews[34] in the neuropil in a case of subacute demyelinating MS-like disease. Mycoplasmas are the smallest free living organisms and an important pathogen in poultry, cattle, swine, rodents, goats and man. They share a sufficient number of properties with viruses. There are different subspecies of mycoplasmas, some of them (*Mycoplasma neurolyticum, Mycoplasma gallisepticum*) produce neurotoxins[35]. Sumi and Reifel[36] found such mycoplasma-like intranuclear inclusions of osmiophilic droplets or granular material surrounded by a filamentous ring in a subependymal giant-cell astrocytoma from a patient with tuberous sclerosis. They were morphologically very similar to the present finding, but their significance remains unknown.

CONCLUSIONS

The nuclear and cytoplasmic alterations observed in the present case of a patient who died during a relapse were previously described in other acute cases as well as in chronic cases of MS. Most of those alterations have been considered as virus-like particles, but they are not specific for MS and even their viral nature is very questionable. However, absence of evidence is not evidence of absence and if viruses are involved in the pathogenesis of the disease, it could be that they exist in a genomic form that cannot be demonstrated by morphologic or immunologic techniques. There is still a possibility that recently developed hybridization methods will be more successful than ultra-structural studies in solving the problem of the relationship between viruses and MS development.

On the other hand, large 'globular nuclear bodies' resembled mycoplasma-like membrane-bound bodies previously described in a subacute demyelinating MS-like disease[34]. This may be related to the recently reported case of post-infectious demyelinating perivenous leukoencephalomyelitis associated with pneumonia due to *Mycoplasma pneumoniae*[37].

ACKNOWLEDGEMENTS

We gratefully acknowledge Mrs Nadine Joseph and Mr Yves De Craeye for their excellent technical assistance.

References

1. Andrews, J.M. (1972). The ultrastructural neuropathology of multiple sclerosis. In Wolfgram, F., Ellison, G. W., Stevens, J. G. and Andrews, J. M. (eds.). *Multiple sclerosis, Immunology, Virology and Ultrastructure*, pp. 23-52. (New York, London: Academic Press)
2. Mirra, S.S. and Takei, Y. (1976). Ultrastructural identification of virus in human central nervous system disease. In Zimmerman, H.M. (ed.). *Progress in Neuropathology III.* pp. 69-88 (New York: Grune and Stratton)
3. Narang, H.K. (1981). Comparative morphology of measles virus and paramyxovirus-like tubules in multiple sclerosis using ruthenium red stain. *Neuropathol. Appl. Neurobiol.*, **7**, 411
4. Narang, H.K. and Field, E.J. (1973a). Paramyxovirus like tubules in multiple sclerosis biopsy material. *Acta Neuropathol.*, (Berlin) **25**, 281
5. Prineas, J.W. (1972). Paramyxovirus-like particles associated with acute demyelination in chronic relapsing multiple sclerosis. *Science*, **178**, 760
6. Prineas, J.W. (1975). Pathology of the early lesion in multiple sclerosis. *Hum. Pathol.*, **6**, 531
7. Tanaka, R., Iwasaki, Y. and Koprowski, H. (1975). Paramyxovirus-like structures in brains of multiple sclerosis patients. *Arch. Neurol.*, **32**, 80
8. Hirano, A. and Zimmerman, H.M. (1967). Some new cytological observations of the normal rat ependymal cell. *Anat. Rec.*, **158**, 293
9. Popoff, N. and Stewart, S. (1968). The fine structure of nuclear inclusions in the brain of experimental golden hamster. *J. Ultrastruct. Res.*, **23**, 347
10. Raine, C.S. and Field, E.J. (1968). Nuclear structures in nerve cells in multiple sclerosis. *Brain Res.*, **10**, 266
11. Bauer, H.J., ter Meulen, V., Koprowski, H., Argyrakis, A. and Orthner, H. (1975). Early sterile autopsy in etiological studies on multiple sclerosis. *J. Neurol.*, **208**, 159
12. Kirk, J. and Hutchinson, W.M. (1978). The fine structure of the CNS in multiple sclerosis. I. Interpretation of cytoplasmic papovavirus-like and paramyxovirus-like inclusions. *Neuropathol. Appl. Neurobiol.*, **4**, 343
13. Hayano, M., Sung, J.H. and Mastri, A.R. (1976). 'Paramyxovirus-like' intranuclear inclusions occurring in the nervous system in diverse unrelated conditions. *J. Neuropathol. Exp. Neurol.*, **35**, 287
14. Lhermitte, F., Escourolle, R., Cathala, F., Hauw, J.J. and Marteau, R. (1973). Etude neuropathologique d'un cas de sclérose en plaques. Discussion de la nature virale de particules observées en microscopie électronique sur une biopsie cérébrale et sur cultures cellulaires. *Rev. Neurol.*, **129**, 3
15. Narang, H.K. and Field, E.J. (1973b). An electron-microscopic study of multiple sclerosis biopsy material: some unusual inclusions. *J. Neurol. Sci.*, **18**, 287
16. Narang, H.K. and Field, E.J. (1973c). Letter in *J. Neurol. Sci.*, **20**, 471
17. Raine, C.S., Prineas, J.W., Sheppard, R.D., Bornstein, M.B. and Dubois-Dalcq, M. (1977). Immunocytochemical studies for the localisation of measles antigens in multiple sclerosis plaques and measles virus-infected CNS tissue. *J. Neurol. Sci.*, **33**, 13
18. Tanaka, R., Iwasaki, Y. and Koprowski, H. (1974). Unusual intranuclear filaments in multiple sclerosis brain. *Lancet*, **i**, 1236
19. Tanaka, R., Santoli, D. and Koprowski, H. (1976a). Unusual intranuclear filaments in the circulating lymphocytes of patients with multiple sclerosis and optic neuritis. *Am. J. Pathol.*, **83**, 245
20. Tanaka, R., Iwasaki, Y. and Koprowski, H. (1976b). Intracisternal virus-like particles in brain of a multiple sclerosis patient. *J. Neurol. Sci.*, **28**, 121

21. Watenabe, I. and Okazaki, H. (1973). Virus-like structure in multiple sclerosis. *Lancet*, **ii**, 569

22. Dubois-Dalcq, M., Schumacher, G. and Sever, J. L. (1973). Acute multiple sclerosis: Electron-microscopic evidence for and against a viral agent in the plaques. *Lancet*, **ii**, 1408

23. Kirk, J. (1979a). Pseudoviral hollow-cored vesicles in multiple sclerosis brain. *Acta Neuropathol.* (Berlin), **48**, 63

24. Kirk, J. (1979b). The fine structure of the CNS in multiple sclerosis. II. Vesicular demyelination in an acute case. *Neuropathol. Appl. Neurobiol.*, **5**, 289

25. Raine, C. S., Powers, J. M. and Suzuki, K. (1974). Acute multiple sclerosis. Confirmation of 'paramyxovirus-like' intranuclear inclusions. *Arch. Neurol.*, **30**, 39

26. Hill, T. J. (1973). Letter in *J. Neurol. Sci.*, **20**, 471

27. Raine, C. S., Schaumburg, H. H., Snyder, D. H. and Suzuki, K. (1975). Intranuclear 'paramyxovirus-like' material in multiple sclerosis, adreno-leukodystrophy and Kuf's disease. *J. Neurol. Sci.*, **25**, 29

28. Karasek, J. (1975). Ultrastructural nuclear changes of extranucleolar ribonucleoprotein structures during autolysis of normal liver cells. *Virch. Arch. B Cell. Path.*, **18**, 337

29. Lampert, F. and Lampert, P. (1975). Multiple sclerosis. Morphological evidence of intranuclear paramyxovirus or altered chromatin fibers? *Arch. Neurol.*, **32**, 425

30. Shaw, C. and Sumi, S. H. (1975). Nonviral intranuclear filamentous inclusions. *Arch. Neurol.*, **33**, 428

31. Toga, M., Dubois, D., Bérard, M., Tripier, M. F., Cesarini, J. P. and Choux, R. (1969). Etude ultrastructurale de quatre cas de leucoencéphalite sclérosante subaiguë. *Acta Neuropathol.*, (Berlin), **14**, 1

32. Schremmer, C. N. (1970). Zum Vorkommen von 'nuclear bodies' in verschiedenen gut- und bösartigen Neubildungen des Menschen. *Arch. Geschwulstforsch.*, **36**, 360

33. Büttner, D. W. and Horstmann, E. (1967). Das Sphaeridion, eine weit verbreitete Differenzierung des Karyoplasma. *Z. Zellforsch.*, **77**, 589

34. Andrews, J. M. and Andrews, R. L. (1973). The significance of dense core particles in subacute demyelinating disease in an adult. *Lab. Invest.*, **28**, 236

35. Thomas, L. (1967). The neurotoxins of *M. neurolyticum* and *M. gallisepticum*. *Ann. NY Acad. Sci.*, **143**, 218

36. Sumi, S. M. and Reifel, E. (1971). Unusual nuclear inclusions in astrocytoma. *Arch. Pathol.*, **92**, 14

37. Fisher, R. S., Clark, A. W., Wolinsky, J. S., Parhad, I. M., Moses, H. and Mardiney, M. R. (1983). Postinfectious leukoencephalitis complicating *Mycoplasma pneumoniae* infection. *Arch. Neurol.*, **40**, 109

Author Index

Subject Index